PHOTOGRAPHIC MANUAL
of
REGIONAL ORTHOPAEDIC
and
NEUROLOGICAL TESTS

· THIRD EDITION ·

Rick Krebs   September 2002

PHOTOGRAPHIC MANUAL
of
REGIONAL ORTHOPAEDIC
and
NEUROLOGICAL TESTS

• THIRD EDITION •

JOSEPH J. CIPRIANO, D.C.
Atlanta, Georgia

with contributions by

WARREN T. JAHN, SR., D.C., F.A.C.O.
Associate Professor
Clinical Orthopaedics and Sports Injury
Logan College of Chiropractic
St. Louis, Missouri

MARK E. WHITE, D.C.
Atlanta, Georgia

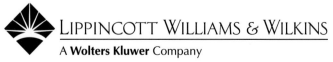
LIPPINCOTT WILLIAMS & WILKINS
A **Wolters Kluwer** Company
Philadelphia • Baltimore • New York • London
Buenos Aires • Hong Kong • Sydney • Tokyo

Editor: Rina Steinhauer
Managing Editor: Linda S. Napora
Production Coordinator: Raymond E. Reter
Copy Editor: Kathleen A. Gilbert
Designer: P. Fry
Illustration Planner: Wayne Hubbel
Cover Designer: Thomas Scheuerman
Typesetter: Bi-Comp, Inc., York, Pennsylvania
Printer & Binder: R. R. Donnelley & Sons Co., Crawfordsville, Indiana
Digitized Illustrations: Bi-Comp, Inc., York, Pennsylvania

351 West Camden Street
Baltimore, Maryland 21201-2436 USA

530 Walnut Street
Philadelphia, Pennsylvania 19106-3621 USA

Printed in the United States of America

First Edition, 1985
Second Edition, 1991

Library of Congress Cataloging-in-Publication Data

Cipriano, Joseph J.
    Photographic manual of regional orthopaedic and neurological tests / Joseph J. Cipriano; with contributions by Warren T. Jahn, Sr., Mark E. White.—3rd ed.
        p. cm.
    Includes bibliographical references and index.
    ISBN 0-683-18100-9
    1. Physical orthopaedic tests—Atlases.   2. Neurologic examination—Atlases.   I. Jahn, Warren T.   II. White, Mark E.   III. Title.
    [DNLM: 1. Neurologic Examination—atlases. 2. Orthopaedics—methods—atlases. WE 17 C577p 1997]
RD734.5.P58C57   1997
617.3—dc20
DNLM / DLC
for Library of Congress   96-43896
                                                                                                                        CIP

The publishers have made every effort to trace the copyright holders for borrowed material. If they have inadvertently overlooked any, they will be pleased to make the necessary arrangements at the first opportunity.

To purchase additional copies of this book, call our customer service department at **(800) 638-3030** or fax orders to **(301) 824-7390.** For other book services, including chapter reprints and large quantity sales, ask for the Special Sales Department. International customers should call **(301) 714-2324.**

Visit Lippincott Williams & Wilkins on the Internet: http://www.lww.com. Lippincott Williams & Wilkins customer service representatives are available from 8:30 am to 6:00 pm, EST.

01 02 03
3 4 5 6 7 8 9 10

To

Mom and Cathy
and
in memory of

Dad

Without their support
there would be
no manual

PREFACE

Photographic Manual of Orthopaedic and Neurological Tests was written to assist the attending physician and student of orthopaedics and neurology in the proper performance and evaluation of standard orthopaedic and neurological tests. The tests are categorized in terms of anatomic application and subcategorized in terms of diagnostic entities. This arrangement facilitates the use of these procedures in evaluating various orthopaedic and neurological conditions.

This text has been designed to be reader-friendly. Each test is accompanied by appropriate photographs that illustrate performance of the test. All of the information is on one page or two facing pages. Where needed, appropriate anatomic illustrations enhance clarity of concept.

There are numerous additions and changes in this Third Edition. As a result of reviewers' comments, the table of contents has been restructured to flow more cohesively by separating the upper and lower extremities. Additionally, the orthopaedic chapters now include palpation of each joint, and discussion of the biomechanical principles has been expanded. The new flow charts at the beginning of each chapter show the logical progression of the decision-making process. The Third Edition includes 60 new tests along with anatomic illustrations and photographs demonstrating the procedures. The overall number of illustrations has nearly doubled.

This Third Edition will keep readers abreast of new tests and changing approaches in assessment. I believe this material will assist in the expedient evaluation of the various orthopaedic and neurological conditions and will enhance your clinical skills. Ultimately, the benefit will be the enhanced well-being of the patients who have sought our help.

ACKNOWLEDGMENTS

I thank the following people for their contributions to this book:

Warren T. Jahn, Sr., D.C., F.A.C.O. and Mark E. White, D.C.—their technical review of the manuscript and suggestions have been greatly appreciated.

Steve Hite, Dr. L.F. Jernigan, and Michelle Larson—their expertise is evident in the 600 photographs that enhance the accuracy of this text.

John Michie, Barry Silverstein, Joseph Castellana, Mark E. White, and Lucas Wells—their time and professionalism as models have my gratitude.

Lydia V. Kibiuk—50 additional illustrations further enhance the readers' comprehension of anatomy throughout the book.

Linda Napora, Managing Editor, Eileen McDonald-Muse, Editorial Assistant, Ray Reter, Production Coordinator, and the staff at Williams & Wilkins—their patience and support were constant during the publication process.

CONTENTS

x   Contents

1
CLINICAL ASSESSMENT PROTOCOL

To accurately evaluate orthopaedic and orthopaedic related neurological conditions, the clinician must have a thorough understanding of basic anatomic and biomechanical principles. These basic skills are required to understand the relationship between structure and function and the role it plays in assessing orthopaedic and neurological dysfunction. The examiner must also be familiar with anatomical and biomechanical variants that may be normal to a particular patient.

The chapters throughout this text will deal primarily with physical examination procedures, which are an integral part of any orthopaedic or orthopaedic-related neurologic examination. The reader must understand that complete patient assessment is not limited to physical examination, but includes other standard procedures, such as radiography, CT scans, and MRI. The clinician must perform the appropriate protocol on the presenting patient to completely evaluate the patient's condition.

This chapter discusses the appropriate protocol for evaluating orthopaedic and orthopaedic-related neurologic problems. These procedures, when followed properly, allow the clinician to assemble parts of a puzzle so that he or she can visualize the "picture," or in this case, the patient's condition. Each piece of the puzzle is analogous to the information gathered by each particular procedure involved in the clinical assessment protocol.

HISTORY

A complete history is one of the most important aspects of the clinical assessment protocol. A complete and thorough history is invaluable in assessing the patient's condition. At times, a history alone may lead us to a proper diagnosis. This history should concentrate on, but not be limited to, the patient's chief complaint, past history, family history, occupational history, and social history. History taking should be accomplished in two steps:

Closed-Ended History

The first step is a closed-ended question and answer format in which the patient answers direct, pointed questions. This step can be accomplished in a written form that the patient fills out.

Open-Ended History

After the close-ended history is complete, an open-ended history should take place, in which patient and examiner engage in an open dialog to discuss the patient's condition. A closed-ended history may lead the examiner to the patient's problem but may not address the patient's fears or concerns regarding this condition. The patient may also have other problems either directly or indirectly related to the presenting complaint that may not be addressed by a closed-ended history.

An open-ended history may take on a discussion-type format in which both the examiner and patient ask questions of each other. In this way, the examiner acquires extra needed information about the patient and the patient's complaint. All aspects of the patient's complaint should be explored and evaluated to its fullest. The following pneumonic OPQRST may be incorporated into this evaluation:

Onset of complaint

Provoking or palliative concerns

Quality of pain

Radiating to a particular area

Site and severity of complaint

Time frame of complaint

Once we have determined all aspects of the presenting complaint, we then focus on the past history of the patient. We need to determine if the patient had prior problems with the presenting complaint or any other complaint. This determination may help us in both assessing the problem and giving us insight on how to treat the problem.

Family history can give us a clue about the patient's propensity of inheriting familial diseases. A significant number of neurological problems and many orthopaedic problems can be traced to family members.

Occupational and social history are also important because it may lead us to a factor causing the patient's problem (such as an overuse syndrome). It can also help us to determine if the patient's condition will respond more favorably if the patient refrains from performing certain work functions or social functions. For example, lifting, bending, and playing tennis or golf may be contraindicated for the patient. The patient may also need to be retrained for other types of work.

OBSERVATION/INSPECTION

Observe the patient for general appearance and functional status. Note the body type, such as slim, obese, short, or tall, and postural deviations for general appearance, gait, muscle guarding, compensatory or substitute movements, and assistive devices for functional status.

Inspection should be divided into three layers: skin, subcutaneous soft tissue, and bony structure. Each layer has its own special characteristic for determining underlying pathology or dysfunction.

Skin

Skin assessment should begin with common and obvious findings, such as bruising, scarring, and evidence of trauma or surgery. Then proceed to look for changes in color, either from vascular changes accompanying inflammation or from vascular deficiency, such as pallor or cyanosis. Large, brownish, pigmented areas and/or hairy regions, especially on or near the spine, may indicate a bony defect such as spina bifida. Changes in texture may accompany reflex sympathetic dystrophies. Open wounds need to be evaluated for either traumatic or insidious origin, which may accompany diabetes.

Subcutaneous Soft Tissue

Subcutaneous soft tissue abnormalities usually involve either inflammation and swelling or atrophy. When evaluating for an increase in size, you should attempt to determine between edema, articular effusion, muscle hypertrophy, or other hypertrophic changes.

Also note the presence of any nodules, lymph nodes, or cysts. The presence of inflammation should be determined by comparing bilateral symmetry for the torso and circumferential measurements for the extremities.

Bony Structure

Bony structure should be evaluated, especially when the patient presents with a functional abnormality such as a gait deviance or an altered range of motion. Bony inspection in the spine should focus on areas such as scoliosis, pelvic tilt, and shoulder height. In the extremities, malformations that may be congenital or trauma related should be noted and possibly measured. Two examples of congenital malformations are genu varus and genu valgus. Trauma related malformations include a healed Colles' fracture with residual angulation. All bony structures should be visualized for abnormalities and documented.

PALPATION

Palpation should be performed in conjunction with inspection because the structures being inspected are the same ones that should be palpated. The layers are the same for palpation as they are for inspection, skin, subcutaneous soft tissue, and bony structures.

When palpating the skin, begin with a light touch, especially if nerve pressure is suspected. Pressure on a nerve may result in dysesthesia, which may feel like an exaggerated burning sensation to the patient.

Skin

Skin temperature should be evaluated first. An increase in the skin temperature may indicate an underlying inflammatory process. A decrease in skin temperature may indicate a vascular deficiency. Skin mobility should also be evaluated for adhesions, especially after surgery or trauma.

Subcutaneous Soft Tissue

The subcutaneous soft tissue consists of fat, fascia, tendons, muscles, ligaments, joint capsules, nerves, and blood vessels. These structures are to be palpated with increased pressure from that of skin palpation. Tenderness is a subjective complaint that should be noted. It may be caused by (a) injury, (b) pathology that correlates directly to the tenderness, such as tenderness at the supraspinatus ligament for supraspinatus tendinitis, or (c) a referred component, such as tenderness in the buttock area from a lumbar injury or pathology.

Swelling or edema is to be evaluated according to its origin. Determine if the inflammation is intra-articular or extra-articular. In intra-articular effusion, the fluid is confined to the joint capsule. In extra-articular effusion, the fluid is in the surrounding tissues. Various palpation techniques are discussed in detail in the regional chapters.

Pulse

Pulse amplitude in certain arteries is an important procedure. It is used to assess the vascular integrity of an area and plays an integral part in certain tests for thoracic outlet syndrome, arterial insufficiency, and vertebrobasilar compromise.

Bony Structures

Bony structure palpation is critical for the detection of alignment problems, such as dislocations, luxations, subluxations, and fractures. When you palpate bony structures, you must also identify the ligaments and tendons that attach to those structures. Tenderness is a major palpatory finding in bony palpation. It may indicate periosteoligamentous sprain. It also may indicate fracture. Bony enlargements usually are associated with healing of fractures and degenerative joint disease.

RANGE OF MOTION

Range of motion evaluation is not only a measurement of function but an important part of biomechanical analysis as well. Range of motion is evaluated for three separate types of functions: passive motion, active motion, and resisted motion.

Passive Range of Motion

In passive motion, the examiner moves the body part for the patient without the patient's help. Passive range of motion testing can yield a significant amount of information about the underlying pathology. The goal obviously depends on which joint is being tested and what pathology or injury is suspected. In evaluating such motion, first note whether the movement is normal, increased, or decreased, and in which planes. Secondly, the presence of pain should be noted. Classically, pain on passive range of motion is indicative of a capsular or ligamentous lesion on the side of movement and/or a muscle lesion on the opposite side of movement. Various other problems may be detected, depending on the degree of mobility and the presence of pain. The following are six possible variations:

1. **Normal mobility with no pain**—a normal joint with no lesion present.
2. **Normal mobility with pain elicited**—may indicate a minor sprain of a ligament or capsular lesion.
3. **Hypomobility with no pain elicited**—may indicate an adhesion of a particular tested structure.
4. **Hypomobility with pain elicited**—may indicate a more acute sprain of a ligament or capsular lesion. When an injury is severe, hypomobility and pain may also be a sign of muscle spasm caused by guarding or by muscle strain that is opposite the side of movement.
5. **Hypermobility with no pain elicited**—suggests a complete tear of a structure where there are no fibers intact where pain can be elicited. It may also be normal if other joints in the absence of trauma are also hypermobile.
6. **Hypermobility with pain elicited**—indicates a partial tear with some fibers still intact. Normal pressure by the weight of structure that is attached to the ligament

or capsule is being exerted. This pressure on the intact fibers can cause pain to be elicited.

Active Range of Motion

Active range of motion is basically performed to evaluate the physical function of a body part. This type of range will yield general information regarding the patient's general ability and willingness to use the part. If a patient is asked to move a joint through a full arc of movement and is unable to move it in its full plane, you are unable to distinguish if the loss of function is caused by pain, weakness caused by a neurological motor dysfunction, stiffness, or the conscious unwillingness of the patient to perform the full function. Therefore, the assessment value of active range of motion in and of itself is vague and limited. Active motion is a basic test for the integrity of the muscle or muscles used in the action and the nerve supply attached to the muscle. Obviously, the integrity of the joint being tested must be intact to evaluate muscular or neurological dysfunction. This integrity is best evaluated by passive range of motion.

When evaluating active motion, you should note the degree of motion in the tested plane as well as any pain associated with the movement. The pain should be correlated with the movement, such as pain in the full arc or only in the extreme range of motion. Crepitus should also be noted when performing active range of motion. Crepitus is a crackling sound that usually indicates a roughening of joint surfaces or an increased friction between a tendon and its sheath (cause by swelling or roughening).

Joint range of motion should be measured and recorded by commonly accepted reproducible means. To measure the range of motion of the spine, the most accurate instrument is the inclinometer (Fig. 1.1). This instrument measures angular displacement relative to gravity as opposed to arcs like a goniometer (Fig. 1.2). The reason for inclinometer measurement of the spine is that the spine is composed of multiple joints that function in unison to produce movement. An arc-type measuring device like a goniometer cannot distinguish the difference between sacral flexion and lumbar flexion in the lower back when the patient is bending forward. In this particular instance, the inclinometer is able to distinguish between true lumbar flexion and sacral or hip flexion (see inclinometer range of motion in cervical, thoracic, and lumbar chapters). Goniometers are best suited to measure extremity range of motion.

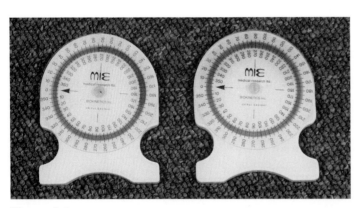

Figure 1.1

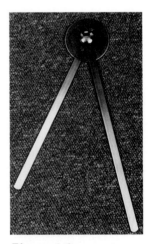

Figure 1.2

Resisted Range of Motion

Resisted range of motion is useful in assessing musculotendinous and neurological structures. It is primarily used to test neurological function (see nerve root lesions). The tests are graded on a scale of 5 to 0, which are adopted by the American Academy of Orthopaedic Surgeons:

5 Complete range of motion against gravity with full resistance
4 Complete range of motion against gravity with some resistance
3 Complete range of motion against gravity
2 Complete range of motion with gravity eliminated (movement in the horizontal plane)
1 Evidence of slight contractility
0 No evidence of contractility

Musculotendinous injuries are generally more painful than they are weak. Neurological lesions are generally more weak than they are painful. The four general pain related reactions to resisted range of motion testing are as follows:

1. Strong with no pain elicited is normal and not indicative of any lesions.
2. Strong with pain elicited may indicate a minor lesion of the muscle or tendon.
3. Weak and painless may indicate a neurological lesion, which will then need to be evaluated with the previous chart. It may also indicate a complete rupture of a tendon or muscle because there are no fibers intact from which pain can be elicited.
4. Weak and painful may indicate a partial rupture of a muscle or tendon because there are fibers which are still intact that may be stressed and could produce pain. Fracture, neoplasm, or acute inflammation may also be possibilities.

SPECIAL PHYSICAL, ORTHOPAEDIC, AND NEUROLOGICAL TESTING

Special physical, orthopaedic, and neurological testing is designed to functionally stress isolated tissue structures in terms of the underlying pathology. Positive physical testing is not diagnostic in itself but rather a biomechanical assessment to be used as part of a complete clinical evaluation.

Before performing certain special testing procedures, you must determine if these special tests will be detrimental to the presenting patient's condition. If it is determined that special physical testing may indeed harm the patient, structural and or functional testing, such as radiography, CT scan, MRI, or EMG, should be employed before any physical testing.

The following chapters contain a collection of special physical orthopaedic and neurological tests organized anatomically and subcategorized by diagnostic entity. This system is best suited for expedient evaluation of musculoskeletal and orthopaedically related neurological conditions. Each test illustrates and discusses the procedures involved for correct performance of the test. Each test is accompanied by an explanation that indicates what the positive indicators for that test are and what they may mean in terms of an underlying pathology or injury. Biomechanical considerations that may not be evident in the classical interpretation of a particular test are also explored.

DIAGNOSTIC IMAGING AND OTHER SPECIALIZED STRUCTURAL TESTING

Diagnostic imaging or structural testing involves the use of specialized equipment to visualize certain anatomical structures. The most common diagnostic imaging procedures include: plain film radiology (x-ray); computed tomography (CT); magnetic resonance imaging (MRI); and skeletal scintigraphy (bone scan). Each individual type of structural test may be best suited to visualize different structures in different ways.

Plain Film Radiology

Plain film radiology dates back to 1895, and its fundamentals are still used in practice today. X-rays are a form of radiant energy that have a short wavelength and are able to penetrate many substances (Fig. 1.3). The x-ray is produced by bombarding a tungsten target with an electron beam within an x-ray tube. Plain film radiography demonstrates five basic densities: air, fat, subcutaneous tissue, bone, and metal. Anatomical structures are seen on radiographs as outlines in whole or part of different tissue densities. These differences in densities are the key in determining the normal or pathologic state of tissues visualized on radiographic film. Bone is the best-visualized tissue on plain film radiography.

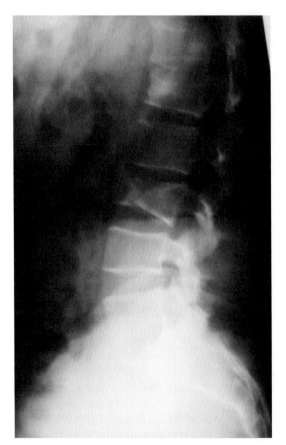

Figure 1.3

Computed Tomography

Computed tomography is a cross-sectional imaging technique that uses x-ray as its energy (Fig. 1.4). A computer is used to reconstruct a cross-sectional image from measurements of x-ray transmission. Most CT units allow for a slice thickness between 1 and 10 mm and are generally limited to the axial plane. CT is best used for bone detail and demonstration of calcifications. Intervertebral disc defects may also be visualized on CT scan (but not as well as with MRI).

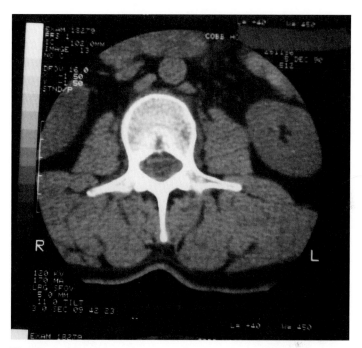

Figure 1.4

Magnetic Resonance Imaging

Magnetic resonance imaging (MRI) is also a cross-sectional imaging technique (Fig. 1.5). This technique uses magnetic fields and radio waves instead of x-ray to produce its images. MRI is based on the ability of the body to absorb and emit radio waves when the body is placed within a strong magnetic field. The absorption and release of this energy is different and detectable in each individual type of tissue. Hence, MRI is invaluable in contrasting soft tissue structures in many different planes without the use of ionizing radiation. It poorly demonstrates bone density detail or calcifications (this is the advantage of the CT scan). It is superior in visualizing an intervertebral disc or other soft tissue structure for pathology.

Patients with any metallic implants or metal fragments (e.g., cardiac pacemakers, insulin pumps, vascular clips, skin staples, bullets, and shrapnel) are advised not to undergo MRI because of the strong magnetic field emitted by the scanner. This field may move or dislodge metallic implants or objects in an individual whose body is being scanned.

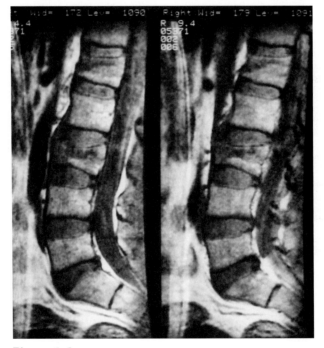

Figure 1.5

Skeletal Scintigraphy

1

Skeletal scintigraphy, or bone scan, is an imaging procedure that uses an intravenous radiopharmaceutical (Technetium-99M) which is attracted to osteoblastic activity in bone tissue and is detected by a gamma camera (Fig. 1.6). Vigorous osteoblastic activity, such as healing fractures and pathologic conditions, stimulate skeletal blood flow and bone repair. In turn, more of the radiopharmaceutical attaches to the area, marking the increased activity for evaluation. Bone scans are best suited for undetectable fractures on x-ray and arthropathies, such as early degenerative changes in joints, osteomyelitis, bony dysplasias, primary bone tumors, and metastatic malignancy.

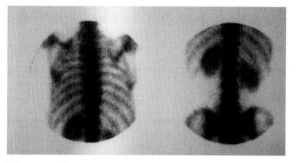

Figure 1.6

FUNCTIONAL TESTING

Functional testing for musculoskeletal and neurological pathology involves testing neurological function by assessing electrical activity of specific neurological structures, such as electroencephalography (EEG), electromyography (EMG), and somatosensory evoked potential studies (SSEP).

Electroencephalography

Electroencephalography (EEG) records the electrical activity of the brain through the skull by surface electrodes. Abnormal electrical activity could possibly indicate cerebral pathology (such as epilepsy, inflammatory encephalopathies, infarction, trauma, or tumor) that may not be detectable by structural testing.

Electromyography

Electromyography (EMG) measures the electrical activity of contracting muscles and is recorded either by surface electrodes or through needles inserted directly into the muscle itself. The surface electrodes record and average the activity from many motor units, whereas needle EMG can detect the activity from a single motor unit. The recordings are used to detect the cause of muscle weakness. They are also useful in detecting neuropathies, denervation, and entrapment syndromes.

Somatosensory Evoked Potential

Somatosensory evoked potential studies (SSEP) measures electrical activity from a distal nerve to a more proximal point on the nerve, spinal cord, or brain stem. A stimulus is given peripherally and responses are recorded and averaged proximal to the stimulated area. The purpose of the test is to determine and quantify nerve, cord, or brain stem lesions. It is used most commonly to detect trauma, tumors, and demyelinating diseases of the nervous system.

In conclusion, the examining clinician should employ the techniques discussed in this chapter to assess the presenting patient's condition. All segments of the clinical assessment protocol need not be employed for each presenting patient and complaint. History, inspection, palpation, range of motion, and physical testing are core requirements. Diagnostic imaging and functional testing are performed based on the outcomes of the core requirements and the clinical judgement and experience of the examiner.

General References

Adams JC, Hamblen DL. Outline of orthopaedics. 11th ed. Edinburgh: Churchill Livingstone, 1990.

American Academy of Orthopeadic Surgeons. The clinical measurement of joint motion. Chicago: American Academy of Orthopaedic Surgeons, 1994.

Bates B. A guide to the physical examination. 4th ed. Philadelphia: JB Lippincott, 1987.

Corrigan B, Maitland GD. Practical orthopaedic medicine. London: Butterworths, 1983.

Cyriax J. Textbook of orthopaedic medicine. Volume one. Diagnosis of soft tissue lesions. 8th ed. London: Bailliere Tindall, 1982.

Endow AJ, Swisher SN. Interviewing and patient care. New York: Oxford University Press, 1992.

Kessler RM, Hertling D. Management of common musculoskeletal disorders. Philadelphia: Harper & Row, 1983.

Krejci VP. Koch muscle and tendon injuries. Chicago: Year Book Medical Publishers, 1979.

Magee DJ. Orthopaedic physical assessment. 2nd ed. Philadelphia: WB Saunders, 1992.

Mooney V. Where is the pain coming from? Spine 1989;12:8:754–759.

Nordin M, Frankel VH. Basic biomechanics of the musculoskeletal system. 2nd ed. Philadelphia: Lea & Febiger, 1989.

Salter RB. Textbook of disorders and injuries of the musculoskeletal system. 2nd ed. Baltimore: Williams & Wilkins, 1983.

2
CERVICAL ORTHOPAEDIC TESTS

2

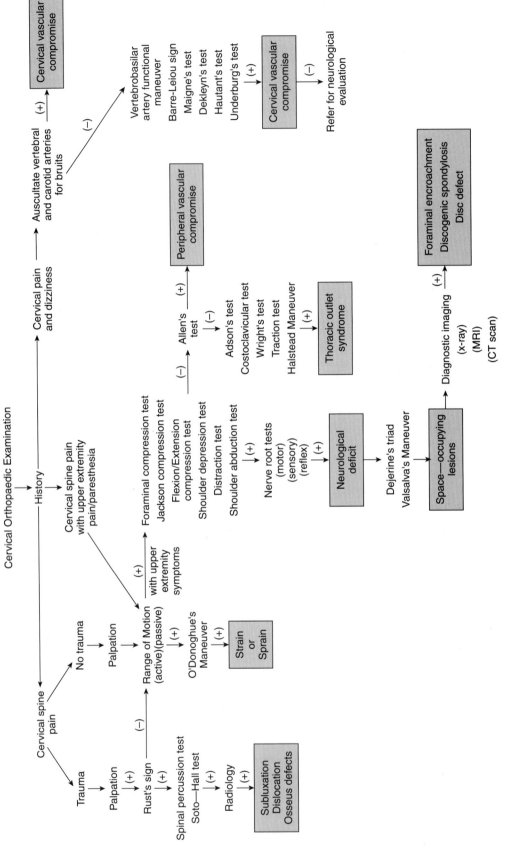

Cervical Orthopaedic Examination

History

Cervical pain and dizziness → Auscultate vertebral and carotid arteries for bruits — (+) → **Cervical vascular compromise**

(−) →

Vertebrobasilar artery functional maneuver
Barre-Leiou sign
Maigne's test
Dekleyn's test
Hautant's test
Underburg's test

(+) → **Cervical vascular compromise** — (−) → Refer for neurological evaluation

Cervical spine pain with upper extremity pain/paresthesia

Foraminal compression test
Jackson compression test
Flexion/Extension compression test
Shoulder depression test
Distraction test
Shoulder abduction test

(−) → Allen's test — (+) → **Peripheral vascular compromise**

(−) →

Adson's test
Costoclavicular test
Wright's test
Traction test
Halstead Maneuver

(+) → **Thoracic outlet syndrome**

Nerve root tests
(motor)
(sensory)
(reflex)

(+) → **Neurological deficit**

(+) → Dejerine's triad
Valsalva's Maneuver → **Space—occupying lesions** → Diagnostic imaging
(x-ray)
(MRI)
(CT scan) — (+) → **Foraminal encroachment
Discogenic spondylosis
Disc defect**

Cervical spine pain

Trauma

Palpation

(+) →

Rust's sign

(+) →

Spinal percussion test
Soto—Hall test

(+) →

Radiology

(+) →

**Subluxation
Dislocation
Osseus defects**

No trauma

Palpation

(−) →

Range of Motion (active)(passive)

(+) with upper extremity symptoms →

(+) →

O'Donoghue's Maneuver

(+) →

**Strain
or
Sprain**

14

CERVICAL PALPATION

Anterior Aspect

Sternocleidomastoid Muscle

2

DESCRIPTIVE ANATOMY:

The sternocleidomastoid muscle extends from the mastoid process of the temporal bone down to the clavicle and sternum (Fig. 2.1). It divides the neck into anterior and posterior triangles. Its action is to laterally flex the head to the same side and rotate it to the opposite side. Both muscles acting together flex the neck forward.

SCM actions (3)

PROCEDURE:

Instruct the patient to turn his head to one side. Pinch the muscle on the same side of head rotation between your thumb and forefinger, traveling from the clavicle upward to the mastoid (Fig. 2.2). Compare each muscle bilaterally, noting any inflammation, palpable bands, and tenderness. Palpable bands are hyperirritable spots within a taut band of skeletal muscle or fascia. *↳ a trgg. points*

Inflammation and tenderness secondary to trauma usually is associated with cervical acceleration/deceleration type injuries (CAD). Torticollis may also cause local inflammation and tenderness. Palpable bands may indicate a myofascial trigger point. These trigger points may be caused by overuse, trauma, or chilling. They may also be indicative of arthritic joints or emotional distress.

CN XI innerv.

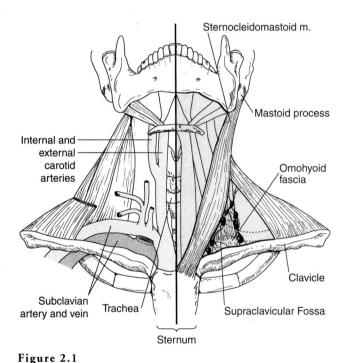

Sternocleidomastoid m.

Mastoid process

Internal and external carotid arteries

Omohyoid fascia

Subclavian artery and vein   Trachea   Clavicle

Supraclavicular Fossa

Sternum

Figure 2.1

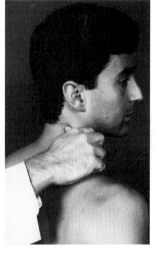

Figure 2.2

torticollis : stiff neck ∝ mm. spasm → lat. flex.
•congen o̅ acquired •aff. CN XI -inner. mm.
•C⁷ : scars, cerv. vert D., adenitis

Carotid Arteries

DESCRIPTIVE ANATOMY:

The carotid arteries are located lateral to the trachea and medial to the sternocleidomastoid muscle. These arteries branch to form the internal and external carotid arteries, which supply blood to the brain (Fig. 2.1).

PROCEDURE:

With your first and second digit, lightly press on the carotid artery against the transverse process of the cervical vertebra (Fig. 2.3). Palpate each artery individually and assess amplitude equality.

A difference in the strength of the pulses may indicate carotid artery stenosis or compression. If carotid artery stenosis or compression is suspected, auscultate the carotid arteries for bruits and evaluate the vertebrobasilar circulation.

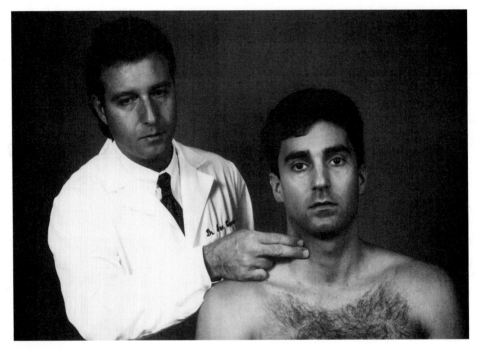

Figure 2.3

Supraclavicular Fossa

DESCRIPTIVE ANATOMY:

The supraclavicular fossa is located superior to the clavicle. It contains the omohyoid fascia, the lymph nodes, and the pressure point for the subclavian artery. It is usually a smooth, contoured depression (Fig. 2.1).

2

PROCEDURE:

Palpate each fossa for swelling, tenderness, and any abnormal bony or soft tissue masses (Fig. 2.4). Pain and tenderness associated with swelling secondary to trauma may indicate a fractured clavicle. Abnormal bony tissue may indicate the presence of a cervical rib, which may cause neurological or vascular symptoms in the upper extremity. If an extra rib is suspect, evaluate for thoracic outlet syndrome (see Chapter 4). An abnormal soft tissue mass may indicate a lymph adenopathy or tumor.

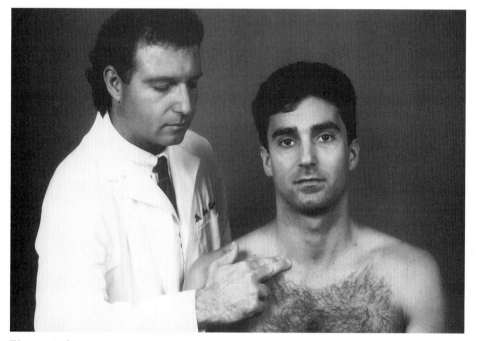

Figure 2.4

Posterior Aspect

Trapezius Muscle

DESCRIPTIVE ANATOMY:

The trapezius muscle is a large, triangular-shaped muscle that extends from the occiput and spinous processes of the cervical and thoracic vertebra to the acromion process of the clavicle and spine of the scapula (Fig. 2.5). Its superior fibers elevate the shoulders, the middle fibers retract the scapula, and the inferior fibers depress the scapula and lower the shoulders.

PROCEDURE:

Palpate each muscle from the superior aspect just below the occiput downward, continuing to the superior aspect of the spine of the scapula, then lateral to the acromion process (Fig. 2.6). From the inferior, palpate from the spinous processes of the thoracic vertebra lateral and superior toward the acromion process (Fig. 2.7).

Inflammation and tenderness secondary to trauma may indicate muscle spasm caused by torn muscle fibers associated with edema. Inflammation and tenderness that are not trauma related may be indicative of fibrosis of muscle tissue or fibromyalgia. Palpable bands are indicative of myofascial trigger points that may be caused by overuse, overload, trauma, or chilling. These palpable bands may also be indicative of arthritic joints or emotional distress.

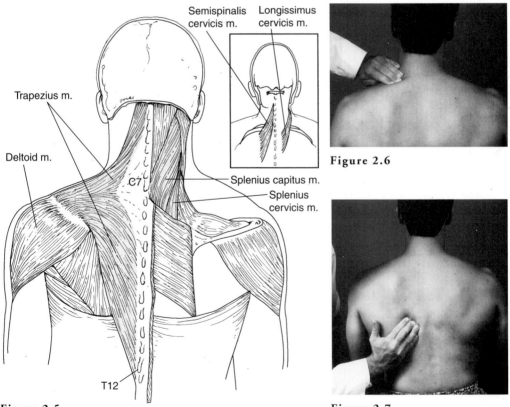

Figure 2.5

Figure 2.6

Figure 2.7

Cervical Intrinsic Musculature

DESCRIPTIVE ANATOMY:

The palpable intrinsic spinal muscles in the cervical spine consist of splenius capitus and cervicis, longissimus cervicis, and semispinalis cervicis. These muscles are used for the maintenance of posture and movements of the cervical spine and are arranged in layers. The superficial layer consists of the splenius capitus and cervicis, and the intermediate layer consists of the longissimus and semispinalis cervicis. These muscles stretch from the base of the occiput to the upper aspect of the thoracic spine (Fig. 2.5). The deep muscle on the cervical spine are difficult at best to palpate and are not discussed here.

PROCEDURE:

The superficial layer is palpated by moving the fingers in a transverse fashion over the belly of the muscle with the cervical spine in slight extension (Fig. 2.8). Note any abnormal tone, tenderness, or palpable bands. The intermediate layer is palpated with the finger tips directly adjacent to the spinous processes also with the cervical spine in slight extension (Fig. 2.9). Note any abnormal tone, tenderness, or palpable bands. Any abnormal tone or tenderness may be indicative of an inflammatory process in the muscle, such as muscle strain, myofascitis, or fibromyalgia. Palpable bands are indicative of myofascial trigger points, which may be caused by overuse, overload, trauma, or chilling. They may also be indicative of arthritic joints or emotional distress.

[handwritten notes]
longissimus : costovert → occiput
semi spin cerv : thor. tvp → cerv sp.
splenius cap : sp (~C7) → mastoid
splenius cerv : (sp thor) → cerv. tvp.

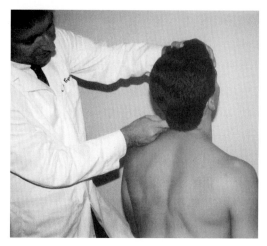

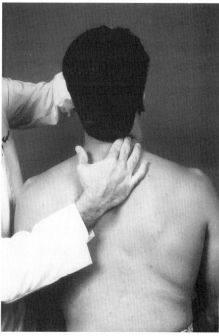

Figure 2.8   **Figure 2.9**

Spinous Process/Facet Joints

DESCRIPTIVE ANATOMY:

The C1 or atlas vertebra has a posterior arch rather than a spinous process which is difficult at best to palpate. The C2 to C7 vertebra have relatively prominent spinous processes that are easily palpable. Slightly lateral to the spinous processes lie the facet joints. Each facet joint is composed of a posterior inferior articular processes and a posterior superior articular process from congruent vertebra (Fig. 2.10).

PROCEDURE:

With the patient seated and his head slightly flexed, palpate each spinous process with your index and/or middle finger. Each spinous should be palpated individually, and you should note any pain and/or tenderness (Fig. 2.11). Also, each spinous should be evaluated while moving the cervical spine in flexion and extension to determine hypomobility versus hypermobility (Fig. 2.12).

Again, with the patient's head slightly flexed, using your thumb and index finger, palpate the facet joints bilaterally both in a static position (Fig. 2.13) and in a flexed position while performing extension movements simultaneously (Fig. 2.14). Tenderness at the spinous and/or facet joint is indicative of an inflammatory process taking place at the respective sites. The inflammation is usually secondary to subluxation or trauma, i.e., hyperflexion/hyperextension injuries. Crepitus on movement may indicate degenerative joint disease.

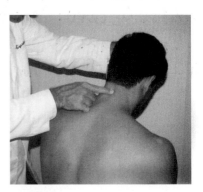

Figure 2.11

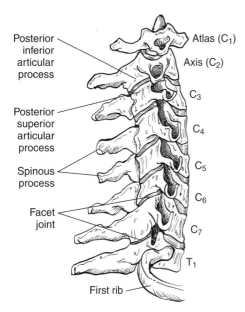

Posterior inferior articular process

Posterior superior articular process

Spinous process

Facet joint

Atlas (C_1)

Axis (C_2)

C_3

C_4

C_5

C_6

C_7

T_1

First rib

Figure 2.10

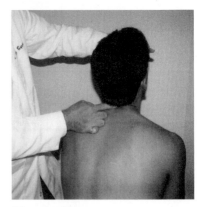

Figure 2.12

2

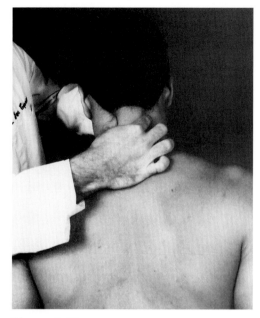

Figure 2.13

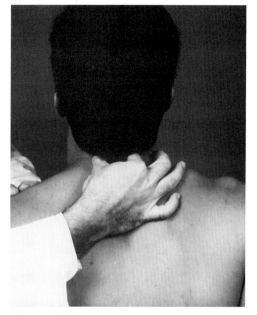

Figure 2.14

CERVICAL RANGE OF MOTION

Cervical range of motion should be evaluated only after taking a proper and thorough history to rule out any contraindications that, by performing these movements, will adversely affect the patient. Severe trauma causing a fracture or dislocation, or cervical vascular compromise should be considered before performing these movements. You should not only note limited motion in the cervical spine but also the presence of pain along with its location and character. The most painful movements should be performed last so that no residual pain is carried over from the previous movement. Crepitus should also be noted upon movement; it may indicate degenerative changes in the cervical spine.

Spinal range of motion is measured using inclinometers, with the patient performing the movements actively and passively. Inclinometers are the preferred instrument for measuring spinal range of motion because they measure angular displacement relative to gravity. For continuity of reporting and for evaluating patient compliance, the movements should be performed three times. The three measurements must be between 5° or within 10% of each other for a valid reporting criteria. Note that the full arc of motion is paramount to the evaluation of range of motion in the cervical spine. Adding the opposing measurements to determine the full arc of movement is the most objective way to assess cervical spine movement. For example, the patient carries his head in 10° of flexion, which for him is the neutral position. When you measure cervical flexion on this individual, cervical flexion may be reduced 10° from average. If you then measure extension, you may possibly have an increase of 10°. This increase may be caused by the 10° flexion angle, which is the neutral position for that patient. If you take each measurement individually, you have a deficit movement in flexion and an increase in movement in extension. If you add both movements, you see that his full arc is within normal limits.

perform t. 3x & need w/in 5° avg ō 10% of each other

Flexion (Inclinometer Method) (1,2)

With the patient seated and the cervical spine in the neutral position, place one inclinometer over the T1 spinous process in the sagittal plane. Place the second inclinometer at the superior aspect of the occiput also in the sagittal plane (Fig. 2.15). Zero out both inclinometers. Instruct the patient to flex his head forward, and then record both angles (Fig. 2.16). Subtract the T1 inclination from the occipital inclination to obtain the active *cervical flexion angle.*

NORMAL RANGE

60° or greater from the neutral or 0 position for active movement.

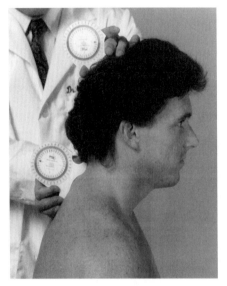

Figure 2.15

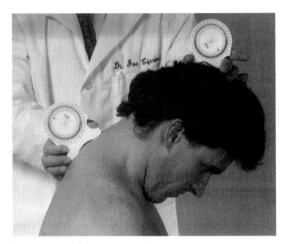

Figure 2.16

Extension (Inclinometer Method) (1,2)

With the patient seated and the cervical spine in the neutral position, place one inclinometer slightly lateral to the T1 spinous process in the sagittal plane. Place the second inclinometer at the superior aspect of the occiput also in the sagittal plane (Fig. 2.17). Zero out both inclinometers. Instruct the patient to extend his head backward, and then record both inclinations (Fig. 2.18). Subtract the T1 inclination from the occipital inclination to obtain the active *cervical extension angle*.

NORMAL RANGE

<u>75° or greater</u> from the neutral or 0 position for active movement.

Full Arc of Active Flexion and Extension •

135°

Full Arc of Passive Flexion/Extension (3) •

← active vs. passive ROM

Age	Degrees
20–29	151 ± 17
30–49	141 ± 35
> 50	129 ± 14

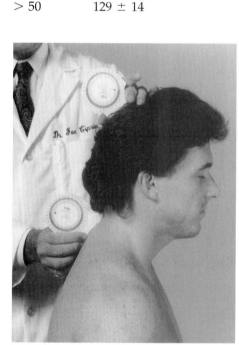

Figure 2.17

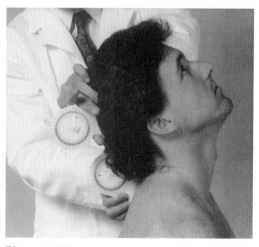

Figure 2.18

Lateral Flexion (Inclinometer Method) (1,2)

With the patient seated and the cervical spine in the neutral position, place one inclinometer flat on the T1 spinous process in the coronal plane. Place the second inclinometer at the superior aspect of the occiput also in the coronal plane (Fig. 2.19). Zero out both inclinometers. Instruct the patient to flex his head to one side, and then record both inclinations (Fig. 2.20). Subtract the T1 inclination from the occipital inclination to obtain the active *cervical lateral flexion angle*. Repeat with flexion to the opposite side.

NORMAL RANGE

45° or greater from the neutral or 0 position for active movement. *(each side)*

Full Arc of Active Right and Left Lateral Flexion

90°

Full Arc of Passive Right and Left Lateral Flexion (3)

Age	Degrees
20–29	101 ± 11
30–49	93 ± 13
> 50	80 ± 17

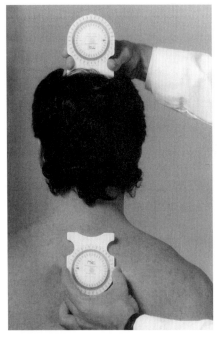

Figure 2.19

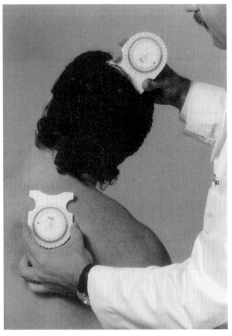

Figure 2.20

2

Rotation (Inclinometer Method) (1,2)

With the patient in the supine position, place the inclinometer at the crown of the head in the transverse plane (Fig. 2.21). Zero out the inclinometer. Instruct the patient to rotate his head to one side, and then record your findings (Fig. 2.22). Repeat the procedure with the patient's head rotated to the opposite side.

NORMAL RANGE

80° or greater from the neutral or 0 position for active movement.

Full Arc of Active Right and Left Rotation

160°

Full Arc of Passive Right and Left Rotation (3)

Age	Degrees
20–29	183 ± 11
30–49	172 ± 13
> 50	155 ± 15

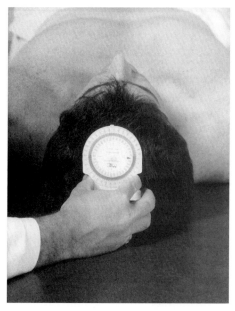

Figure 2.21

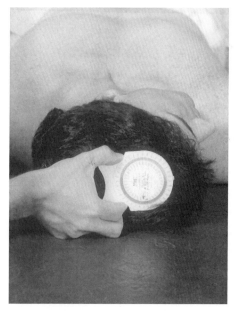

Figure 2.22

CERVICAL RESISTIVE ISOMETRIC MUSCLE TESTING

The same movements that were previously tested and measured can also be tested for resistive strength. Contraindications such as fracture, dislocation, or cervical vascular compromise must be considered before testing for resistive strength.

Flexion

With the patient seated and in the neutral position, instruct him to flex his head forward against your resistance, making sure that there is no patient movement and only muscle contraction (Fig. 2.23).

Muscles Involved in Action	Nerve Supply
1. Longus colli	C2–C5
2. Scalenus anterior	C4–C6
3. Scalenus medius	C3–C8
4. Scalenus posterior	C6–C8
5. Sternocleidomastoid	Accessory, C2

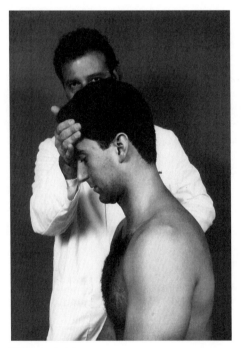

Figure 2.23

Extension

With the patient seated and in the neutral position, instruct him to extend his head backward against your resistance, making sure that there is no patient movement and only muscle contraction (Fig. 2.24).

Muscles Involved in Action	Nerve Supply
1. Splenius cervicis	C6, C7, C8
2. Semispinalis cervicis	C1–C6, C7, C8
3. Longissimus cervicis	C6–C8
4. Levator scapulae	C3–4
5. Iliocostalis cervicis	C6, C7, C8
6. Spinalis cervicis	C6, C8
7. Multifidus	C1–C6, C7, C8
8. Interspinalis cervicis	C1–C8
9. Trapezius (Upper)	C3, C4
10. Rectus capitus posterior major	C1
11. Rotatores breves	C1–C8
12. Rotatores longi	C1–C8

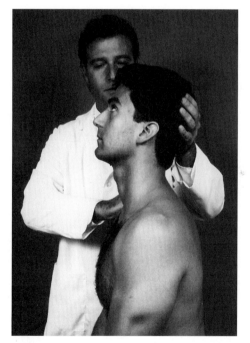

Figure 2.24

Lateral Flexion

With the patient seated and in the neutral position, instruct him to bend his head to one side against your resistance, making sure that there is no patient movement and only muscle contraction (Fig. 2.25). This action should be performed bilaterally.

Muscles Involved in Action	Nerve Supply
1. Levator scapulae	C3–C4
2. Splenius cervicis	C4–C6
3. Iliocostalis cervicis	C6—C8
4. Longissimus cervicis	C6–C8
5. Semispinalis cervicis	C1–C8
6. Multifidus	C1–C8
7. Intertransversarii	C1–C8
8. Scaleni	C3–C8
9. Sternocleidomastoideus	C2
10. Obliquus capitus inferior	C1
11. Rotatores breves	C1–C8
12. Rotatores longi	C1–C8
13. Longus colli	C2–C6
14. Trapezius	C3–C4

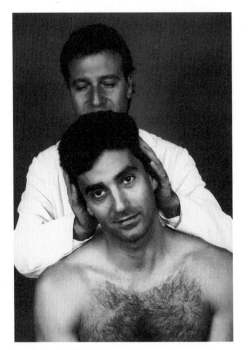

Figure 2.25

2

Rotation

With the patient seated and in the neutral position, instruct him to rotate his head to one side against your resistance, making sure that there is no patient movement and only muscle contraction (Fig. 2.26). This action should be performed bilaterally.

Muscles Involved in Action	Nerve Supply
Moves Face to Same Side	
1. Levator scapulae	C3–C4
2. Splenius cervicis	C4–C6
3. Iliocostalis cervicis	C6–C8
4. Longissimus cervicis	C6–C8
5. Intertransversarii	C1–C8
6. Obliquus capitis inferior	C1
7. Rotatores breves	C1–C8
8. Rotatores longi	C1–C8
Moves Face to Opposite Side	
1. Multifidus	C1–C8
2. Scaleni	C3–C8
3. Sternocleidomastoideus	C2

RATIONALE:

Pain on resistive isometric contraction may indicate a musculotendinous strain of one or more of the muscles involved in the action. Weakness may indicate a neurological disruption to the muscle or muscles involved in the action.

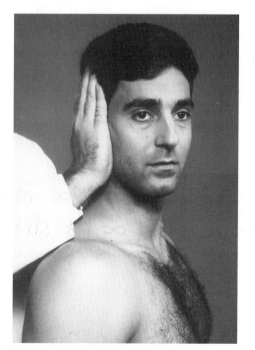

Figure 2.26

DIFFERENTIAL DIAGNOSIS: STRAIN VERSUS SPRAIN

O'Donoghue Maneuver (4)

PROCEDURE:

With the patient in the seated position, put the cervical spine through resisted range of motion (Fig. 2.27), then through passive range of motion (Fig. 2.28). See "Cervical Range of Motion" and "Cervical Resistive Isometric Muscle Testing" in this chapter.

RATIONALE:

Pain during resisted range of motion or isometric muscle contraction signifies muscle strain. Pain during passive range of motion may indicate a ligament sprain.

NOTE:

This maneuver can be applied to any joint or series of joints to determine ligamentous or muscular involvement. By remembering that resistive range of motion mainly stresses muscles and that passive range of motion mainly stresses ligaments, you should be able to determine between strain and sprain or a combination thereof.

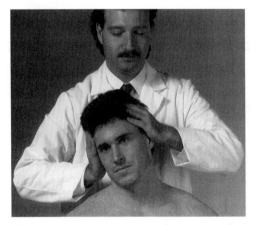

Figure 2.27

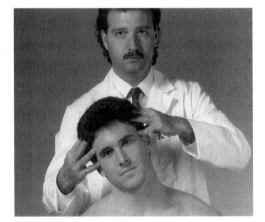

Figure 2.28

pn during resisted motion ∝ mm strain
pn c̄ passive RoM ∝ lig. strain

VERTEBROBASILAR CIRCULATION ASSESSMENT

Vascular insufficiency may be aggravated by positional change in the cervical spine. Assessment of vertebrobasilar circulation must be done if cervical adjustment/manipulation is to be performed. Absolute contraindications and risks of cervical adjustment/manipulation can be minimized significantly, even though reportedly small, with proper diagnostic evaluation. These risks and contraindications may be predicted in some cases by functional or provocative testing and by adequate history (familial history of stroke or cardiovascular disease, hypertension, smoking, cervical spondylosis/arthrosis, bleeding disorders, medication, and/or anatomical anomaly/pathology). Vascular accidents may still occur with no evidence of vascular insufficiency, deficit, and negative provocative procedures.

bw.
CVA

All of the following tests incorporate a positional change in the cervical spine. The rotation aspect of this change is the common denominator of all the following tests. Rotation of C1 on C2 between 30 and 45° causes the vertebral artery at the atlantoaxial junction to become compressed on the opposite side of head rotation, subsequently reducing blood flow to the basilar artery (Fig. 2.29) (5,6). In the normal patient, this diminution of blood flow caused by positional change of the cervical spine will not cause any neurological symptoms, such as dizziness, nausea, tinnitus, faintness, or nystagmus. This lack of symptoms is a result of the normal flow of collateral circulation by the opposite vertebral artery, common carotid arteries, and a communicating cerebral arterial circle (Circle of Willis) (Fig. 2.30).

Rotational instability in the upper cervical spine caused by trauma, arterial artery disease, and/or degenerative joint disease in the cervical spine may lead to a mechanical reduction of blood flow to an area, causing neurological symptoms. This reduction of blood flow must be so severe that the collateral circulation may not be sufficient to sustain normal function to the brain. Therefore, when you positionally stress a vessel in the cervical spine, you are testing the integrity of the collateral circulation supplied to the area (which is normally supplied by the vessel being stressed).

Assessment of the vertebrobasilar circulation by provocative or functional testing stresses seven areas of possible compression. These areas are (Fig 2.31) as follows:

1. Between C1–2 transverse processes, where the vertebral arteries are relatively fixed at the C1 and C2 transverse foramina.
2. C2–3 at the level of the superior articular facet of C3 on the ipsilateral side to head rotation.
3. The C1 transverse process and the internal carotid artery.
4. The atlanto-occipital aperture by the posterior arch of atlas and the rim of foramen magnum, or anteriorly by folding of the atlanto-occipital joint capsule and posteriorly by the atlanto-occipital membrane.
5. C4–5 or C5–6 levels because of arthrosis of the joints of von Luschka with compression on the ipsilateral side to head rotation.
6. At the transverse foramina of the atlas or axis between the obliquus capitis inferior and intertransversarii during rotatory movements.
7. Before entering the C6 transverse process by the longus colli muscle or by tissue communicating between the longus colli and scalenus anterior muscles.

testing collateral circulation c̄ positional stress

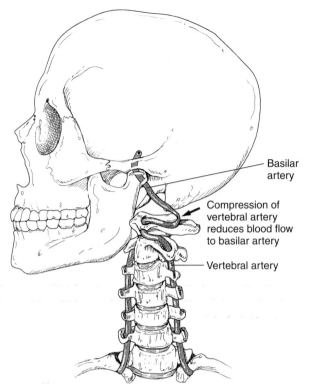

Basilar
artery

Compression of
vertebral artery
reduces blood flow
to basilar artery

Vertebral artery

Figure 2.29

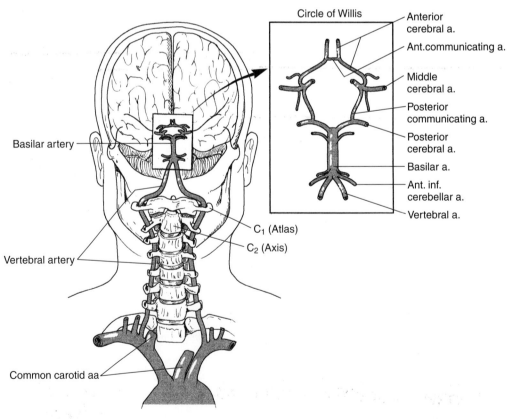

Circle of Willis

Anterior
cerebral a.

Ant.communicating a.

Middle
cerebral a.

Posterior
communicating a.

Posterior
cerebral a.

Basilar a.

Ant. inf.
cerebellar a.

Vertebral a.

Basilar artery

C₁ (Atlas)

C₂ (Axis)

Vertebral artery

Common carotid aa

Figure 2.30

2

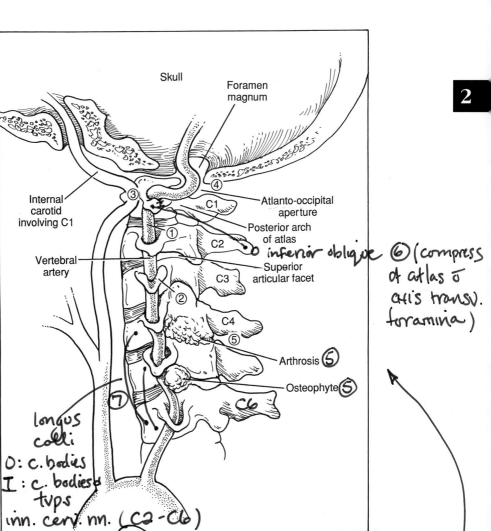

Figure 2.31

Handwritten annotations on figure:

O inferior oblique ⑥ (compress of atlas ō atl's transv. foramina)

Arthrosis ⑤

Osteophyte ⑤

longus colli
O: c. bodies
I: c. bodies & tvps
inn. cerv. nn. (C2-C6)

seven areas of possible compression:

Printed figure labels:

Skull

Foramen magnum

Atlanto-occipital aperture

Internal carotid involving C1

Posterior arch of atlas

Vertebral artery

Superior articular facet

C1

C2

C3

C4

C6

Barre-Leiou Sign (7)

PROCEDURE:

With the patient seated, instruct him to rotate his head to one side and then the other (Fig. 2.32).

RATIONALE:

Rotating the head causes compression of the vertebral artery opposite the side of head rotation (see Fig. 2.29). Therefore, you are testing the patency of the vertebral artery on the same side of head rotation. Vertigo, dizziness, visual blurring, nausea, faintness, and nystagmus are all signs of a positive test. This sign is indicative of buckling vertebral artery syndrome. Also, consideration must be given to the patency of the carotid arteries and a communicating cerebral arterial circle.

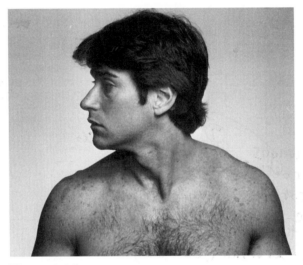

Figure 2.32

2

Vertebrobasilar Artery Functional Maneuver (8)

PROCEDURE:

With the patient in the seated position, palpate and auscultate the carotid (Fig. 2.33) and subclavian arteries (Fig. 2.34) for pulsations or bruits. When auscutating, instruct the patient to hold his breath. If either of these are not present, instruct the patient to rotate and hyperextend his head to one side and then the other (Fig. 2.35). If pulsations or bruits are present, DO NOT PERFORM the rotation and hyperextension portion of the test.

RATIONALE:

If pulsations or bruits are present at the carotid or subclavian arteries, this test is considered positive. It may indicate a compression or stenosing of the carotid or subclavian arteries. The rotation and hyperextension portion of the test places a motion-induced compression on the vertebral artery opposite the side of head rotation (see Fig. 2.29). Vertigo, dizziness, visual blurring, nausea, faintness, and nystagmus are all signs of a positive test. A positive result is indicative of vertebral or basilar artery stenosis or compression at one of the seven sites discussed at the beginning of this chapter. Consideration must also be given to the patency of the carotid arteries and a communicating cerebral arterial circle.

NOTE:

Vertebrobasilar Artery Functional Maneuver and George's Screening Procedure are both subsections of the "George's Cerebrovascular Craniocervical Functional Test."

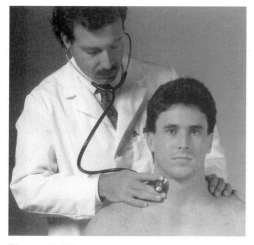

Figure 2.33

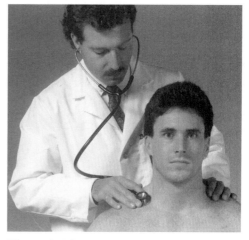

Figure 2.34

Figure 2.35

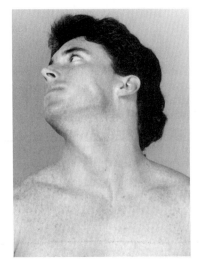

Maigne's Test (9)

PROCEDURE:

With the patient in the seated position, instruct the patient to extend and rotate his head and hold that position for 15 to 40 seconds (Fig. 2.36). Repeat the test with the patient's head rotated to the opposite side.

RATIONALE:

Rotation and extension of the head places a motion-induced compression on the vertebral artery on the opposite side of head rotation (see Fig. 2.29). Vertigo, dizziness, visual blurring, nausea, faintness, and nystagmus are all signs of a positive test. This test is indicative of vertebral, basilar, or carotid artery stenosis or compression at one of the seven sites discussed at the beginning of this section. Consideration must also be given to the patency of the carotid arteries and a communicating cerebral arterial circle.

Figure 2.36

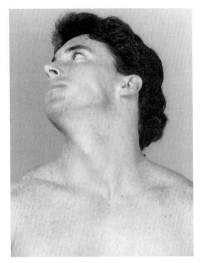

Dekleyn's Test (10,11)

PROCEDURE:

With the patient in the supine position and the patient's head off the table, instruct the patient to hyperextend and rotate the head and hold for 15 to 40 seconds (Fig. 2.37). Repeat with the head rotated and extended to the opposite side.

RATIONALE:

Rotation and hyperextension of the head places a motion-induced compression on the vertebral arteries on the opposite side of head rotation (see Fig. 2.29). Vertigo, dizziness, visual blurring, nausea, faintness, and nystagmus are all signs of a positive test. This test is indicative of vertebral, basilar, or carotid artery stenosis or compression at one of the seven sites discussed at the beginning of this section. Consideration must also be given to the patency of the carotid arteries and a communicating cerebral arterial circle.

Figure 2.37

Hautant's Test

PROCEDURE:

With the patient seated and the patient's eyes closed, instruct the patient to extend his arms out in front of him with his palms up. Instruct the patient to extend and rotate his head to one side (Fig. 2.38). Repeat with the head rotated and extended to the opposite side.

RATIONALE:

A patient with stenosis or compression to the vertebral, basilar, or subclavian arteries without sufficient collateral circulation will tend to lose his balance, drop his arms, and pronate his hands. If this occurs, then suspect a vertebral, basilar, or carotid artery stenosis or compression at one of the seven sites discussed at the beginning of this section.

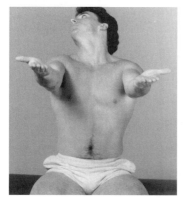

Figure 2.38

Underburg's Test

PROCEDURE:

With the patient standing, instruct him to outstretch his arms, supinate his hands, and close his eyes. Then instruct the patient to march in place (Fig. 2.39). Next, instruct the patient to extend and rotate his head while continuing to march in place (Fig. 2.40). Repeat with the patient's head rotated and extended to the opposite side.

RATIONALE:

Marching in place increases the heart rate, which causally increases the rate of blood flow through the suspected vessels. Extension and rotation of the head places a motion-induced compression on the vertebral arteries on the opposite side of head rotation (see Fig. 2.29). Vertigo, dizziness, visual blurring, nausea, faintness, and nystagmus are all signs of a positive test. This test is indicative of vertebral, basilar, or carotid artery stenosis or compression at one of the seven sites discussed at the beginning of this section. Consideration must also be given to the patency of the carotid arteries and a communicating cerebral arterial circle.

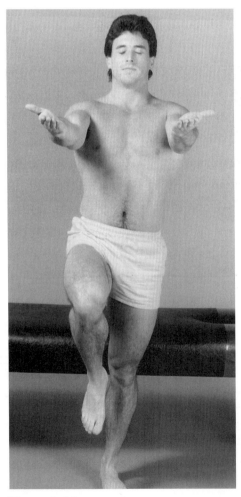

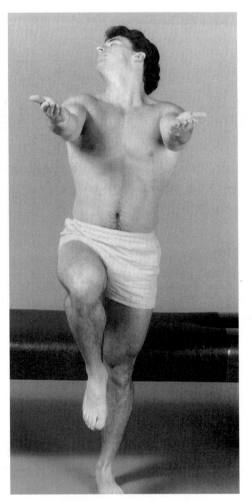

Figure 2.39   Figure 2.40

2

Hallpike Maneuver

PROCEDURE:

Put the patient in the supine position with his head extending off the examination table. Support the patient's head and move the head into extension (Fig. 2.41). Then rotate and laterally flex the head to one side (Fig. 2.42) and hold for 15 to 45 seconds. Repeat the test to the opposite side. Finally, slowly release the head and allow it to hang free in hyperextension (Fig. 2.43).

RATIONALE:

Rotation hyperextension and lateral flexion of the head places a motion-induced compression on the vertebral arteries on the opposite side of head rotation (see Fig. 2.29). Vertigo, dizziness, visual blurring, nausea, faintness, and nystagmus are all signs of a positive test. This test is indicative of vertebral, basilar, or carotid artery stenosis or compression at one of the seven sites discussed at the beginning of this section. Consideration must also be given to the patency of the carotid arteries and a communicating cerebral arterial circle.

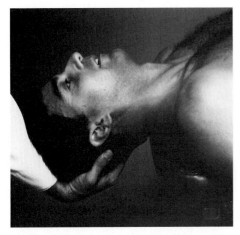

Figure 2.41

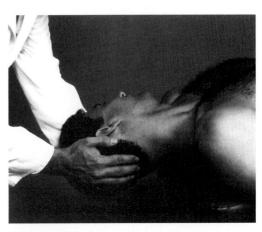

Figure 2.42

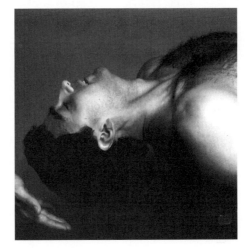

Figure 2.43

SUBCLAVIAN ARTERY COMPROMISE

George's Screening Procedure (8)

PROCEDURE:

With the patient seated, take the patient's blood pressure bilaterally and record the findings (Fig. 2.44). Determine the character of the patient's radial pulse bilaterally (Fig. 2.45).

RATIONALE:

A difference of 10 mm Hg between the two systolic blood pressures and a feeble or absent radial pulse is suggestive of a possible subclavian artery stenosis on the side of the feeble or absent pulse.

NOTE:

If the test is negative, place a stethoscope over the supraclavicular fossa and auscultate the subclavian artery for bruits (Fig. 2.46). If bruits are present, a possible subclavian artery stenosis or compression is suspect.

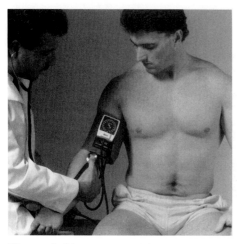

Figure 2.44

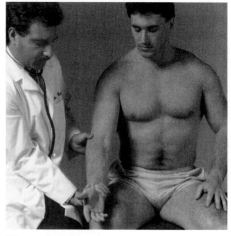

Figure 2.45

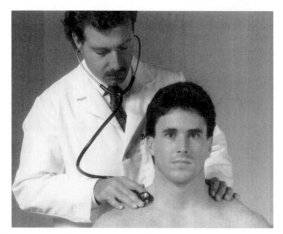

Figure 2.46

CERVICAL FRACTURES

Spinal Percussion Test (4,12)

PROCEDURE:

With the patient sitting and the head slightly flexed, percuss the spinous process (Fig. 2.47) and associated musculature (Fig. 2.48) of each of the cervical vertebrae with a neurological reflex hammer.

RATIONALE:

Evidence of localized pain may indicate a possible fractured vertebra. Evidence of radicular pain indicates a possible disc lesion. If a fracture is suspected, full cervical x-ray series is indicated. If radicular pain is elicited, a posterior disc lesion may be suspected. Refer to Chapter 3 to assess which neurological level is affected.

NOTE:

Because of the nonspecificity of this test, other conditions will also elicit a positive pain response. A ligamentous sprain will elicit a positive sign when percussing the spinous processes. Percussing the paraspinal musculature will elicit a positive sign for muscular strain.

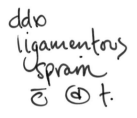

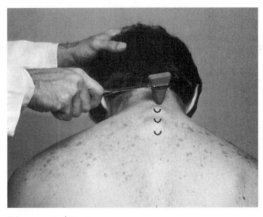

Figure 2.47

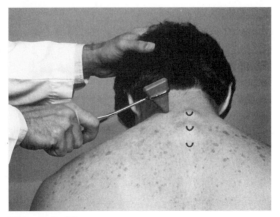

Figure 2.48

Soto-Hall Test (13)

PROCEDURE:

With the patient in the supine position, apply pressure on the patient's sternum with one hand. With the other hand, passively flex the patient's neck to his chest (Fig. 2.49).

RATIONALE:

Evidence of localized pain may indicate ligament, muscular, osseous pathology or injury, or cervical cord disease.

This test is nonspecific; it merely isolates the cervical spine in passive flexion. If the patient reports radicular symptoms in the upper extremity on passive flexion, then a disc defect may be suspect. When the cervical spine is flexed forward, the intervertebral disc is compressed at the anterior and stretched at the posterior (Fig. 2.50). The dura is also tractioned at the posterior. If the patient has a posterior disc defect, this movement may exacerbate the defect, resulting in spinal cord or nerve root compression.

Figure 2.49

flexion will exaccerbate poss Posterior disk lesion & reprod. pn ⟶

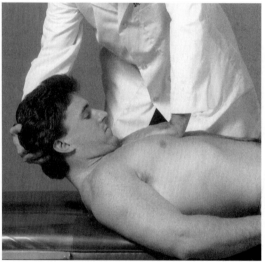

Figure 2.50

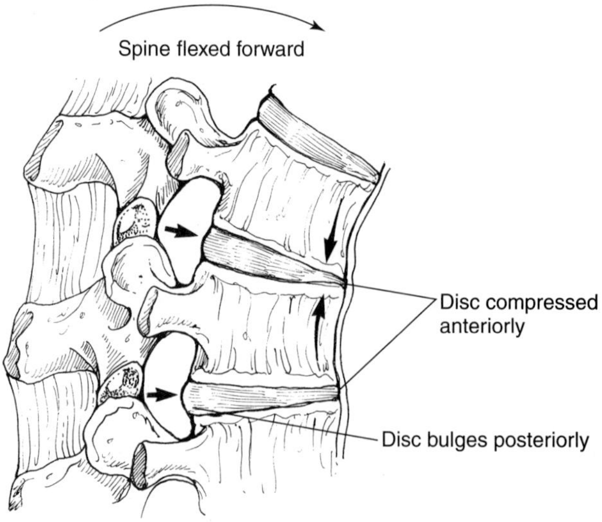

Spine flexed forward

Disc compressed anteriorly

Disc bulges posteriorly

Rust's Sign

PROCEDURE:

A patient with severe injury to the cervical spine will present with the patient grasping the head with both hands to support the weight of the head on the cervical spine (Fig. 2.51). If the patient is supine, he will support his head while attempting to raise his trunk to rise from the supine position.

RATIONALE:

The patient with a severe upper cervical injury, such as severe muscular sprain, ligamentous instability, posterior disc defect, upper cervical fracture, or dislocation, is subject to guarded movements, including stabilization of the head with slight traction to reduce the pain.

note pt.
supporting
head c̄
cervical
L.

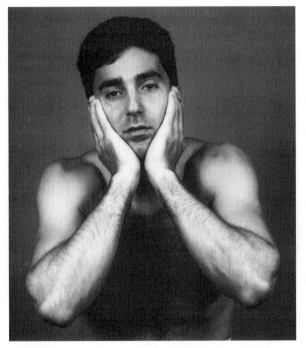

Figure 2.51

SPACE-OCCUPYING LESIONS

Valsalva's Maneuver (14)

PROCEDURE:

With the patient in the seated position, instruct him to bear down as if defecating but concentrating the bulk of the stress at the cervical region (Fig. 2.52). Ask the patient if he feels any increased pain and if so, have him point to its location. This test is very subjective and requires an accurate response from the patient.

RATIONALE:

This test increases intrathecal pressure in the entire spine, but the patient should be able to localize the stress to the cervical spine. Localized pain secondary to the increased pressure may indicate a space-occupying lesion (e.g., disc defect, mass, osteophyte) in the cervical canal or foramen.

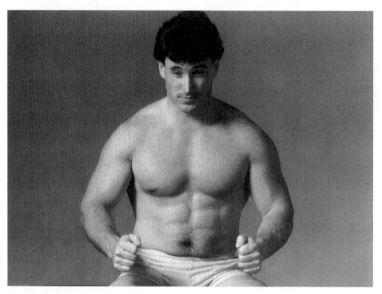

Figure 2.52

Dejerine's Sign

PROCEDURE:

With the patient seated, instruct the patient to cough, sneeze, and bear down as if defecating (Valsalva's maneuver).

RATIONALE:

Pain, either localized or radiating to the shoulders or upper extremities after any of the above actions, indicates an increase in the intrathecal pressure. This pain may be caused by a space-occupying lesion, such as a disc defect, osteophyte, or mass.

2

Swallowing Test (14)

PROCEDURE:

With the patient seated, instruct him to swallow (Fig. 2.53).

RATIONALE:

Pain upon swallowing is usually indicative of esophageal or pharyngeal injury, dysfunction, or pathology. Pain upon swallowing has an orthopaedically related significance. Because of the close proximity of the esophagus to the anterior longitudinal ligament in the cervical spine, anterior pathology of the cervical spine, such as anterior disc defect, osteophyte, mass, or muscle spasm, may compress or irritate the esophagus and cause pain upon swallowing.

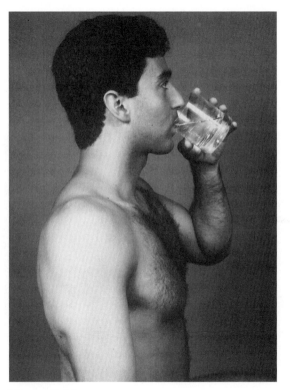

Figure 2.53

CERVICAL NEUROLOGICAL COMPRESSION AND IRRITATION

Foraminal Compression Test (15, 16,17)

PROCEDURE:

With the patient in the seated position and the patient's head in the neural position, exert strong downward pressure on his head (Fig. 2.54). Repeat the test with the head rotated bilaterally (Fig. 2.55).

RATIONALE:

When downward pressure is applied to the head, the following biomechanical considerations take place: 1) narrowing of the intervertebral foramina; 2) compression of the apophyseal joints in the cervical spine; and 3) compression of the intervertebral discs in the cervical spine.

Localized pain may indicate foraminal encroachment without nerve root pressure or apophyseal capsulitis. Radicular pain may indicate pressure on a nerve root by a decrease in the foraminal interval (foraminal encroachment) or by a disc defect.. If nerve root involvement is suspected, see Chapter 3 to evaluate the neurological level involved.

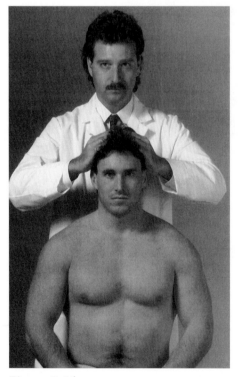

Figure 2.54

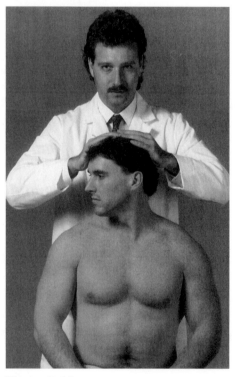

Figure 2.55

Jackson Compression Test (18)

Procedure:

With the patient seated, laterally flex his neck and exert strong downward pressure on his head. Perform this test bilaterally (Fig. 2.56).

2

Rationale:

With the neck laterally flexed and downward pressure applied, the following biomechanical considerations take place: 1) narrowing of the intervertebral foramina on the side of lateral bending; 2) compression of the facet joints on the side of lateral bending; and 3) compression of the intervertebral discs in the cervical spine.

Localized pain may indicate foraminal encroachment without nerve root pressure or apophyseal joint pathology. Radicular pain may indicate pressure on a nerve root by a decrease in the foraminal interval (foraminal encroachment) or a disc defect. If nerve root involvement is suspected, see Chapter 3 to evaluate the neurological level involved.

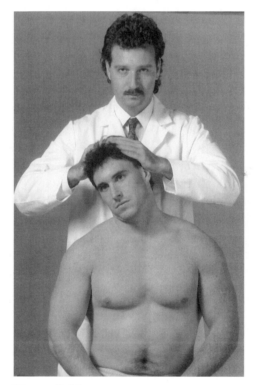

Figure 2.56

Extension Compression Test (19)

PROCEDURE:

With the patient in the seated position, instruct the patient to extend his head approximately 30°. Then place downward pressure on the patient's head (Fig. 2.57).

RATIONALE:

When pressure is applied to the patient's head with the cervical spine in extension, the cervical intervertebral disc space is decreased posteriorly and increased vertically and anteriorly with an increased load on the posterior apophyseal joints (Fig. 2.58). If a decrease in the patient's symptoms occur, then a posterolateral disc defect is suspect because of the anterior and vertical displacement of discal material away from the nerve root or spinal cord. Downward pressure on the head also compresses the posterior apophyseal joints, which, if irritated, can cause localized cervical pain.

An increase in upper extremity radicular symptoms may indicate a pathology in the intervertebral foramina, such as an osteophyte or mass or a degenerating cervical intervertebral disc. This pathology is possible because the pressure on the head decreases the intervertebral foraminal interval.

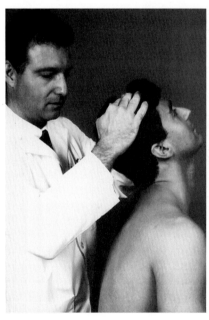

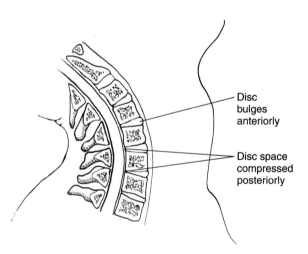

Disc
bulges
anteriorly

Disc space
compressed
posteriorly

Figure 2.57   **Figure 2.58**

Flexion Compression Test (19)

PROCEDURE:

With the patient in the seated position, instruct the patient to flex his head forward. Then place downward pressure on the patient's head (Fig. 2.59).

RATIONALE:

When the patient flexes his head forward and pressure is applied to his head, the intervertebral disc is compressed anteriorly and the load is placed on the intervertebral disc. This pressure also causes the posterior aspect of the disc to bulge posteriorly (Fig. 2.60). An increase in cervical and or radicular symptoms may indicate a discal defect. Flexion of the cervical spine and compression on the head also reduces the load on the posterior apophyseal joints. A decrease in localized scleratogenous pain may be indicative of apophyseal joint injury or pathology.

Figure 2.59

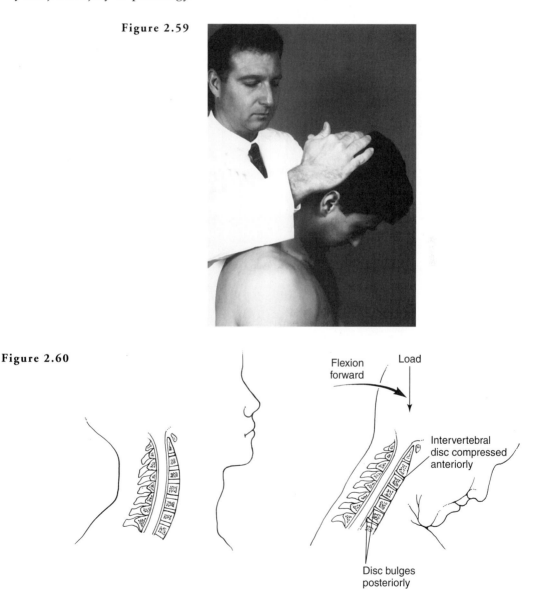

Figure 2.60

Spurling's Test (15)

PROCEDURE:

With the patient in the seated position, laterally flex the patient's head and gradually apply strong downward pressure on his head (Fig. 2.61). If pain is elicited, the test is considered positive; do not continue with the next procedure. If no pain is elicited, put the patient's head in a neutral position and deliver a vertical blow to the upper-most portion of the patient's head (Fig. 2.62).

RATIONALE:

Localized pain may indicate facet joint involvement either from the strong downward pressure placed on the head or from the vertical blow to the head. Radicular pain may indicate foraminal encroachment, degenerating cervical intervertebral disc, or disc defect with nerve root pressure. This test may also indicate a lateral disc defect.

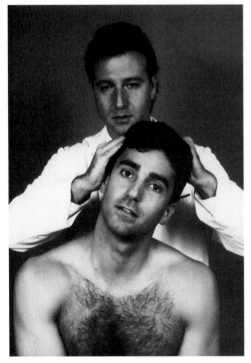

Figure 2.61

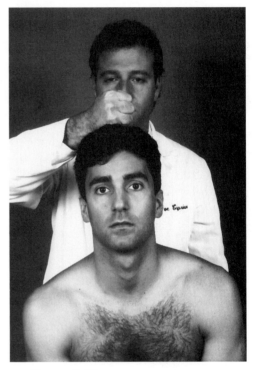

Figure 2.62

Maximal Foraminal Compression Test

PROCEDURE:

With the patient in the seated position, instruct the patient to approximate his chin to his shoulder and extend his neck. Perform this test bilaterally (Fig. 2.63).

RATIONALE:

Rotation of the head and hyperextension of the neck causes the following biomechanical considerations take place: 1) narrowing of the intervertebral foramina on the side of head rotation; 2) compression of the facet joints on the side of head rotation; and 3) compression of the intervertebral discs in the cervical spine. Pain on the side of head rotation with a radicular component may indicate nerve root compression caused by a pathology or decrease interval in the foramina, such as an osteophyte or mass. Local pain with no radicular component may indicate apophyseal joint pathology on the side of head rotation and neck extension. Pain on the opposite side of head rotation is indicative of muscular strain or ligament sprain.

If nerve root compression is suspected, see Chapter 3 to evaluate the neurological level of the suspected pathology.

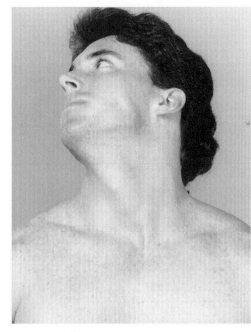

Figure 2.63

L'hermitte's Sign (20, 21)

PROCEDURE:

With the patient in the seated position, passively flex the patient's chin to his chest (Fig. 2.64)

RATIONALE:

When the cervical spine is flexed forward, the spinal cord and its coverings are tractioned at the posterior, and the intervertebral disc is compressed at the anterior and bulged at the posterior (Fig. 2.65). If the patient has a posterior disc defect, this movement may exacerbate the defect resulting in spinal cord or nerve root compression. Cervical cord disease, meningitis, osteophytes, and masses may cause local and/or radicular pain into the upper and/or lower extremities. A sudden electrical tingling felt in the spine and/or extremities during neck flexion may indicate cervical myelopathy or multiple sclerosis.

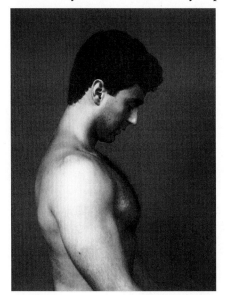

Figure 2.64

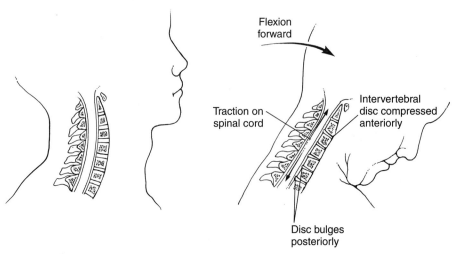

Figure 2.65

Shoulder Depression Test (18)

PROCEDURE:

With the patient seated, place downward pressure on the shoulder while laterally flexing the patient's head to the opposite side (Fig. 2.66).

RATIONALE:

When pressure is applied to the shoulder and the head is slightly flexed to the opposite side, the muscles, ligaments, nerve roots, nerve root coverings, and the brachial plexus are stretched and the clavicle is depressed approximating the first rib. Local pain on the side being tested indicates shortening of the muscles, muscular adhesions, muscle spasm, or ligamentous injury. Radicular pain may indicate compression of the neurovascular bundle, adhesion of the dural sleeve, or thoracic outlet syndrome (TOS). On the opposite side being tested, the foraminal interval is decreased, the apophyseal joints are compressed, and the intervertebral disc is compressed. If pain is elicited on the opposite side being tested, it may indicate a pathological decrease in the foraminal interval, facet pathology, or disc defect.

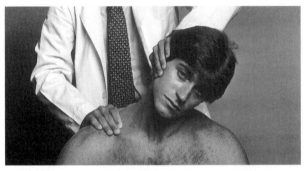

Figure 2.66

Distraction Test (14)

PROCEDURE:

With the patient in the seated position, grasp beneath the mastoid processes and exert upward pressure on the patient's head. This removes the weight of the patient's head on his neck (Fig. 2.67).

RATIONALE:

When the head is distracted, the cervical muscles, ligaments, and apophyseal joint capsules are stretched. If local pain is increased on distraction, then muscle strain, spasm, ligamentous sprain, or facet capsulitis is suspect. Also, when the head is distracted, the interforaminal and intervertebral interval are increased. Relief of local or radicular pain is indicative of either foraminal encroachment or a disc defect.

Figure 2.67

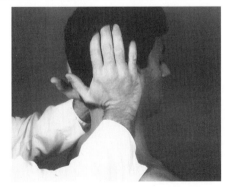

Shoulder Abduction Test (Bakody Sign) (22)

PROCEDURE:

With the patient in the seated position, instruct the patient to abduct his arm and place his hand on top of his head (Fig. 2.68).

RATIONALE:

By placing the hand above the head, the suprascapular nerve is elevated, reducing the traction on the lower trunk of the brachial plexus. This procedure subsequently reduces the traction on a compressed nerve. A decrease or relief of the patient's symptoms is indicative of a cervical extradural compression problem such as a herniated disc, epidural vein compression, or nerve root compression, usually in the C5–C6 area.

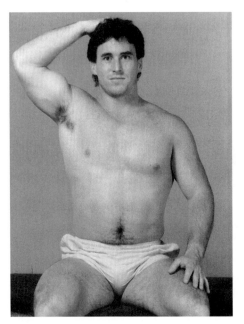

Figure 2.68

References

1. American Medical Association. Guides to the evaluation of permanent impairment. 3rd ed. Chicago: American Medical Association, 1988.
2. American Academy of Orthopaedic Surgeons. The clinical measurement of joint motion. Chicago: American Association of Orthopaedic Surgery, 1994.
3. Dvorak J, Antinnes JA, Panjabi M, et al. Age and gender normal motion of the cervical spine. Spine 1992;17(suppl 10):S393–S398.
4. O'Donoghue D. Treatment of injuries to athletes. 4th ed. Philadelphia: WB Saunders, 1984.
5. Okawara S, Nibbelink D. Vertebral artery occlusion following hyperextension and rotation of the head. Stroke 1974;5;640–642.
6. White AA, Panjabi MM. Clinical biomechanics of the spine. Philadelphia: JB Lippincott, 1978.
7. Barre JA. Le syndrome sympathique cervical posterieur. Rev Neurol 1926;33:248–249.
8. George PE, Silverstein HT, Wallace H, et al. Identification of the high risk pre-stroke patient. J Chiropractic 1981;15:26–28.
9. Maigne R. Orthopaedic medicine. A new approach to vertebral manipulations. Springfield, IL: Charles C. Thomas, 1972:155.
10. deKleyn A, Versteegh C. Ueber verschiendene Formen von Menieres Syndrom. Deutsche Ztschr 1933;132:157.
11. deKleyn A, Nieuwenhuyse P. Schwindelandfaelle und Nystagmus beieiner bestimmten Stellung des Kopfes. Acta Otolaryng 1927;11:555.
12. Turek SL. Orthopaedics. 3rd ed. Philadelphia: JB Lippincott, 1977.
13. Soto-Hall R, Haldeman K. A useful diagnostic sign in vertebral injuries. Surg Gynecol Obstet 827–831.
14. Hoppenfeld S. Physical examination of the spine and extremities. New York: Appleton-Century-Crofts, 1976:127.
15. Spurling RG, Scoville WB. Lateral rupture of the cervical IVDs—a common cause of shoulder and arm pain. Surg Gynecol Obstet 1944;78:350–358.
16. Harris NM. Cervical spine dysfunction. GP 1967;32(4):78–88.
17. Depalma A, Rothman RH. The intervertebral disc. Philadelphia: WB Saunders, 1970:88.
18. Jackson R. The cervical syndrome. 3rd ed. St. Louis: Mosby, 1985.
19. Gerard J, Kleinfeld S. Orthopaedic testing. New York: Churchill Livingstone, 1993.
20. L'hermitte J. Etude de la commotion de la moella. Rev Neurol (Paris), 1:210, 1932.
21. Chermitte J, Bollak P, Nicholas M. Les douleurs a type de decharge electrique dans la sclerose en plaques. Un cas e forme sensitive de la sclerose multiple.
22. Davidson RI, Dunn EJ, Metzmater JN. The shoulder abduction test in the diagnosis of radicular pain in cervical extradural compressive monoradiculopathies. Spine 1981; 6:441.

General References

Clarkson HM, Gilewich GB. Musculoskeletal assessment: joint range of motion and manual muscle strength. Baltimore: Williams & Wilkins, 1989.

Cyriax J. Textbook of orthopaedic medicine. Vol. 1. Diagnosis of soft tissue lesions. London: Bailliere Tindall, 1982.

Edwards BC. Combined movements in the cervical spine (C2-7): their value in examination and technique choice. Aust J Physiother 1980;26:165.

Foreman SM, Croft AC. Whiplash injuries: the cervical acceleration/deceleration syndrome. 2nd ed. Baltimore: Williams & Wilkins, 1995.

Kapandji IA. The physiology of joints. Vol. 3. The trunk and the vertebral column. New York: Churchill Livingstone, 1974.

Naffzinger HC, Grant WT. Neuritis of the brachial plexus mechanical in origin: the scalenus syndrome. Clin Orthop 1967;51:7.

Neviaser JS. Musculoskeletal disorders of the shoulder region causing cervicobrachial pain: differential diagnosis and treatment. Surg Clin North Am 1963;43:1703.

Nichols HM. Anatomic structures of the thoracic outlet. Clin Orthop 1967;51:17.

Norkin CC, Levangie PK. Joint structure and function: a comprehensive analysis. Philadelphia: FA Davis, 1983.

Terrett AGJ. Importance and interpretation of tests designed to predict susceptibility to neurocirculatory accidents from manipulation. J Aust Chiropr Assoc 1983;13(2):29–34.

3

CERVICAL NERVE ROOT LESIONS

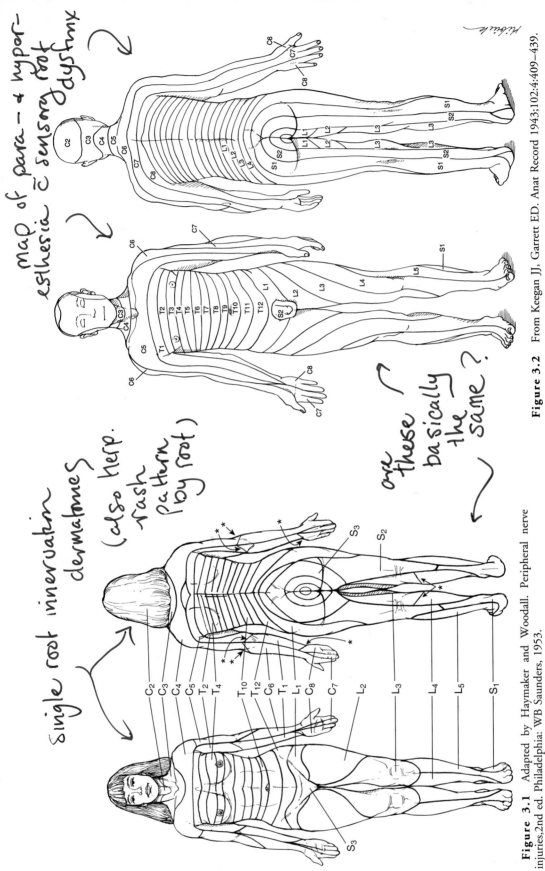

map of para- & hyper-esthesia & sensory root dysfunx

single root innervatin dermatomes
(also herp. rash pattern by root)

are these basically the same?

Figure 3.1 Adapted by Haymaker and Woodall. Peripheral nerve injuries, 2nd ed. Philadelphia: WB Saunders, 1953.

Figure 3.2 From Keegan JJ, Garrett ED. Anat Record 1943;102:4:409–439.

If a nerve root lesion is suspect, you must evaluate three important clinical aspects of the neurological examination: sensory, motor, and reflex dysfunction.

Sensory testing attempts to delineate the segmental cutaneous innervation to the skin. It is tested with a sterile or disposable neurotip or pinwheel in specific dermatomal patterns. Two dermatomal maps are provided here. Figure 3.1 is based on: the body areas of intact sensation when roots above and below an isolated root were interrupted; sensation loss when one or more continuous roots were interrupted; or the pattern of herpetic rash and hypersensitivity in isolated root involvment. Figure 3.2 is based on the hyposensitivity to pin scratch in various root lesions and is consistant with electrical skin resistance studies showing axial dermatomes extending to the distal extremities. This pattern is useful in evaluating paresthesias and hyperesthesias secondary to root irritation. This is the pattern that I will delineate to evaluate sensory root dysfunction. A fair amount of segmental overlap exists; therefore, a single unilateral lesion may affect more than one dermatomal level. Motor function will be evaluated by testing the muscle strength of specific muscles innervated by a particular nerve root or roots using the muscle grading chart adopted by the American Academy of Orthopaedic Surgeons (Fig. 3.3). The reflex arc will be tested by evaluating the superficial stretch reflex associated with the particular nerve root. These arcs are graded by the Wexler Scale (Fig. 3.4).

3

testing
mm.
funk.

5	Complete range of motion against gravity with full resistance.
4	Complete range of motion against gravity with some resistance.
3	Complete range of motion against gravity.
2	Complete range of motion with gravity eliminated.
1	Evidence of slight contractility. No joint motion.
0	No evidence of contractility.

Figure 3.3 Muscle grading chart.

each dermatome
chart will
be
different   testing
reflex
funx →

0	No response
+1	Hyporeflexia
+2	Normal
+3	Hyperreflexia
+4	Hyperreflexia with transient clonus
+5	Hyperreflexia with sustained clonus

Figure 3.4 Wexler scale.

The clinical presentation of nerve root lesions depend on two important factors: location and severity of the injury or pathology. The combination of these two factors will determine the injury's clinical presentation. The possibilities are endless and can range from no clinical presentation or slight clinical manifestation, such as slight loss of sensation and pain, to total denervation with loss of total function to the structures innervated by that nerve root (motor, sensory, and reflex).

Each nerve root will have its own sensory distribution, muscle test or tests, and a stretch reflex; these will be grouped together to facilitate the identification of the suspected level.

Remember that the clinical evaluation is not made solely on one aspect of the "Neurological Package" but is instead determined by the combination of history, inspection, palpation, the three individual tests (motor, reflex, and sensory) and appropriate diagnostic imaging and/or functional neurological testing, such as EMG. We must also realize that the injury or pathology we are attempting to evaluate may not necessarily be affecting a nerve root but it may be affecting the brachial plexus, a trunk of that plexus, or a named nerve. Depending on the severity and location of the injury or pathology, various combinations of neurological dysfunction may be elicited.

I. C5

The C5 nerve root exits the spinal canal between the C4 and C5 vertebrae and may be affected by the C4 intervertebral disc (Fig. 3.5).

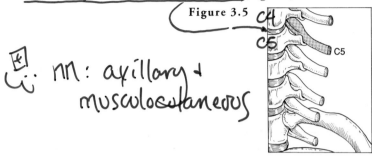

Figure 3.5

Handwritten: nn: axillary + musculocutaneous

A. Motor

Deltoid Muscle (C5-Axillary Nerve Innervation)

PROCEDURE:

With the patient in the seated position, stand behind the patient and place your hand at the lateral aspect of the elbow. Instruct the patient to abduct his arm against resistance (Fig. 3.6). Grade the strength according to the muscle grading chart. Perform this test bilaterally and compare each side. *(0–5)*

RATIONALE:

A grade 0 to 4 unilaterally may indicate a neurological deficit of the C5 nerve root, upper trunk of the brachial plexus, or the axillary nerve. A weak or strained deltoid muscle may be suspected if the sensory and reflex portions of the C5 "Neurological Package" are intact.

Handwritten: motor dysfunc only...

Handwritten: 0-4 grade indic. neurolog. deficit in any of (3) areas

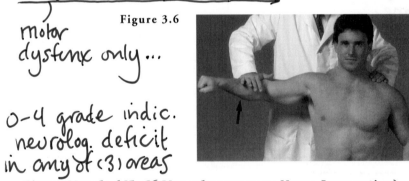

Figure 3.6

Biceps Muscle (C5, C6-Musculocutaneous Nerve Innervation)

PROCEDURE:

With the patient in the seated position and the forearm flexed, stabilize the patient's elbow with one hand, and grasp the anterior aspect of the patient's wrist with your opposite hand. Instruct the patient to flex his forearm against resistance (Fig. 3.7). Grade the strength according to the muscle grading chart and compare each side.

RATIONALE:

A grade 0 to 4 unilaterally may indicate a neurological deficit of the C5 or C6 nerve roots, upper trunk of the brachial plexus, or musculocutaneous nerve. A weak or strained biceps muscle may be suspected if the sensory and reflex portions of the C5 "Neurological Package" are intact.

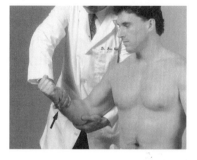

Figure 3.7

B. Reflex

Biceps Reflex (C5, C6-Musculocutaneous Nerve Innervation)

PROCEDURE:

Place the patient's arm across your opposite arm with your thumb on the biceps tendon. Strike your thumb with the narrow end of the reflex hammer (Fig. 3.8). The biceps muscle should contract slightly under your thumb. Grade your response according to the reflex chart and evaluate bilaterally.

RATIONALE:

Hyporeflexia may indicate a C5, C6 nerve root deficit. Loss of reflex may indicate an interruption of the reflex arc (lower motor neuron lesion). Hyperreflexia may indicate an upper motor neuron lesion.

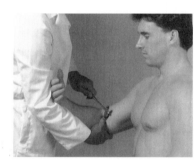

Figure 3.8

reflex :
• loss : lower m.n. L.
• hypo~ : C5, C6 n.root l.
• hyper~ : upper m.n. l.

C. Sensory

PROCEDURE:

With a pin, stroke the lateral aspect of the arm (Fig. 3.9).

RATIONALE:

Unilateral hypoesthesia may indicate a neurological deficit of the C5 nerve root or the axillary nerve.

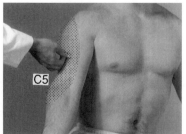

Figure 3.9

C5

II. C6

The C6 nerve root exits the spinal canal between the C5 and C6 vertebrae and may be affected by the C5 intervertebral disc (Fig. 3.10).

Figure 3.10

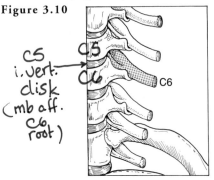

(handwritten:) C5 i.vert. disk (mb aff. C6 root)

A. Motor

(1) Biceps Muscle (C5, C6-Musculocutaneous Nerve Innervation)

See Figure 3.7 and accompanying text.

(2) Wrist Extensor Group: Extensor Carpi Radialis, Longus, and Brevis (C6, C7-Radial Nerve Innervation)

PROCEDURE:

With the patient seated, stabilize the patient's forearm by grasping the patient's elbow with your hand. Instruct the patient to make a fist, and dorsiflex his wrist (Fig. 3.11). With your opposite hand, grasp the patient's fist and attempt to force the wrist into flexion against patient resistance (Fig. 3.12). Evaluate according to the muscle grading chart and compare bilaterally.

RATIONALE:

(handwritten:) i.e., these form rad. n

A grade 0 to 4 unilaterally may indicate a neurological deficit of the C6 or C7 nerve root. A weak or strained wrist extensor may be suspected if the sensory and reflex portions of the C6 and C7 "Neurological Packages" are intact.

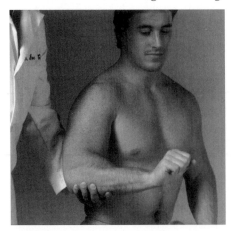

Figure 3.11

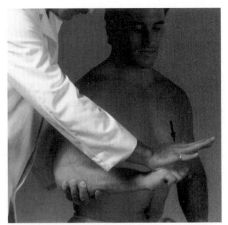

Figure 3.12

(handwritten:) 0-4 on mm. grade chart ∞ n. root (neurolog.) deficit.

B. Reflex

Brachioradialis Reflex (C5, C6-Radial Nerve Innervation)

PROCEDURE:

Place the patient's arm across your opposite arm and tap the brachioradialis tendon at the distal aspect of the forearm with the neurological reflex hammer (Fig. 3.13). The brachioradialis muscle should contract slightly on your arm. Grade your response according to the reflex chart and evaluate bilaterally.

RATIONALE:

Hyporeflexia may indicate a nerve root deficit. Loss of reflex may indicate an interruption of the reflex arc (lower motor neuron lesion). Hyperreflexia may indicate an upper motor neuron lesion.

Figure 3.13

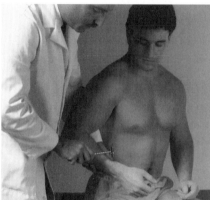

hyporeflex: n. root lesion
areflexia: reflex arc prob.
hyperreflex: upper m.n.
lesion

C. Sensory

PROCEDURE:

With a pin, stroke the lateral aspect of the forearm, thumb, and index finger (Fig. 3.14).

RATIONALE:

Unilateral hypoesthesia may indicate a neurological deficit of the C6 nerve root or the musculocutaneous nerve.

Figure 3.14

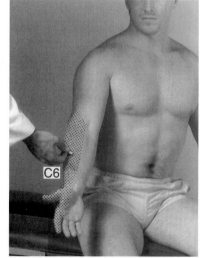

C6

Hypoesth. ∞
neurolog.: C6
δ
musculo cut. n.
deficit

C6: 💡 biceps mm, wrist extensors,
+ brachioradialis (flex forearm.)

III.C7

The C7 nerve root exits the spinal canal between the C6 and C7 vertebrae and may be affected by the C6 intervertebral disc (Fig. 3.15).

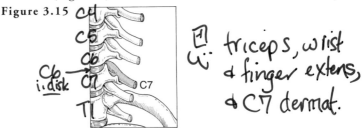

Figure 3.15

(handwritten) C4 C5 C6 C6 i.disk C7 T1 C7

(handwritten right margin) C7: triceps, wrist & finger extens, & C7 dermat.

A. Motor

Triceps Muscle (C7-Radial Nerve Innervation)

PROCEDURE:

With the patient in the supine position, flex the shoulder and elbow to 90°. Grasp the proximal aspect of the arm to stabilize the extremity. With your opposite hand, grasp the patient's wrist and ask the patient to extend his forearm against your resistance (Fig. 3.16). Grade the strength according to the muscle grading chart and compare bilaterally.

RATIONALE:

A grade 0 to 4 unilaterally may indicate a neurological deficit of the C7 nerve root or radial nerve. A weak or strained triceps muscle may be suspected if the sensory and reflex portions of the C7 "Neurological Package" are intact.

Figure 3.16

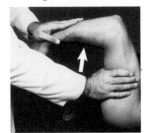

(handwritten left) "0-4" grad. ∝ neurolog. C7 n.r. def. (triceps)

(handwritten right) if S & R ✗, r/o weak triceps m.

(1) *Wrist Flexor Group: Flexor Carpi Radialis (C7-Median Nerve Innervation) and Flexor Carpi Ulnaris (C8-Ulnar Nerve Innervation)*

PROCEDURE:

With the patient seated, stabilize the patient's forearm by grasping the forearm with your hand. Instruct the patient to make a fist and flex his wrist. With your opposite hand, grasp the patient's fist and attempt to force the wrist into extension against patient resistance (Fig. 3.17). Grade according to the muscle grading chart and compare bilaterally.

RATIONALE:

A grade 0 to 4 unilaterally may indicate a neurological deficit of the C7 or C8 nerve root. A weak or strained wrist flexor may be suspected if the sensory and reflex portions of the C7 and C8 "Neurological Packages" are intact.

Figure 3.17

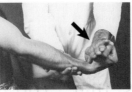

(handwritten) "0-4" ∝ neuro. def of C7 ō C8

(2) ***Finger Extensor Group: Extensor Digitorum Communis,***
Extensor Digiti Indicis, Extensor Digiti Minimi (C7-Radial
Nerve Innervation)

"0-4" indic: siu. deficit (C7 õ C8 n.r.)

PROCEDURE:

With the patient's wrist in the neutral position, grasp the patient's wrist with your hand. Have the patient extend his metacarpal-phalangeal joints and flex his proximal and distal interphalangeal joints (Fig. 3.18). Place your hand on the distal aspect of the proximal phalanges and attempt to force the metacarpal-phalangeal joints into flexion against patient resistance (Fig. 3.19). Grade according to the muscle grading chart and evaluate bilaterally.

3

RATIONALE:

A grade 0 to 4 unilaterally may indicate a neurological deficit of the C7 or C8 nerve root. A weak or strained finger extensor may be suspected if the sensory and reflex portions of the C7 and C8 "Neurological Packages" are intact.

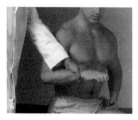

Figure 3.18

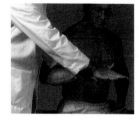

Figure 3.19

B. **Reflex**

Triceps Reflex (C7-Radial Nerve Innervation)

PROCEDURE:

Flex the patient's arm across your opposite arm and tap the triceps tendon at the olecranon fossa with the neurological reflex hammer (Fig. 3.20). The triceps muscle should contract slightly. Grade your response according to the reflex chart and evaluate bilaterally.

RATIONALE:

Unilateral hyporeflexia may indicate a nerve root deficit. Loss of reflex unilaterally may indicate an interruption of the reflex arc (lower motor neuron lesion). Unilateral hyper-reflexia may indicate an upper motor neuron lesion.

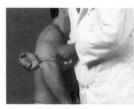

Figure 3.20

hyporef.: C7 prob.
areflex: ↓ lower m.n.
hyperref: upper m.n. prob.

C. **Sensory**

PROCEDURE:

With a pin, stroke the palmar surface of the middle finger (Fig. 3.21).

RATIONALE:

Unilateral hypoesthesia may indicate a neurological deficit of the C7 nerve root or the radial nerve.

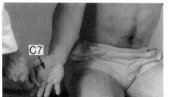

Figure 3.21

C7

IV. C8

The C8 nerve root exits the spinal canal between the C7 and T1 vertebrae and may be affected by the C7 intervertebral disc (Fig. 3.22).

Figure 3.22

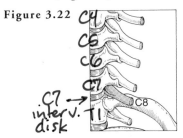

[handwritten labels:] C4, C5, C6, C7, C8, C7→T1 interv. disk

A. Motor

(1) ***Finger Flexor Group: Flexor Digitorum Superficialis (C7, C8-Median Nerve Innervation) and Flexor Digitorum Profundis (C7, C8-Median and Ulnar Nerve Innervation)***

PROCEDURE:

With the patient seated, grasp the patient's wrist with one hand to stabilize the hand. Curl your fingers into the patient's fist and attempt to pull the fingers out of flexion against patient resistance (Fig. 3.23). Grade according to the muscle grading chart and compare bilaterally.

RATIONALE:

A grade 0 to 4 unilaterally may indicate a neurological deficit of the C8 nerve root. A weak or strained finger flexor group muscle may be suspected if the sensory portion of the C8 "Neurological Package" is intact.

[handwritten:] "0-4" ∝ C8 neurolog. def.

Figure 3.23

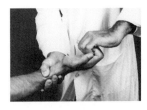

[handwritten:] "DAB" dorsal inkross. & abduction

(2) ***Finger Abductor Group: Dorsal Interossei, Abductor Digiti Minimi (C8, T1-Ulnar Nerve Innervation)***

PROCEDURE:

With the patient's hand pronated, instruct him to abduct his fingers. The examiner is to take each pair of fingers and pinch them together against patient resistance (Fig. 3.24). Grade your findings according to the muscle grading chart and compare bilaterally.

RATIONALE:

A grade 0 to 4 unilaterally may indicate a neurological deficit of the C8 or T1 nerve root. A weak or strained finger abductor may be suspected if the sensory portion of the C8 and T1 "Neurological Packages" is intact.

Figure 3.24

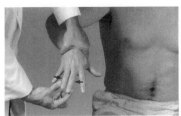

[handwritten:] "0-4" grade ∝ C8 ō T1 deficit; r/o weak phal. abductors if (R) S ok.

66

(3) ***Palmar Interossei (C8, T1-Ulnar Nerve Innervation)***

"PAD" = palmar intero.
& adduction.

PROCEDURE:

With the patient's hand pronated, have the patient adduct all his fingers. The examiner is to grasp each pair of the patient's fingers and attempt to pull them apart against patient resistance (Fig. 3.25). Grade according to the muscle grading chart and compare bilaterally.

RATIONALE:

A grade 0 to 4 unilaterally may indicate a neurological deficit of the C8 or T1 nerve root. A weak or strained finger adductor may be suspected if the sensory portion of the C8 and T1 "Neurological Packages" is intact.

3

Figure 3.25

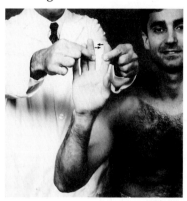

"0-4" ∝ C8 & T1
deficit
(cm. phal.
abd. grp.)
(2)

B. Reflex

None !

C. Sensory

PROCEDURE:

With a pin, stroke the palmar surface of the last two digits and the ulnar aspect of the forearm (Fig. 3.26).

RATIONALE:

Unilateral hypoesthesia may indicate a neurological deficit of the C8 nerve root or the ulnar nerve.

Figure 3.26

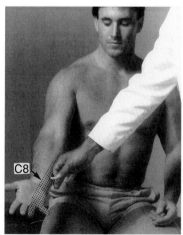

δ: check C8 &
ulnar n.
integrity

V. T1

The T1 nerve root exits the spinal canal between the T1 and T2 vertebrae and may be affected by the T1 intervertebral disc (Fig. 3.27).

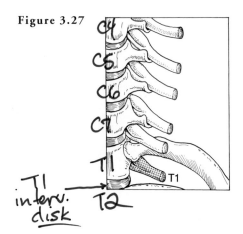

Figure 3.27

A. Motor

Finger Abductor and Adductor Groups (cm. C8 tests 1 d 2)

See C8 Neurological Level

B. Reflex

None !

Brachial plexus :

Sensory

PROCEDURE:

With a pin, stroke the medial proximal aspect of the arm and forearm (Fig. 3.28).

RATIONALE:

Unilateral hypoesthesia may indicate a neurological deficit of the T1 nerve root or the medial brachial cutaneous nerve.

3

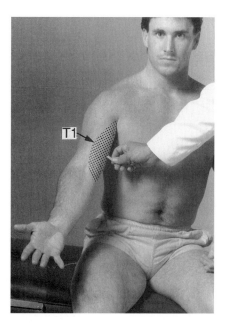

Figure 3.28

hypoesth. ∝
T1 &/ō
med. brachial
cutaneous n.

General References

Bronisch FW. The clinically important reflexes. New York: Grune & Stratton, 1952.

Chusid JG. Correlative neuroanatomy and functional neurology. 17th ed. Los Altos, CA: Lange Medical Publishers, 1976.

DeJong RN. The neurologic examination. 4th ed. Hagerstown, MD: Harper & Row, 1979.

Hoppenfeld S. Physical examination of the spine and extremities. New York: Appleton-Century-Croft, 1976:127.

Kendall FP, McCreary EK, Provance PG. Muscles, testing and function. 4th ed. Baltimore: Williams & Wilkins, 1993.

Mancall E. Essentials of the neurologic examination. 2nd ed. Philadelphia: FA Davis, 1981.

Parsons N. Color atlas of clinical neurology. Chicago: Year Book Medical Publishers, 1989.

VanAllen MW, Rodnitzky RL. Pictorial manual of neurologic tests. 2nd ed. Chicago: Year Book Medical Publishers, 1981.

4

SHOULDER ORTHOPAEDIC TESTS

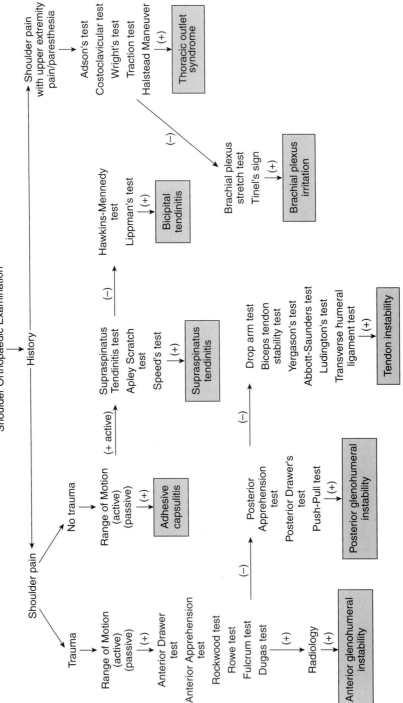

Shoulder Orthopaedic Examination

History

Shoulder pain

Trauma

Range of Motion
(active)
(passive)
(+)

Anterior Drawer
test
Anterior Apprehension
test
Rockwood test
Rowe test
Fulcrum test
Dugas test
(+)

Radiology
(+)

Anterior glenohumeral instability

(−)

Posterior
Apprehension
test
Posterior Drawer's
test
Push-Pull test
(+)

Posterior glenohumeral instability

(−)

Drop arm test
Biceps tendon
stability test
Yergason's test
Abbott-Saunders test
Ludington's test
Transverse humeral
ligament test
(+)

Tendon instability

No trauma

Range of Motion
(active)
(passive)
(+)

Adhesive capsulitis

(+ active)

Supraspinatus
Tendinitis test
Apley Scratch
test
Speed's test
(+)

Supraspinatus tendinitis

(−)

Hawkins-Mennedy
test
Lippman's test
(+)

Bicipital tendinitis

Shoulder pain
with upper extremity
pain/paresthesia

Adson's test
Costoclavicular test
Wright's test
Traction test
Halstead Maneuver
(+)

Thoracic outlet syndrome

(−)

Brachial plexus
stretch test
Tinel's sign
(+)

Brachial plexus irritation

SHOULDER PALPATION

Anterior Aspect

Clavicle, Sternoclavicular and Acromioclavicular Joints

DESCRIPTIVE ANATOMY:

The clavicle is located slightly anterior and inferior to the top of the shoulder. The sternoclavicular joint is located at the medial end of the clavicle and attaches the clavicle to the sternum. The acromioclavicular joint is lateral and attaches the clavicle to the acromion process of the scapula (Fig. 4.1).

PROCEDURE:

With your finger tips, palpate the length of the clavicle from the medial aspect at the sternoclavicular joint to the lateral aspect at the acromioclavicular joint (Fig. 4.2). Note any abnormal tenderness or bumps along the length of the clavicle that would indicate a fracture secondary to recent trauma or a healed fracture with callous formation. Compare both clavicles for symmetry and placement. Next, palpate the sternoclavicular joint (Fig. 4.3) and acromioclavicular joint (Fig. 4.4) for tenderness with your index and middle fingers. If the affected clavicle and respective joint is more anterior, posterior, or superior than the nonaffected clavicle, then a subluxation or dislocation of the clavicle at the affected joint may be suspect. By flexing and extending the shoulder during acromioclavicular joint palpation, crepitus may be felt (Fig. 4.5). Crepitus is secondary to joint inflammation such as osteoarthritis.

4

Figure 4.1

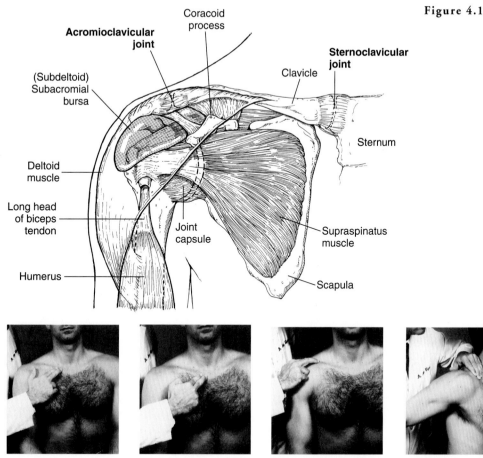

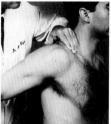

Figure 4.2   Figure 4.3   Figure 4.4   Figure 4.5

Subacromial (Subdeltoid) Bursa

DESCRIPTIVE ANATOMY:

The subacromial portion of the bursa is a fluid-filled sac that extends over the supraspinatus tendon and beneath the acromion process. The subdeltoid portion is beneath the deltoid muscle (Fig. 4.6) and separates the deltoid muscle from the rotator cuff.

PROCEDURE:

With one hand, extend the patient's arm. With your opposite hand, palpate for tenderness, masses, and thickening of both subacromial (Fig. 4.7) and subdeltoid (Fig. 4.8) portions of the bursa. Subacromial or subdeltoid bursitis is suspect if tenderness of the bursa is present. Tenderness may also be associated with restriction of motion and crepitus of the shoulder especially in abduction and forward flexion.

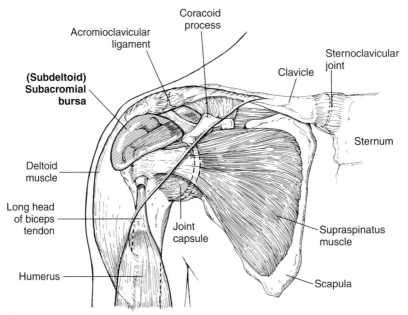

Figure 4.6

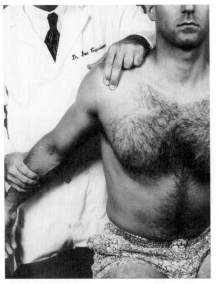

Figure 4.7

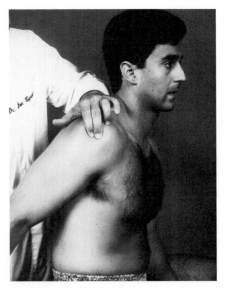

Figure 4.8

Rotator Cuff

DESCRIPTIVE ANATOMY:

The rotator cuff is composed of four muscles—three that are palpable and one that is not. The three palpable muscle are: supraspinatus, which lies above the spine of the scapula and whose tendon lies under the acromion process; infraspinatus, which lies posterior to the supraspinatus; and teres minor, which is posterior to the infraspinatus (Figs. 4.9 and 4.10). The forth muscle is the subscapularis, which is under the scapula and is not palpable. The rotator cuff holds the humerus into the glenoid cavity and blends with the articular capsule to provide dynamic stabilization.

4

PROCEDURE:

With the examiner sitting behind the patient, take one hand and grasp the patient's arm and extend it backwards 20°. With the opposite hand, palpate inferior to the anterior border of the acromion process (Fig. 4.11). Note any tenderness, swelling, nodular masses, or gaps in the cuff. Tendinitis, tears, abnormal calcium deposits, and degeneration in the cuff may elicit tenderness and pain upon palpation. A palpable gap may indicate a ruptured tendon.

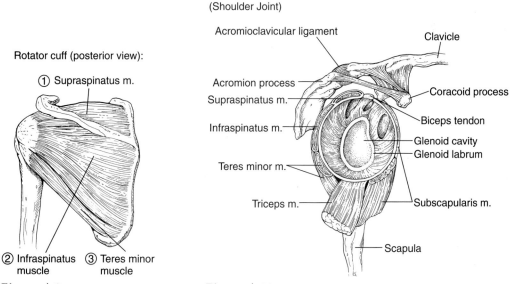

(Shoulder Joint)

Rotator cuff (posterior view):

① Supraspinatus m.

② Infraspinatus muscle   ③ Teres minor muscle

Acromioclavicular ligament

Clavicle

Acromion process

Supraspinatus m.

Coracoid process

Infraspinatus m.

Biceps tendon

Glenoid cavity

Glenoid labrum

Teres minor m.

Triceps m.

Subscapularis m.

Scapula

Figure 4.9   **Figure 4.10**

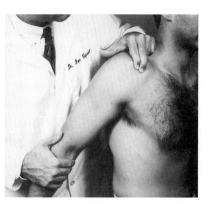

Figure 4.11

Bicipital Groove

DESCRIPTIVE ANATOMY:

The bicipital groove is located anterior and medial to the greater tuberosity of the humerus. The tendon of the long head of the biceps and its synovial sheath are located in its groove. The tendon is held in place by the transverse humeral ligament (Fig. 4.12).

PROCEDURE:

With one hand, locate the inferior tip of the acromion process, then move inferiorly to the greater tuberosity of the humerus. With your opposite hand, grasp the patient's arm and externally rotate it (Fig. 4.13). You will feel the bicipital groove slip under your fingers. Note any tenderness, which may indicate a tenosynovitis of the bicipital tendon and its sheath. Also note any excessive movement of the tendon in its groove; it may indicate a predisposition of the tendon to dislocate out of the bicipital groove or a torn or ruptured transverse humeral ligament.

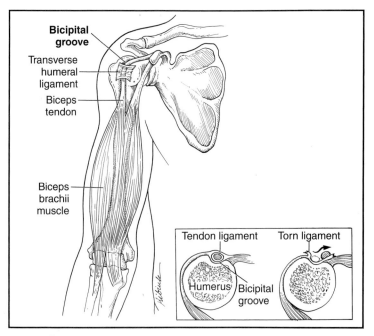

Figure 4.12

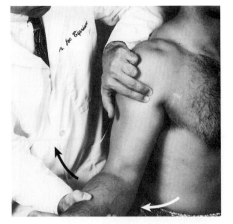

Figure 4.13

Biceps Muscle

DESCRIPTIVE ANATOMY:

The biceps muscle has two heads that originate from two different areas. The long head originates from the tuberosity above the glenoid cavity, and the short head originates from the coracoid process of the scapula. They both insert into the bicipital tuberosity of the radius (Fig. 4.12).

PROCEDURE:

4

With the elbow flexed to 90°, begin palpating distally from the bicipital tuberosity of the radius upward to the bicipital groove (Fig. 4.14). Note any tenderness, spasm, or muscle mass. Tenderness at the proximal end may indicate a tenosynovitis of the biceps tendon. Tenderness at the belly of the muscle may indicate muscle strain or an active trigger point. If a curling of the muscle is evident at the mid-arm secondary to overload, then a rupture of the biceps tendon from its origin may be suspect.

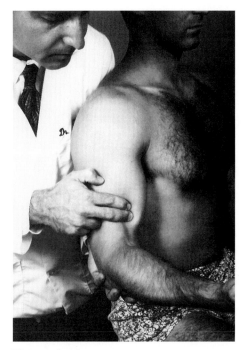

Figure 4.14

Deltoid Muscle

DESCRIPTIVE ANATOMY:

The deltoid muscle originates from the clavicle and acromion process of the scapula and inserts into the deltoid tuberosity of the humerus (Fig. 4.15). The fibers are divided in three different parts: anterior, middle, and posterior. This muscle is capable of acting in parts or as a whole. The anterior part flexes and medially rotates the humerus. The middle part abducts the humerus. The posterior part extends and laterally rotates the humerus.

PROCEDURE:

Begin palpation of the anterior portion of the deltoid muscle from the acromion process inferiorly (Fig. 4.16), then from the lateral aspect of the shoulder (again inferiorly) for the middle part of the deltoid muscle (Fig. 4.17). Finally, the posterior aspect of the deltoid muscle should be palpated from the superior aspect to the inferior aspect with the shoulder extended (Fig. 4.18). Note any tenderness or taught muscle fibers. Tenderness at the lateral aspect of the deltoid is associated with subdeltoid bursitis. Tenderness at the anterior aspect of the deltoid may be associated with a pathology or injury in the bicipital groove because the anterior aspect the deltoid muscle covers the groove and its tendon. General tenderness may indicate a strain or active trigger point of the deltoid muscle secondary to overuse, overload, trauma, or chilling.

Figure 4.15

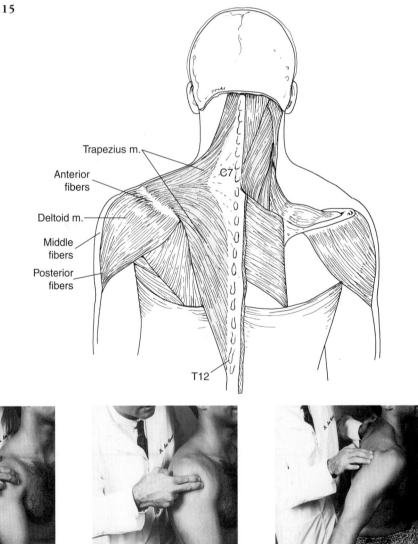

Figure 4.16   **Figure 4.17**   **Figure 4.18**

Posterior Aspect

Scapula

DESCRIPTIVE ANATOMY:

The scapula is located between T2 and T7. It has three borders: a medial border, a lateral border, and a superior border. It also has a sharp ridge that extends from the acromion process, which is the spine of the scapula (Fig. 4.19).

PROCEDURE:

Starting with the medial border of the scapula, palpate all three borders, noting any tenderness (Figs. 4.20–4.22). Next, palpate the spine of the scapula, noting any tenderness and/or abnormality (Fig. 4.23). Finally, palpate the posterior surfaces above the spine of the scapula for the supraspinatus muscle (Fig. 4.24) and below the spine for the infraspinatus muscle (Fig. 4.25). Note any tenderness, palpable bands, atrophy, or spasm. Palpable bands in the supraspinatus and infraspinatus muscle may indicate a myofascial syndrome caused by overuse, overload trauma, or chilling. Atrophy may indicate a disruption of the nerve supply to the suspected muscle.

4

Figure 4.19

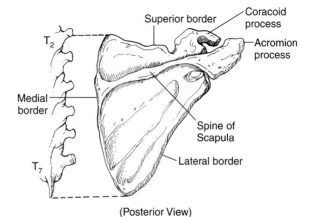

(Posterior View)

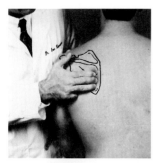

Figure 4.20

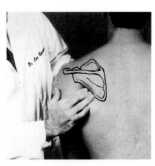

Figure 4.21

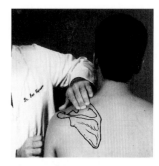

Figure 4.22

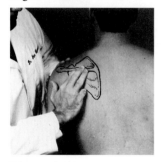

Figure 4.23

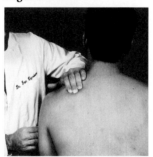

Figure 4.24

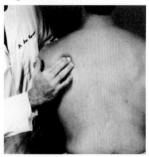

Figure 4.25

Trapezius Muscle

DESCRIPTIVE ANATOMY:

The Trapezius muscle originates from the occiput, ligamentum nuchae, and spine of C7 through T12 vertebra. It inserts into the acromion process and spine of the scapula (Fig. 4.26). The trapezius muscle contains three sets of fibers that perform different actions. The superior fibers elevate the shoulders, the middle fibers retract the scapula, and the inferior fibers depress the scapula and lower the shoulders.

PROCEDURE:

Begin at the origin at the base of the occiput, palpating superior fibers inferior towards the spine of the scapula (Fig. 4.27). Then, from the spine of the scapula, palpate the middle (Fig. 4.28) and inferior (Fig. 4.29) fibers down towards the T12 spinous process. Note any tenderness, spasm, palpable bands, or asymmetry of the muscles. Tenderness and spasm may be present secondary to hyperextension/hyperflexion injuries. Tight palpable bands may be secondary to active myofascial trigger points. According to Travell, myofascial trigger points in muscle are activated directly by trauma, overuse, overload, or chilling. They are activated indirectly by visceral disease, arthritis, and emotional distress.

Figure 4.26

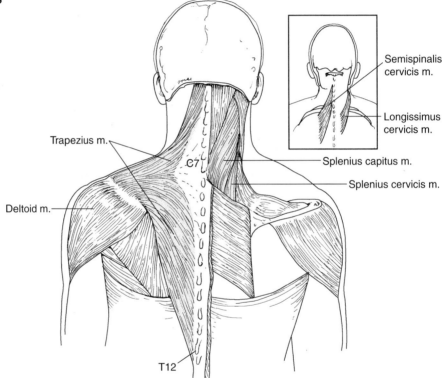

Figure 4.27

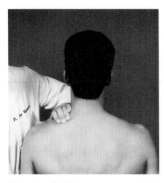

Figure 4.28

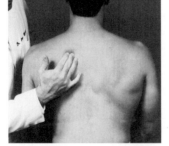

Figure 4.29

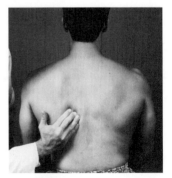

SHOULDER RANGE OF MOTION

Flexion (1,2)

With the patient seated, place the goniometer in the sagittal plane at the level of the glenohumeral joint (Fig. 4.30). Instruct the patient to elevate his arm forward while following his arm with one arm of the goniometer (Fig. 4.31).

NORMAL RANGE:

167° ± 4.7° from the 0 or neutral position.

Note: This expressed degree of motion probably did not permit enough external rotation and abduction to achieve 180° of flexion described by others.

Muscles Involved in Action	*Nerve Supply*
1. Anterior Deltoid	Axillary
2. Pectoralis major	Lateral Pectoral
3. Coracobrachialis	Musculocutaneous
4. Biceps	Musculocutaneous

4

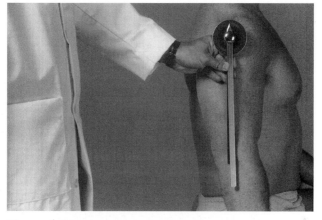

Figure 4.30

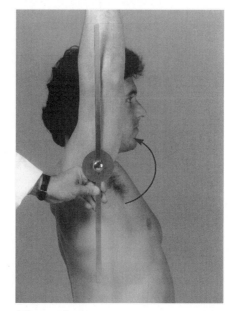

Figure 4.31

Extension (1,2)

With the patient seated, place the goniometer in the sagittal plane at the level of the glenohumeral joint (Fig. 4.32). Instruct the patient to elevate his arm backward while following his arm with one arm of the goniometer (Fig. 4.33).

NORMAL RANGE:

62° ± 9.5° from the 0 or neutral position.

Muscles Involved in Action	Nerve Supply
1. Posterior Deltoid	Axillary
2. Teres major, minor	Subscapular
3. Latissimus dorsi	Thoracodorsal
4. Pectoralis major	Lateral pectoral
5. Triceps	Radial

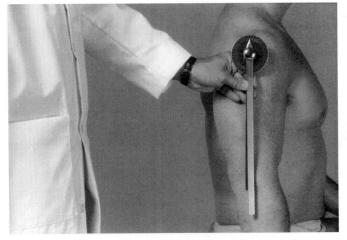

Figure 4.32

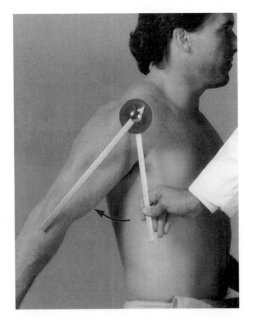

Figure 4.33

Internal Rotation (1,2)

With the patient seated, have the patient abduct his arm to 90° and flex his elbow to 90°. This is the 0 or neutral position for rotation of the shoulder. Place the goniometer in the sagittal plane with the center at the lateral aspect of the elbow (Fig. 4.34). Instruct the patient to rotate his shoulder inward by moving the forearm so that the palm of the hand faces posteriorly, and follow the forearm with one arm of the goniometer (Fig. 4.35).

NORMAL RANGE:

69° ± 4.6° from the 0 or neutral position.

Muscles Involved in Action	*Nerve Supply*
1. Pectoralis major	Lateral pectoral
2. Anterior deltoid	Axillary
3. Latissimus dorsi	Thoracodorsal
4. Teres major	Subscapular
5. Subscapularis	Subscapular

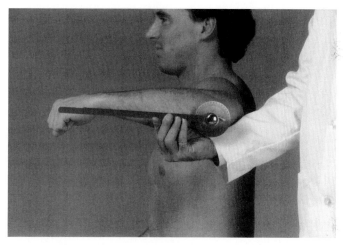

Figure 4.34

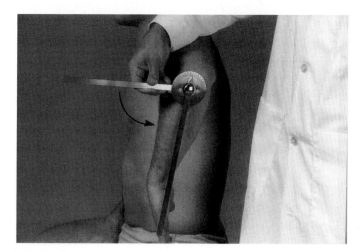

Figure 4.35

External Rotation (1,2)

With the patient seated, have the patient abduct his arm to 90° and flex his elbow to 90°. This is the 0 or neutral position for rotation of the shoulder. Place the goniometer in the sagittal plane with the center at the lateral aspect of the elbow (Fig. 4.36). Instruct the patient to rotate his shoulder outward by moving the forearm so that the palm of the hand faces anteriorly, and follow the forearm with one arm of the goniometer (Fig. 4.37).

NORMAL RANGE:

104° ± 8.5° from the 0 or neutral position.

Muscles Involved in Action	Nerve Supply
1. Infraspinatus	Suprascapular
2. Posterior deltoid	Axillary
3. Teres minor	Axillary

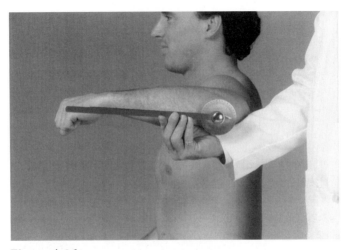

Figure 4.36

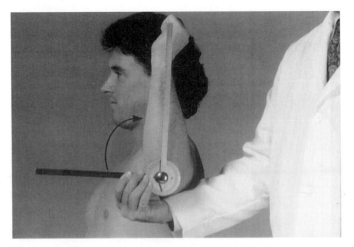

Figure 4.37

Abduction (1,2)

With the patient in the seated position, place the goniometer in the coronal plane with the center at the level of the glenohumeral joint (Fig. 4.38). Instruct the patient to raise his arm laterally while following his arm with one arm of the goniometer (Fig. 4.39).

NORMAL RANGE:

184° ± 7.0 from the 0 or neutral position.

Muscles Involved in Action	Nerve Supply
1. Deltoid	Axillary
2. Supraspinatus	Suprascapular
3. Infraspinatus	Suprascapular
4. Subscapularis	Subscapular
5. Teres minor	Axillary
6. Biceps brachii, long head	Musculocutaneous

4

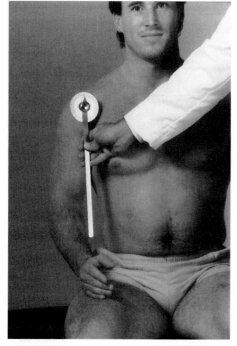

Figure 4.38

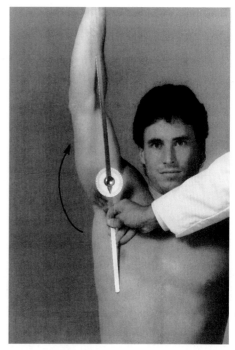

Figure 4.39

Adduction

With the patient in the seated position, place the goniometer in the coronal plane with the center at the level of the glenohumeral joint (Fig. 4.40). Instruct the patient to raise his arm medially while following his arm with one arm of the goniometer (Fig. 4.41).

NORMAL RANGE:

75° or greater from the 0 or neutral position.
Note: Adduction is a composite movement of flexion and adduction. Most sources do not measure composite movements. Clinically, I feel it is an important movement and should be measured.

Muscles Involved in Action	*Nerve Supply*
1. Pectoralis major	Lateral pectoral
2. Latissimus dorsi	Thoracodorsal
3. Teres major	Subscapular
4. Subscapularis	Subscapular

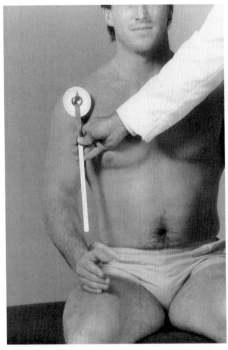

Figure 4.40

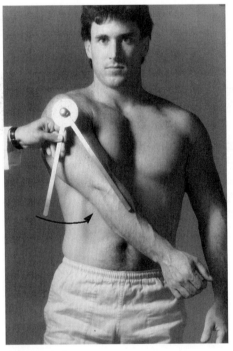

Figure 4.41

TENDINITIS (SUPRASPINATUS)

Supraspinatus Tendinitis Test

PROCEDURE:

With the patient seated, instruct him to abduct his arm to 90° with the arm between abduction and forward flexion. Instruct the patient to abduct his arm against resistance. (Fig. 4.42).

RATIONALE:

Resisting shoulder abduction stresses mainly the deltoid muscle and the supraspinatus muscle and tendon. Pain over the insertion of the supraspinatus tendon may be indicative of degenerative tendinitis of the supraspinatus tendon or a strained deltoid muscle.

4

Figure 4.42

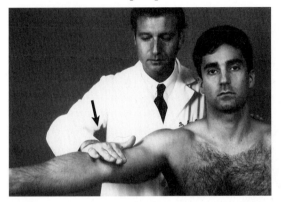

Apley Scratch Test (3)

PROCEDURE:

With the patient seated, instruct him to place his hand on the side of the affected shoulder behind his head and touch the opposite superior angle of the scapula (Fig. 4.43). Then instruct the patient to place his hand behind his back and attempt to touch the opposite inferior angle of the scapula (Fig. 4.44).

RATIONALE:

By actively attempting to touch the opposite superior and inferior aspect of the scapula, stress is being placed on the tendons of the rotator cuff. Exacerbation of the patient's pain indicates degenerative tendinitis of one of the tendons of the rotator cuff, usually the supraspinatus tendon.

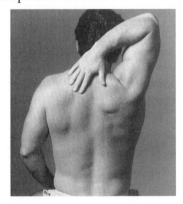

Figure 4.43

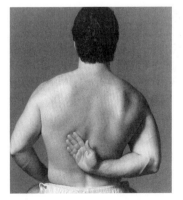

Figure 4.44

Hawkins-Kennedy Impingement Test (4)

PROCEDURE:

With the patient standing, flex the shoulder forward to 90°, then force the shoulder in an internal rotation without patient resistance (Fig. 4.45).

RATIONALE:

This movement pushes the supraspinatus tendon against the anterior surface of the cora-coacromial ligament. Localized pain is indicative of supraspinatus tendinitis.

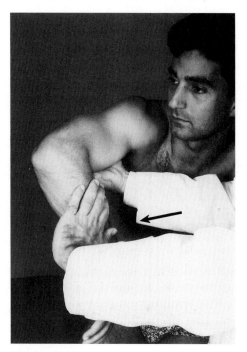

Figure 4.45

TENDINITIS (BICIPITAL)

Speed's Test (3,5)

PROCEDURE:

With the patient's forearm completely extended, supinated, and forward flexed to 45°, place your fingers on the bicipital groove and your opposite hand on the patient's wrist (Fig. 4.46). Instruct the patient to forwardly elevate his arm against your resistance (Fig. 4.47).

RATIONALE:

This test stresses the biceps tendon in the bicipital groove. Pain or tenderness in the bicipital groove is indicative of bicipital tendinitis.

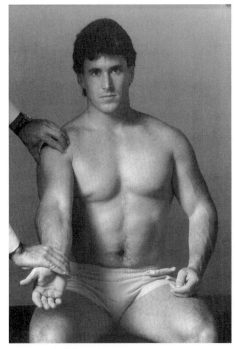

Figure 4.46

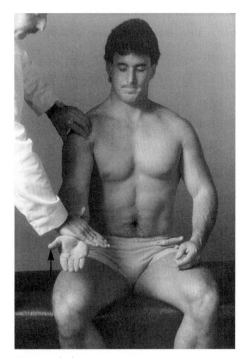

Figure 4.47

Lippman's Test (5)

PROCEDURE:

With the patient sitting, instruct the patient to flex the elbow to 90°; stabilize his elbow with one hand, and with your other hand palpate the biceps tendon and move it from side to side in the bicipital groove (Fig. 4.48).

RATIONALE:

Moving the biceps tendon manually in the bicipital groove stresses the tendon and transverse humeral ligament. Pain is indicative of bicipital tendinitis. Apprehension may indicate a propensity for subluxation or dislocation of the biceps tendon out of the bicipital groove or a ruptured transverse humeral ligament (Fig. 4.49).

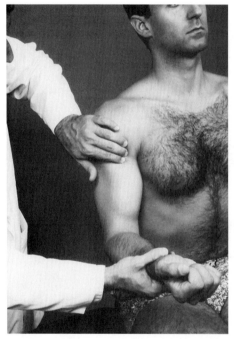

Figure 4.48

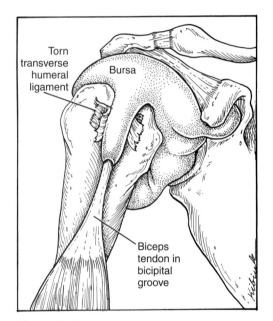

Figure 4.49

BURSITIS

Subacromial Push-Button Sign

PROCEDURE:

With the patient seated, apply pressure to the subacromial bursa (Fig. 4.50).

RATIONALE:

Localized pain is suggestive of inflammation of the subacromial bursa or bursitis (Fig. 4.51).

4

Figure 4.50

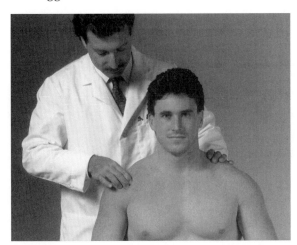

Figure 4.51

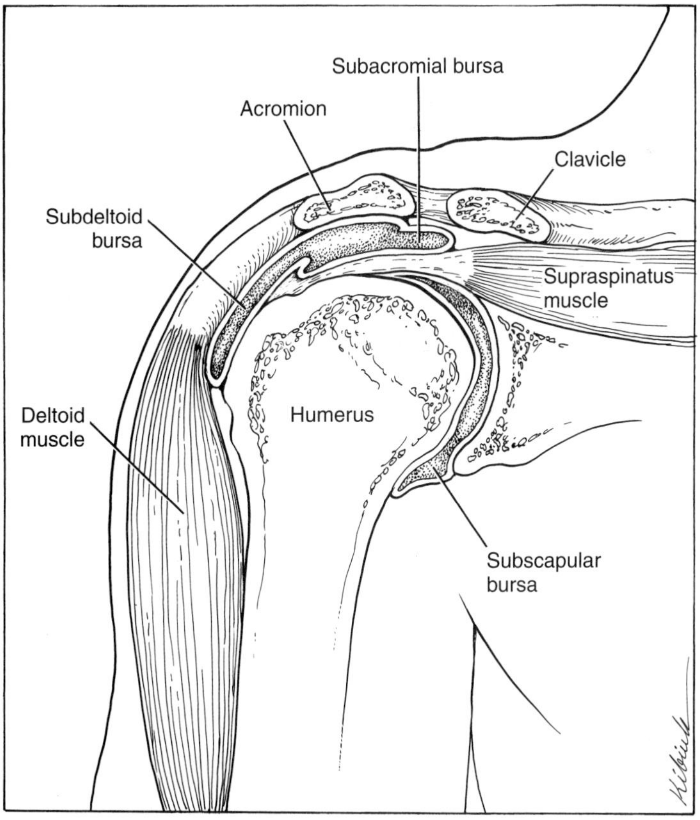

Subacromial bursa

Acromion

Clavicle

Subdeltoid bursa

Supraspinatus muscle

Deltoid muscle

Humerus

Subscapular bursa

Dawbarn's Test (5)

PROCEDURE:

With the patient seated, apply pressure just below the acromion process on the side being tested. Note if there is any pain or tenderness (Fig. 4.52). Then, abduct the patient's arm past 90° with pressure on the spot below the acromion still applied (Fig. 4.53).

RATIONALE:

The spot below the acromion is the palpable portion of the subacromial bursa. Pain and/ or tenderness at that location may indicate an inflammation of the bursa or bursitis. When the arm is abducted, the deltoid muscle will cover that spot below the acromion. By covering that spot, pressure on the bursa will diminish, consequently decreasing the tenderness if inflammation of the bursa is present. A decrease in the tenderness to that point is indicative of subacromial bursitis (Fig. 4.54).

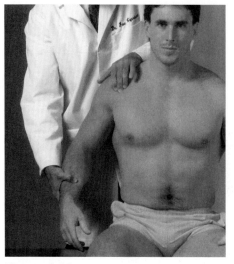

Figure 4.52

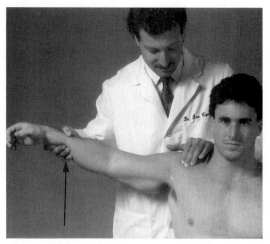

Figure 4.53

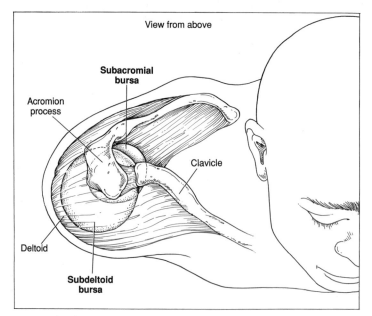

Figure 4.54

92

ANTERIOR GLENOHUMERAL INSTABILITY

Anterior Drawer Test (6)

PROCEDURE:

With the patient in the supine position, place the patient's hand in the examiner's axilla. With your opposite hand, grasp the posterior scapula with your fingers and place your thumb over the coracoid process (Fig. 4.55). Using the arm that is holding the patient's hand, grasp the posterior aspect of the patient's arm and draw the humerus forward (Fig. 4.56).

RATIONALE:

Attempting to move the humerus forward while stabilizing the scapula tests the integrity of the anterior portion of the rotator cuff, which holds the humerus into the glenoid cavity. An abnormal amount of movement and/or a click compared with the normal side is indicative of a anterior instability of the glenohumeral joint.

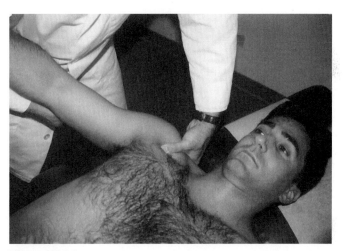

Figure 4.55

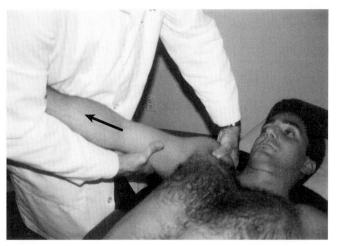

Figure 4.56

Anterior Apprehension Test (3)

PROCEDURE:

With the patient seated, stand behind the patient. Abduct to 90° and externally rotate the affected arm slowly (Fig. 4.57).

RATIONALE:

Localized pain indicates a chronic anterior shoulder dislocation. This test is named apprehension because you should observe for a look of apprehension on the patient's face. The patient may also state that the feeling experienced is what it felt like when the shoulder was previously dislocated.

External rotation of the arm predisposes the humerus to dislocate anteriorly. This test is forcing external rotation to anteriorly dislocate the humerus from the glenoid fossa. If the integrity of the rotator cuff muscles, joint capsule, and the glenoid fossa are sound, then the patient should not experience any pain or apprehension when this test is performed. It is testing the integrity of the inferior glenohumeral ligament, anterior capsule, rotator cuff tendons, and the glenoid labrum.

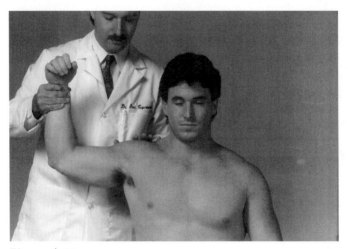

Figure 4.57

Rockwood Test (7)

PROCEDURE:

This test is a variation of the previously described Anterior Apprehension Test. With the patient seated, externally rotate the shoulder with the arm in the neutral position (Fig. 4.58). Repeat the test with the arm at 45° of abduction (Fig. 4.59); then at 90° of abduction (Fig. 4.60); then at 120° of abduction (Fig. 4.61).

RATIONALE:

The patient must show marked apprehension at 90° with pain. At 0° there is rarely any apprehension. At 45° and 120° there should be more pain with slight apprehension. The patient might state that the feeling experienced is what it felt like when the shoulder was previously dislocated. This procedure tests the integrity of the inferior glenohumeral ligament, anterior capsule, rotator cuff tendons, and the glenoid labrum.

4

Figure 4.58

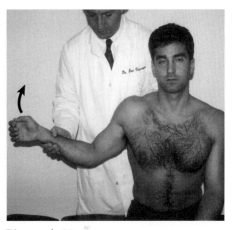

Figure 4.59

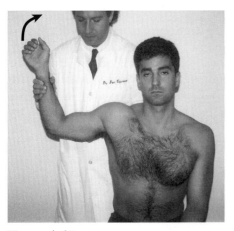

Figure 4.60

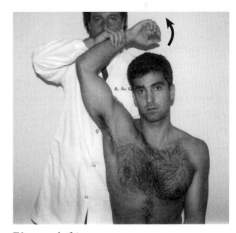

Figure 4.61

Rowe Test for Anterior Instability (8)

PROCEDURE:

With the patient in the sitting position, instruct the patient to place his hand on the side of the affected shoulder behind his head. Then, place your clenched fist against the posterior humeral head and push anteriorly while using your opposite hand to extend the patient's arm (Fig. 4.62).

RATIONALE:

The examiner is attempting to anteriorly dislocate the patient's glenohumeral joint. A look of apprehension is indicative of a positive test. The patient may also state that the feeling experienced is what it felt like when the shoulder was previously dislocated. This procedure tests the integrity of the inferior glenohumeral ligament, anterior capsule, rotator cuff tendons, and the glenoid labrum.

Figure 4.62

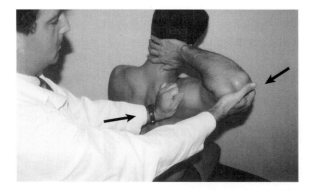

Fulcrum Test (9)

PROCEDURE:

With the patient in the supine position and the arm abducted to 90°, place your hand under the glenohumeral joint. Then, externally rotate the patient's arm over his hand (Fig. 4.63).

RATIONALE:

The examiner is attempting to dislocate the head of the humerus anteriorly. A look of apprehension with pain is a positive sign. The patient may also state that the feeling experienced is what it felt like when the shoulder was previously dislocated. This procedure also tests the integrity of the inferior glenohumeral ligament, anterior capsule, rotator cuff tendons, and the glenoid labrum. A congenital shallow glenoid fossa may also predispose the shoulder to dislocation.

Figure 4.63

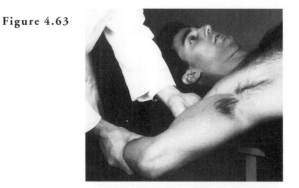

Dugas Test (10,11)

PROCEDURE:

With the patient seated, instruct him to touch the opposite shoulder and bring his elbow to the chest wall (Fig. 4.64).

RATIONALE:

Inability to touch the opposite shoulder because of pain indicates an anterior dislocation of the humeral head out of the glenoid cavity. This dislocation is usually caused by forced external rotation when the arm is abducted. When the humerus is dislocated anteriorly, a characteristic sign is a prominent acromion process.

4

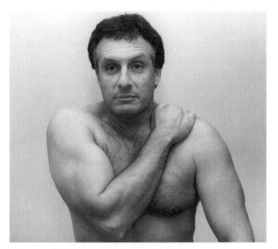

Figure 4.64

POSTERIOR GLENOHUMERAL INSTABILITY

Posterior Apprehension Test (5)

PROCEDURE:

With the patient in the supine position, forwardly flex and internally rotate the patient's shoulder. With your hand, apply posterior pressure on the patient's elbow (Fig. 4.65).

RATIONALE:

This test attempts to dislocate the shoulder posteriorly and stresses the rotator cuff and the posterior joint capsule. Localized pain or discomfort and a look of apprehension on the patient's face indicates a chronic posterior shoulder instability. The patient may also state that the feeling experienced is what it felt like when the shoulder was previously dislocated.

The mechanism of injury is commonly a position of forced adduction with internal rotation in some degree of elevation.

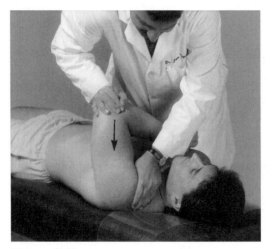

Figure 4.65

Posterior Drawer Test (12)

PROCEDURE:

With the patient in the supine position, grasp the patient's forearm, flex the patient's elbow and abduct and flex the shoulder. With your opposite hand, stabilize the scapula with your index and middle finger on the spine of the scapula and your thumb on the coracoid process (Fig. 4.66). Then, rotate the forearm internally and forwardly flex the shoulder, taking the thumb of your other hand off the coracoid and forcing the humerus posteriorly (Fig. 4.67).

RATIONALE:

Here you are attempting to dislocate the shoulder posteriorly, stressing the rotator cuff and joint capsule. Localized pain and a look of apprehension is the sign of a positive test. This test stresses the rotator cuff and the posterior joint capsule.

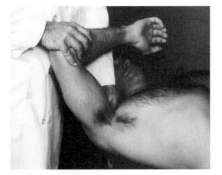

Figure 4.66   Figure 4.67

Norwood Stress Test (13,14)

PROCEDURE:

With the patient in the supine position, instruct the patient to abduct the shoulder to 90°, externally rotate it to 90°, and flex the elbow to 90°. With one hand, stabilize the scapula while palpating the posterior aspect of the humeral head (Fig. 4.68). With your opposite hand, grasp the elbow, bringing the shoulder into forward flexion and forcing the elbow posteriorly (Fig. 4.69).

RATIONALE:

This test is an attempt to dislocate the shoulder posteriorly, stressing the rotator cuff and the posterior joint capsule. A positive test is indicated by the humeral head slipping posteriorly out of the glenoid fossa. When the arm is returned to the starting position, the humeral head should reduce. A clicking sound may be accompanied with the reduction.

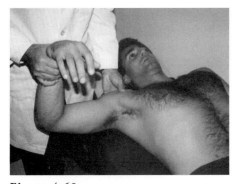

Figure 4.68

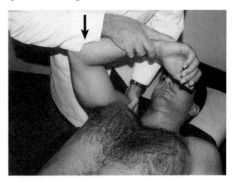

Figure 4.69

Push-Pull Test (9)

PROCEDURE:

With the patient in the supine position, grasp the patient's wrist and abduct the arm to 90° and forward flex it to 30°. With your opposite hand, grasp the arm near the humeral head (Fig. 4.70). Then, pull up on the wrist and push down on the arm (Fig. 4.71).

RATIONALE:

In the normal patient, up to 50% of translation is considered a negative test. More than 50% translation and a look of apprehension is indicative of a positive test. This test is also attempting to dislocate the shoulder posteriorly. It is stressing the rotator cuff and posterior joint capsule.

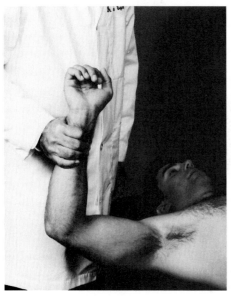

Figure 4.70

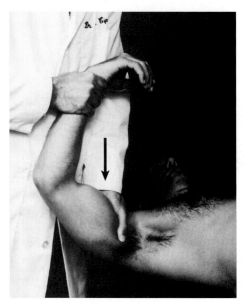

Figure 4.71

MULTIDIRECTIONAL SHOULDER INSTABILITY

Feagin Test (7)

PROCEDURE:

With the patient in the standing position, instruct the patient to abduct his arm and place his hand on your shoulder (Fig. 4.72). With both your hands, grasp the patient's humerus next to the humeral head and exert downward and forward pressure (Fig. 4.73).

RATIONALE:

A look of apprehension on the patient's face signifies a positive test. This is indicative of an anterior inferior shoulder instability. This test is attempting to dislocate the shoulder anteriorly and inferiorly. It is testing the integrity of the inferior glenohumeral ligament, anterior capsule, rotator cuff tendons, and the glenoid labrum.

4

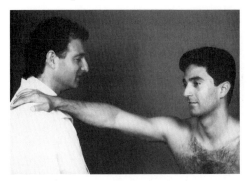

Figure 4.72

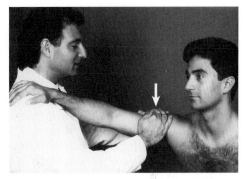

Figure 4.73

Rowe Test for Multidirectional Instability (8)

PROCEDURE:

To test for inferior instability, have the patient standing and flexed forward 45°. Grasp the shoulder with the index and middle finger over the posterior humeral head and the thumb at the anterior humeral head. With your opposite hand, grasp the patient's elbow and pull down on the arm (Fig. 4.74). To test for anterior instability, the humeral head is now pushed anteriorly from behind with your thumb and the patient's arm extended 20 to 30° (Fig. 4.75). To test for posterior instability, push the humeral head posteriorly from the anterior with your index and middle fingers with the patient's shoulder flexed 20 to 30° (Fig. 4.76).

RATIONALE:

This test is attempting to dislocate the humeral head out of the glenoid fossa in various directions. A look of apprehension and/or local discomfort on the patient's face is a positive sign. This test is stressing the glenohumeral ligament, rotator cuff tendons, and the joint capsule.

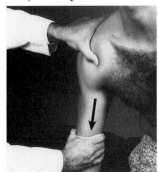

Figure 4.74

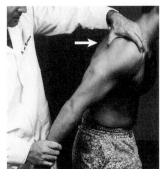

Figure 4.75

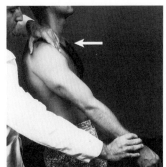

Figure 4.76

TENDON INSTABILITY

Drop Arm Test (2)

PROCEDURE:

With the patient seated, abduct his arm past 90° (Fig. 4.77). Instruct the patient to lower his arm slowly (Fig. 4.78).

RATIONALE:

If the patient is unable to lower his arm slowly or if he drops it suddenly, this is indicative of a rotator cuff tear, usually of the supraspinatus. The supraspinatus muscle acts as an abductor of the arm and holds the head of the humerus in place. A tear of the supraspinatus tendon causes unsteadiness of the humerus in abduction, causing it to suddenly drop.

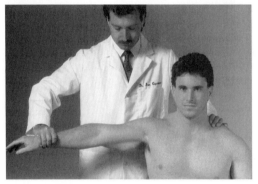

Figure 4.77

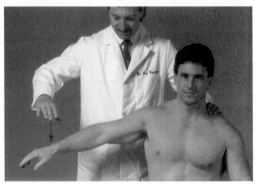

Figure 4.78

Biceps Tendon Stability Test (3,10)

PROCEDURE:

With the patient seated, instruct the patient to flex his elbow. The examiner grasps the patient's wrist and instructs him to continue to flex his elbow and externally rotate it against resistance (Fig. 4.79).

RATIONALE:

Pain localized to the biceps tendon is indicative of instability of or tendinitis of the biceps tendon (Fig. 4.80).

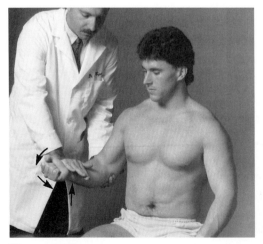

Figure 4.79

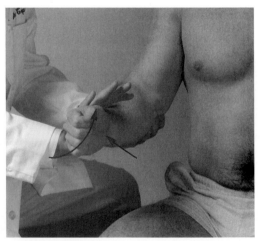

Figure 4.80

Yergason's Test (15)

PROCEDURE:

With the patient seated and the elbow flexed to 90°, stabilize the patient's elbow with one hand (Fig. 4.79). With your opposite hand, grasp the patient's wrist and have the patient externally rotate the shoulder and supinate his forearm against your resistance (Fig. 4.80).

RATIONALE:

Resisted supination of the forearm and external rotation of the shoulder stresses the bicipital tendon and the transverse humeral ligament. Localized pain and/or tenderness in the bicipital tendon indicates an inflammation of the biceps tendon or tendinitis. If the tendon "pops" out of the bicipital groove, then a lax or ruptured transverse humeral ligament or a congenital shallow bicipital groove is suspect, causing the tendon to subluxate (Fig. 4.81).

4

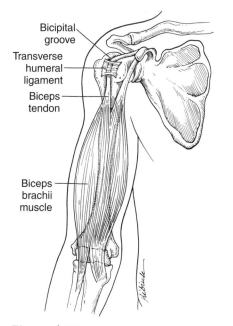

Bicipital groove
Transverse humeral ligament
Biceps tendon
Biceps brachii muscle

Figure 4.81

Abbott-Saunders Test (16)

PROCEDURE:

With the patient in the seated position, abduct and externally rotate maximally the patient's arm (Fig. 4.82). Then lower the arm to the patient's side while palpating the bicipital groove with your opposite hand (Fig. 4.83).

RATIONALE:

Abduction and external rotation of the shoulder stresses the biceps tendon against the transverse humeral ligament. A palpable or audible click at the bicipital groove is indicative of a subluxation or dislocation of the biceps tendon out of the groove caused by a lax or ruptured transverse humeral ligament or congenitally shallow bicipital groove.

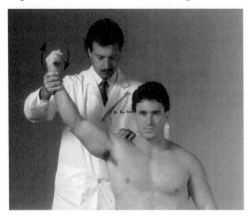
Figure 4.82

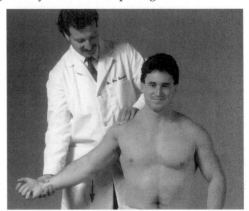
Figure 4.83

Ludington's Test (5)

PROCEDURE:

Instruct the patient to clasp both hands on top of his head while interlocking his fingers (Fig. 4.84). Then instruct the patient to alternately contract and relax the biceps muscle while you palpate the biceps tendon (Fig. 4.85).

RATIONALE:

Placing the hands on the patient's head allows for support of the upper limb and relaxation of the biceps muscle. If the biceps tendon on the affected side is not contracting and palpable, then a rupture of the long head of the biceps tendon is suspect.

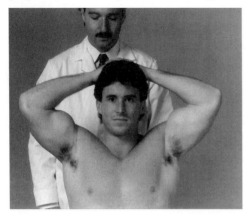
Figure 4.84

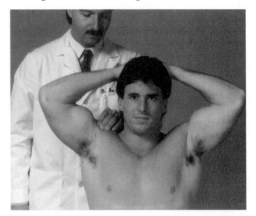
Figure 4.85

Transverse Humeral Ligament Test (5)

PROCEDURE:

With the patient seated, grasp the patient's wrist. Abduct the shoulder to 90° and internally rotate it with one hand. With your opposite hand, palpate the bicipital groove (Fig. 4.86). Then externally rotate the shoulder (Fig. 4.87).

RATIONALE:

External rotation of the shoulder causes the biceps tendon to move in the bicipital groove. If you feel the bicipital tendon snap in and out of the bicipital groove, a torn or lax transverse humeral ligament or shallow bicipital groove is suspect (Fig. 4.88).

4

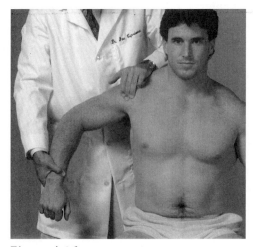

Figure 4.86   Figure 4.87

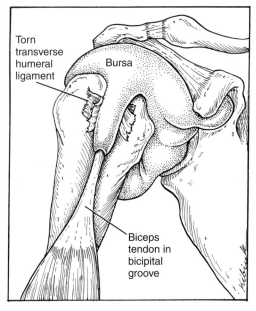

Figure 4.88

THORACIC OUTLET SYNDROME

Adson's Test (17–19)

PROCEDURE:

With the patient in the seated position, establish the amplitude of the radial pulse (Fig. 4.89). Compare the amplitude bilaterally. Instruct the patient to take a deep breath and sustain it while he rotates his head and elevates his chin to the side being tested (Fig. 4.90). If the test is negative, have the patient rotate and elevate his chin to the opposite side (Fig. 4.91).

RATIONALE:

Rotation and extension of the head places a motion-induced compression on the subclavian artery and brachial plexus. A decrease or absence of the amplitude of the radial pulse indicates a compression of the vascular component of the neurovascular bundle (subclavian artery) by a spastic or hypertrophied scalenus anterior muscle, presence of a cervical rib, or a mass, such as a Pancoast tumor. Paresthesias or radiculopathy in the upper extremity is indicative of compression of the neural component of the neurovascular bundle (brachial plexus) (Fig. 4.92).

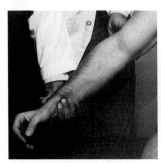
Figure 4.89

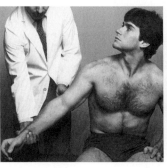
Figure 4.90

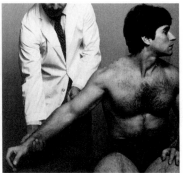
Figure 4.91

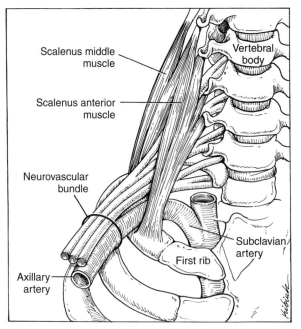
Figure 4.92

Costoclavicular Test (20–22)

PROCEDURE:

With the patient seated, establish a radial pulse (Fig. 4.93). Instruct the patient to force his shoulders posteriorly and have him flex his chin to his chest (Fig. 4.94).

RATIONALE:

Forcing the shoulders posteriorly decreases the space between the clavicle and first rib. The neurovascular bundle (brachial plexus, axillary artery) and the axillary vein runs between a narrow cleft beneath the clavicle and on top of the first rib.

Decrease or absence of the amplitude of the radial pulse indicates a compression to the vascular component of the neurovascular bundle. This compression is caused by a decrease in the space between the clavicle and the first rib. This decrease may be caused by a recent or healed fracture to the clavicle or first rib with or without callous formation, dislocation of the medial aspect of the clavicle, or a spastic or hypertrophied subclavius muscle. Paresthesias or radiculopathy in the upper extremity is indicative of compression to the brachial plexus or compression of the axillary vein (Fig. 4.95). Compression of the brachial plexus is usually localized to a nerve root or peripheral nerve distribution. Compression of the axillary vein typically presents as a diffuse radicular vascular discomfort not localized to a nerve root or peripheral nerve distribution.

4

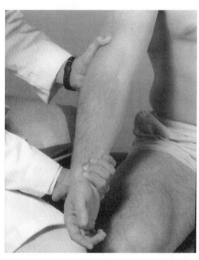

Figure 4.93

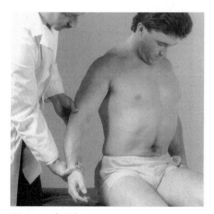

Figure 4.94

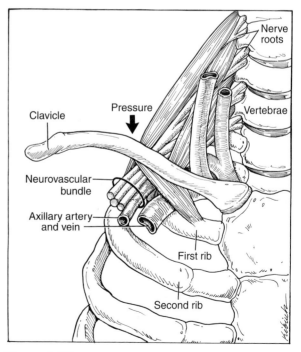

Figure 4.95

Wright's Test (23,24)

P<small>ROCEDURE</small>:

With the patient seated, establish the character of the radial pulse (Fig. 4.96). Hyperabduct the arm and retake the pulse (Fig. 4.97).

R<small>ATIONALE</small>:

The axillary artery, vein, and three cords of the brachial plexus pass under the pectoralis minor muscle on the coracoid process. By abduction of the arm to 180°, these structures are stretched around the tendon of the pectoralis minor muscle and the coracoid process.

Decrease or absence of the amplitude of the radial pulse indicates a compression of the axillary artery by either a spastic or hypertrophied pectoralis minor muscle or by a deformed or hypertrophied coracoid process (Fig. 4.98).

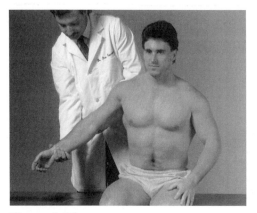

Figure 4.96

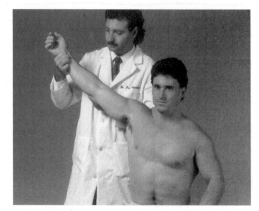

Figure 4.97

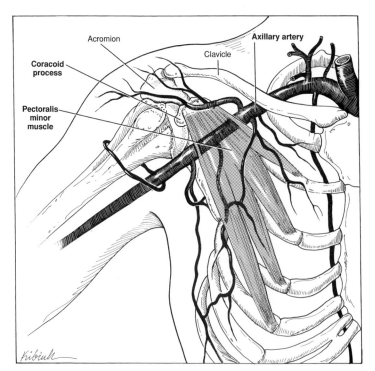

Acromion

Clavicle

Axillary artery

Coracoid process

Pectoralis minor muscle

Figure 4.98

Traction Test (25)

PROCEDURE:

With the patient seated, establish a radial pulse (Fig. 4.99). While maintaining the pulse, extend and apply traction to the arm (Fig. 4.100).

RATIONALE:

Traction and extension of the arm tractions the subclavian artery over the first rib. A decreased or obliterated pulse is nondiagnostic; however, when the test is repeated on the opposite side and reveals no change, the test is indicative of a subluxated or malpositioned first rib or a cervical rib on the side of the decreased or obliterated pulse.

4

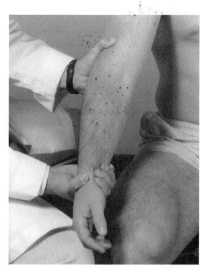

get positive t.
if notice
decreased RP
after checking
bilaterally

Figure 4.99

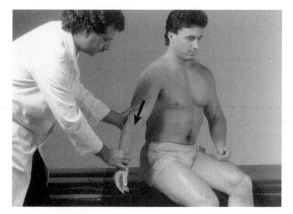

Figure 4.100

Halstead Maneuver (5)

PROCEDURE:

With the patient seated, locate the radial pulse and note the amplitude (Fig. 4.101). With your opposite hand, traction the patient's arm and ask the patient to hyperextend his neck (Fig. 4.102). Repeat the test on opposite arm.

RATIONALE:

A traction pressure on the arm tractions the neurovascular bundle (brachial plexus and axillary artery) over the first rib. Extension of the neck tightens the scalene muscles. A decreased or obliterated pulse amplitude is indicative of the presence of a cervical rib, subluxation, or malposition of the first rib. An upper extremity radicular component indicates compression of the brachial plexus by the scalenus anterior muscle (see Fig. 4.92).

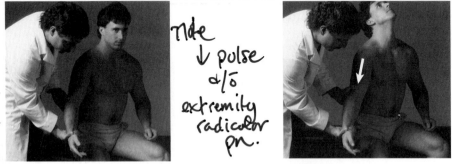

note
↓ pulse
c/ō
extremity
radicular
pn.

Figure 4.101   Figure 4.102

Eden's Test

PROCEDURE:

With the patient sitting, obtain a radial pulse and note the amplitude (Fig. 4.103). Instruct the patient to bring the shoulders back, retracting the scapula. Then put downward pressure on the shoulder (Fig. 4.104). Note any difference in pulse amplitude or increase in radicular symptoms.

RATIONALE:

By abducting the scapula and applying downward pressure to the shoulder, compression of the space between the first rib and clavicle occur. If this space is compromised, a decrease in the amplitude of the radial pulse and/or an increase in radicular symptoms may indicate a compression of the neurovascular bundle. This compression can be caused by an elongated C7 transverse process, a cervical rib, an inflamed subclavius muscle, a displaced or healed fracture, subluxation, or dislocation of the clavicle or first rib.

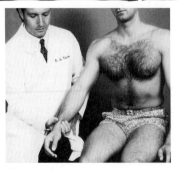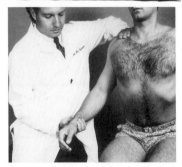

Figure 4.103   Figure 4.104

BRACHIAL PLEXUS IRRITATION

Brachial Plexus Stretch Test

PROCEDURE:

With the patient in the seated position, instruct the patient to laterally flex his head opposite the affected side and extend his shoulder and elbow (Fig. 4.105).

RATIONALE:

This test is similar to a straight leg raising test for the upper extremity. This test stretches the brachial plexus opposite the side of lateral head flexion. Any damage to the plexus will cause pain and/or paresthesia along the distribution of the brachial plexus. Pain and paresthesia on the same side of lateral bending may indicate a nerve root problem. Localized cervical pain on the same side of lateral bending may indicate a cervical facet joint problem because the facets are compressed on the side of lateral bending.

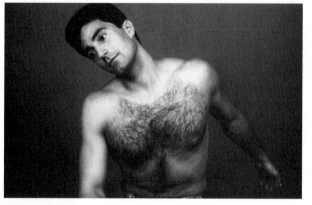

Figure 4.105

Tinnel's Sign (for Brachial Plexus Lesions) (26)

PROCEDURE:

With the patient seated and the head laterally flexed, tap along the trunks of the brachial plexus with your index finger (Fig. 4.106).

RATIONALE:

Localized pain may indicate a cervical plexus lesion. A tingling sensation in the distribution of one of the trunks may indicate a compression or neuroma of one or more of the trunks of the brachial plexus.

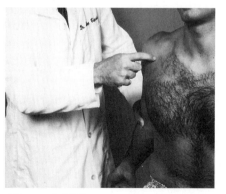

Figure 4.106

References

1. American Academy of Orthopaedic Surgeons. The clinical measurement of joint motion. Chicago American Academy of Orthopaedic Surgeons, 1994.
2. Boons DC, Azen SP. Normal range of motion of joints in male subjects. J Bone Joint Surg Am 1979;61:756–759.
3. Hoppenfeld S. Physical examination of the spine and extremities. New York: Appleton-Century-Crofts, 1976;127.
4. Hawkins RJ, Kennedy JC. Impingement syndrome in athletics. Am J Sports Med 1980;8:151–163.
5. MaGee DJ. Orthopedic physical assessment. 2nd ed. Philadelphia: WB Saunders, 1992.
6. Gerber C, Maitland GD. Practical orthopedic medicine. London: Butterworths, 1969.
7. Rockwood CA. Subluxations and dislocations about the shoulder. In: Rockwood CA, Green DP, eds. Fractures in adults—1. Philadelphia: JB Lippincott, 1984.
8. Rowe CR. Dislocations of the shoulder. In: Rowe CR, ed. The shoulder. Vol 1. Edinburgh: Churchill Livingstone, 1988.
9. Matsen FA, Thomas SC, Rockwood CA. Glenohumeral instability. In: Rockwood CA, Matsen FA, eds. The shoulder. Philadelphia: WB Saunders, 1990.
10. Jahn WT. Standardization of orthopaedic testing of the upper extremity. J Manipulative Physiol Ther 1981;4(2).
11. Stimson BBA. A manual of fractures and dislocations. 2nd ed. Philadelphia: Lea & Febiger, 1946.
12. Gerber C, Ganz R. Clinical assessment of instability of the shoulder. J Bone Joint Surg 1984;66B:551–556.
13. Norwood LA, Terry GC. Shoulder posterior and subluxation. Am J Sports Med 1984;12:25–30.
14. Cofield RH, Irving JF. Evaluation and classification of shoulder instability. Clin Orthop 1987;223:32–43.
15. Yergason RM. Supination sign. J Bone Joint Surg 1931;13:160.
16. Abbott LC, Saunders JB. Acute traumatic dislocation of tendon of long head of biceps brachii: report of cases with operative findings. Surgery 1939;6:817–840.
17. Adson AW. Cervical ribs: symptoms, differential diagnosis and indications for section of the insertion of the scalenus anticus muscle. J Coll Int Surg 1951;106:546.
18. Adson AW, Coffey JR. Cervical rib. Ann Surg 1927;85:839–857.
19. Lord JR, Rosati LM, eds. Thoracic-outlet syndromes. New Jersey, CIBA Pharmaceutical Company, 1971;21(2):9–10.
20. Falconer MA, Li FWP. Resection of first rib in costoclavicular compression of the brachial plexus. Lancet 1962;59(1):63.
21. Falconer MA, Weddel G. Costoclavicular compression of the subclavian artery and vein: relation to scalene anticus syndrome. Lancet 1943;2:542.
22. Devay AD. Costoclavicular compression of brachial plexus and subclavian vessels. Lancet 1945;2:164.
23. Wright JS. The neurovascular syndrome produced by hyperabduction of the arms. Am Heart J 1945;29(1).
24. Wright JS. Vascular diseases in clinical practice, 2nd ed. Chicago: Year Book Medical Publishers, 1952.
25. McRae R. Clinical orthopedic examination. New York: Churchill Livingstone, 1976.
26. Landi A, Copeland S. Value of the Tinel sign in brachial plexus lesions. Ann Roy Coll Surg Eng 1979;61:470–471.

General References

Cailliet R. Shoulder pain. Philadelphia: FA Davis Co., 1966.

Cipriano J. Calcific tendinitis vs. chronic bursitis in shoulder joint pathology. Today's Chiropractic 1986;14(4):15–16.

Cyriax J. Textbook of orthopaedic medicine. Vol. 1. Diagnosis of soft tissue lesions. London: Bailliere Tindall, 1982.

De Palma AF, Flannery GF. Acute anterior dislocations of the shoulder. J Sports Med Phys Fitness 1973;1:6–15.

Kapandji IA. The physiology of the joints. Vol I. Upper limb. New York: Churchill Livingstone, 1970.

Neviaser JS. Musculoskeletal disorders of the shoulder region causing cervicobrachial pain: differential diagnosis and treatment. Surg Clin North Am 1963;43:1703.

Post M. Physical examination of the musculoskeletal system. Chicago: Year Book Medical Publishers, 1987.

Post M, Silver R, Singh M. Rotator cuff tear: diagnosis and treatment. Clin Orthop 1983;173:78.

Yocum LA. Assessing the shoulder: history, physical examination, differential diagnosis, special tests used. Clin Sports Med 1983;2:281.

5

ELBOW ORTHOPAEDIC TESTS

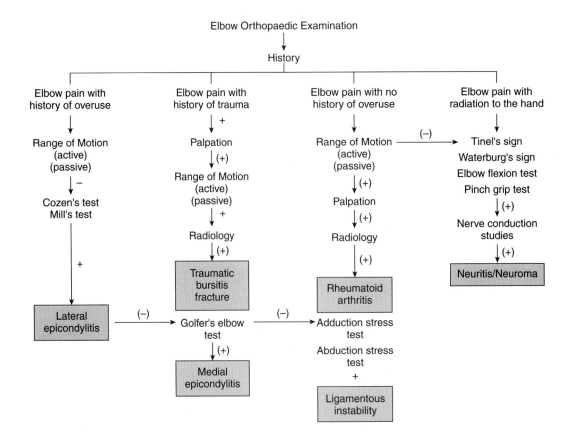

ELBOW PALPATION

Medial Aspect

Ulnar Nerve

DESCRIPTIVE ANATOMY:

The ulnar nerve is a branch of the medial cord of the brachial plexus. It passes in the groove between the medial epicondyle and the olecranon fossa (Fig. 5.1).

PROCEDURE:

With your index finger, palpate the groove between the medial epicondyle and the olecranon process. Note if the nerve is tender to palpation or thickened (Fig. 5.2). This can indicate a nerve compression or scar tissue formation on the nerve leading to paresthesia into the forearm and/or loss of interosseous muscle strength.

5

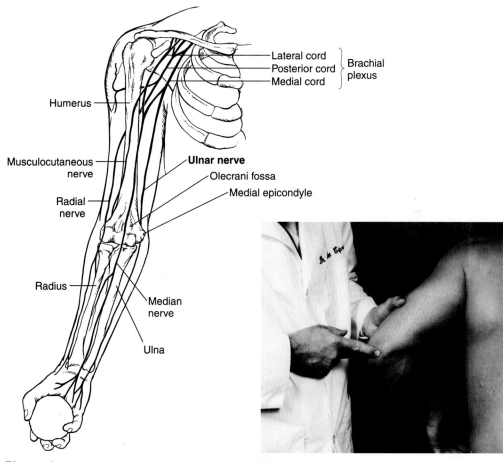

Figure 5.1

Figure 5.2

Medial Epicondyle and Attached Tendons

DESCRIPTIVE ANATOMY:

The medial epicondyle is a relatively large protuberance at the medial distal end of the humerus. Attached to the condyle are the wrist flexor and pronator group muscles. This group consists of the pronator teres, flexor carpi radialis, palmaris longus, and flexor carpi ulnaris. All these muscle originate from the medial epicondyle as a common tendon (Fig. 5.3).

PROCEDURE:

With the elbow flexed to 90° palpate the epicondyle and its tendons with your index finger; look for tenderness, inflammation, and temperature elevation (Fig. 5.4). This may indicate a strain of one or more of the previously mentioned tendons or an inflammation of the medial epicondyle caused by various activities, such as golf or tennis.

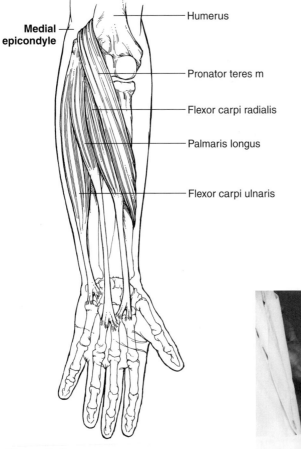

Medial epicondyle

Humerus

Pronator teres m

Flexor carpi radialis

Palmaris longus

Flexor carpi ulnaris

Figure 5.3

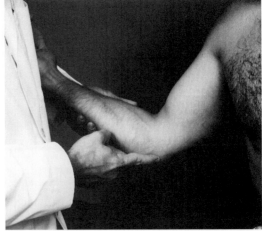

Figure 5.4

Ulnar Collateral Ligament

DESCRIPTIVE ANATOMY:

The ulnar collateral ligament attaches the medial epicondyle to the medial aspect of the ulna at the trochanteric notch (Fig. 5.5). It stabilizes the humeroulnar articulation medially.

PROCEDURE:

With your index finger, palpate the area of the ulnar collateral ligament (Fig. 5.6). Ordinarily it is not palpable. You should check for tenderness, which may indicate a sprain caused by forced valgus stress.

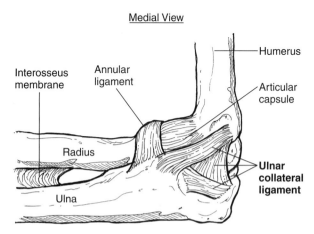

Figure 5.5

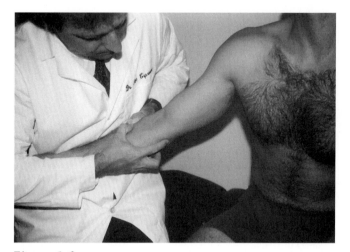

Figure 5.6

Lateral Aspect

Lateral Epicondyle and Wrist Extensor Tendons

DESCRIPTIVE ANATOMY:

The lateral epicondyle is a relatively large protuberance at the lateral distal end of the humerus. Attached to the condyle is the common extensor tendon. From this tendon arises the carpi radialis brevis, extensor digitorum, extensor digiti minimi, and extensor carpi ulnaris. The brachioradialis and extensor carpi radialis longus and brevis is attached superior to the lateral epicondyle at the supracondylar ridge (Fig. 5.7).

PROCEDURE:

With the patient's elbow flexed to 90°, palpate the lateral epicondyle and supracondylar ridge with your index and middle fingers (Fig. 5.8). Note any tenderness, inflammation, and temperature elevation at either location. These signs may indicate an inflammation of the lateral epicondyle (epicondylitis) or a strain of the extensor tendons of the wrist.

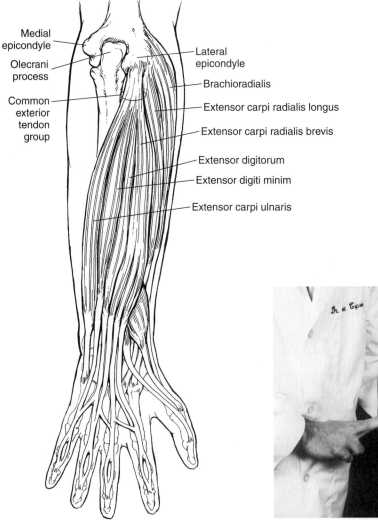

Medial epicondyle

Olecrani process

Common exterior tendon group

Lateral epicondyle

Brachioradialis

Extensor carpi radialis longus

Extensor carpi radialis brevis

Extensor digitorum

Extensor digiti minim

Extensor carpi ulnaris

Figure 5.7

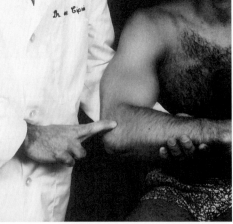

Figure 5.8

Radial Collateral Ligament and Annular Ligament

DESCRIPTIVE ANATOMY:

Radial collateral ligament and annular ligaments are thick structures that extend from the lateral epicondyle of the humerus to the annular ligament and lateral aspect of the ulnar. The annular ligament encircles the radial head (Fig. 5.9). The radial collateral ligament stabilizes the humeroulnar articulation laterally.

PROCEDURE:

With your index and middle fingers, palpate the area of the radial collateral ligament from the lateral epicondyle to the annular ligament (Fig. 5.10). Check for tenderness, which may indicate a sprain caused by forced varus stress.

5

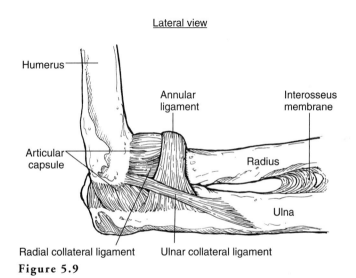

Figure 5.9

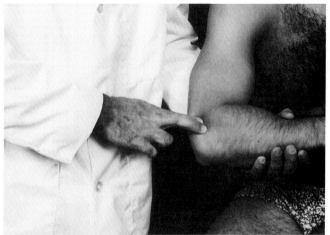

Figure 5.10

Posterior Aspect

Olecranon Process and Bursa

DESCRIPTIVE ANATOMY:

The olecranon process is located posterior to the elbow at the proximal end of the ulnar. It is covered by the olecranon bursa, which is not normally palpable (Fig. 5.11).

PROCEDURE:

With the patient's elbow flexed to 90°, palpate the olecranon process and bursa for tenderness, inflammation, and increased temperature (Fig. 5.12). A thick, boggy feeling may indicate olecranon bursitis. Check the posterior aspect of the olecranon border for rheumatoid nodules, which is indicative of rheumatoid arthritis.

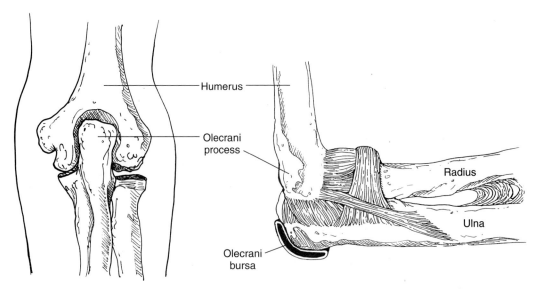

Figure 5.11

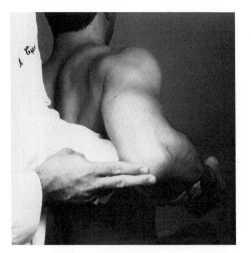

Figure 5.12

Triceps Muscle

DESCRIPTIVE ANATOMY:

The triceps muscle has three heads; the long head crosses both the glenohumeral joint and the elbow joint and it inserts into the olecranon process (Fig. 5.13).

PROCEDURE:

With the patient's elbow slightly flexed, have the patient lean on a table. This will facilitate the palpation of the muscle. With your thumb and index finger, palpate the length of the muscle down to the olecranon process looking for any tenderness or defects secondary to trauma (Fig. 5.14). This could indicate a strain or active trigger points of the triceps muscle. A hard mass may indicate myositis ossificans secondary to repeated trauma.

5

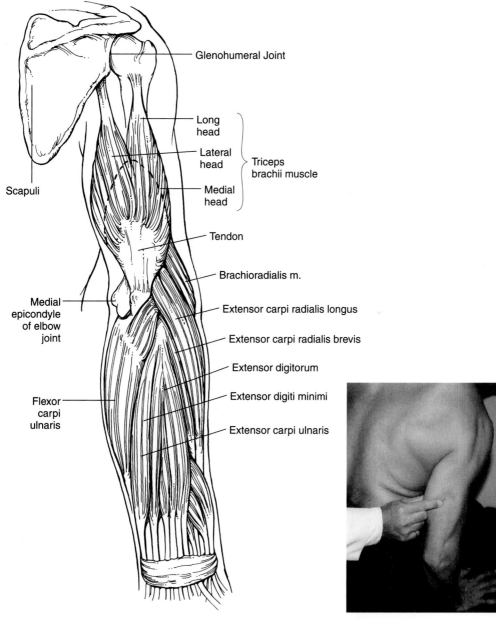

Glenohumeral Joint

Long head

Lateral head

Medial head

} Triceps brachii muscle

Scapuli

Tendon

Brachioradialis m.

Medial epicondyle of elbow joint

Extensor carpi radialis longus

Extensor carpi radialis brevis

Extensor digitorum

Extensor digiti minimi

Flexor carpi ulnaris

Extensor carpi ulnaris

Figure 5.13

Figure 5.14

Anterior Aspect

Cubital Fossa

LOCATION:

The cubital fossa is the triangular space bordered by the brachioradialis laterally and the pronator teres medially. The base is an imaginary line between the two epicondyles. The structures that pass between the fossa are the biceps tendon, brachial artery, median nerve, and musculocutaneous nerve (Fig. 5.15).

PROCEDURE:

With the patient's elbow slightly flexed and the patient resisting flexion, palpate the cubital fossa with your index finger looking for the biceps tendon, which lies medial to the brachioradialis muscle (Fig. 5.16). Tenderness may indicate a strain in the musculotendinous junction. A ruptured tendon would not be palpable in the fossa, and a bulbous gathering of muscle will be evident in the upper arm.

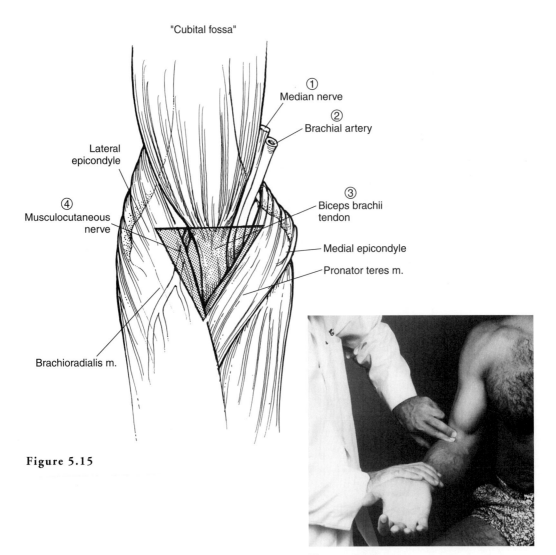

"Cubital fossa"

① Median nerve

② Brachial artery

Lateral epicondyle

④ Musculocutaneous nerve

③ Biceps brachii tendon

Medial epicondyle

Pronator teres m.

Brachioradialis m.

Figure 5.15

Figure 5.16

ELBOW RANGE OF MOTION

Flexion (1)

With the patient seated and his elbow extended, place the goniometer in the sagittal plane with the center at the elbow joint (Fig. 5.17). This is the neutral position for the elbow joint for flexion and extension. Instruct the patient to flex his arm as far as possible while following his forearm with one arm of the goniometer (Fig. 5.18).

NORMAL RANGE:

141 ± 4.9 degrees or greater from the 0 or neutral position (2)

Muscles Involved in Action	*Nerve Supply*
1. Brachialis	Musculocutaneous
2. Biceps brachii	Musculocutaneous
3. Brachioradialis	Radial
4. Pronator teres	Median
5. Flexor carpi ulnaris	Ulnar

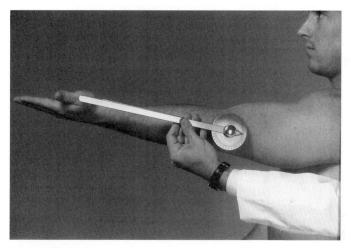

Figure 5.17

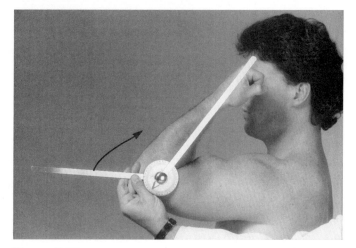

Figure 5.18

Extension (1)

With the elbow in full extension, place the goniometer in the sagittal plane with the center at the elbow joint (Fig. 5.19). Instruct the patient to further extend his elbow while following his forearm with one arm of the goniometer (Fig. 5.20).

NORMAL RANGE:

0.3 ± 2.0 degrees from full extension (2)

Muscles Involved in Action	Nerve Supply
1. Triceps	Radial
2. Anconeus	Radial

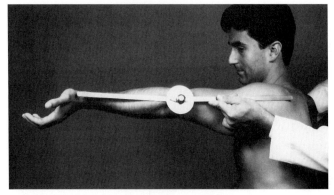

Figure 5.19 & 5.20

Supination (1)

With the patient's elbow in 90° of flexion and the thumb facing upward, place the goniometer in the coronal plane (Fig. 5.21). This is the neutral position for supination and pronation. Instruct the patient to rotate his thumb outward while you follow the thumb with one arm of the goniometer (Fig. 5.22).

NORMAL RANGE:

81 ± 4.0 degrees or greater from the 0 or neutral position (2)

Muscles Involved in Action	Nerve Supply
1. Supinator	Radial
2. Biceps brachii	Musculocutaneous

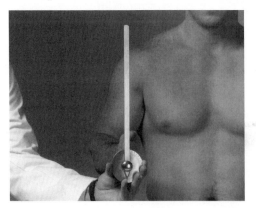
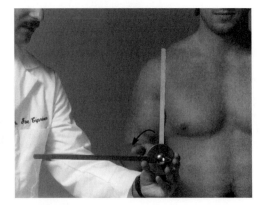

Figure 5.21 **Figure 5.22**

Pronation (1)

With the patient's elbow in 90° of flexion and the thumb facing upward, place the goniometer in the coronal plane (Fig. 5.23). Instruct the patient to rotate his thumb inward while you follow the thumb with one arm of the goniometer (Fig. 5.24).

NORMAL RANGE:

75 ± 5.3 degrees or greater from the 0 or neutral position (2)

Muscles Involved in Action	*Nerve Supply*
1. Pronator quadratus	Median
2. Pronator teres	Median
3. Flexor carpi radialis	Median

5

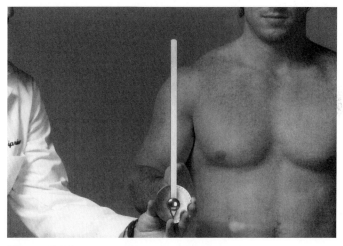

Figure 5.23

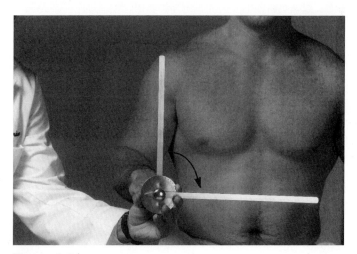

Figure 5.24

LATERAL EPICONDYLITIS (TENNIS ELBOW)

Cozen's Test (3)

PROCEDURE:

With the patient seated, stabilize the patient's forearm. Instruct the patient to make a fist and extend it (Fig. 5.25). Then force the extended wrist into flexion against resistance (Fig. 5.26).

RATIONALE:

The tendons that extend the wrist are attached to the lateral epicondyle (Fig. 5.27). They are the extensor carpi radialis brevis, extensor digitorum, extensor digiti minimi, and extensor carpi ulnaris. If the condyle itself or the common extensor tendons that attach to it are inflamed, then, by forcing the extended wrist into flexion, irritation to the lateral epicondyle and its attaching tendons is reproduced. If pain is elicited at the lateral epicondyle, then inflammation of the lateral epicondyle (epicondylitis) is suspect.

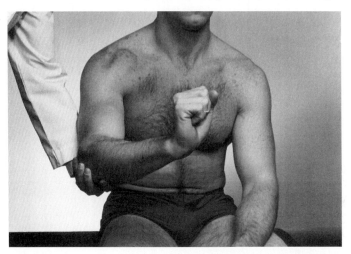

Figure 5.25

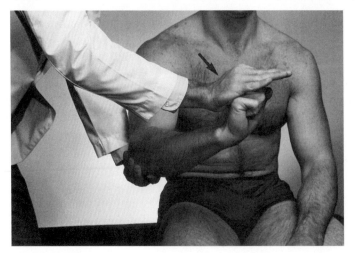

Figure 5.26

5

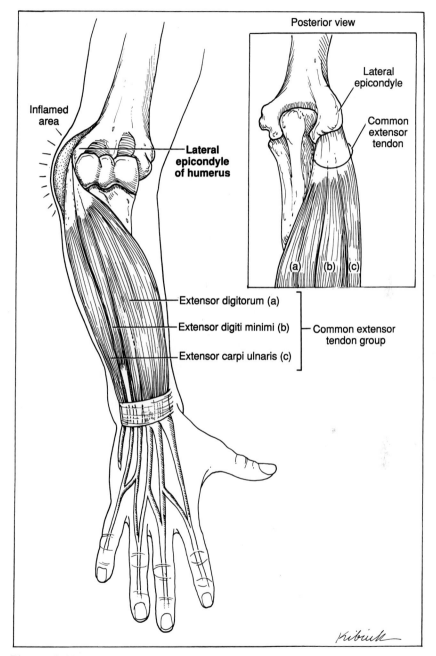

Figure 5.27

Mill's Test (4)

PROCEDURE:

With the patient seated, instruct the patient to pronate the arm and flex the wrist. Then instruct him to supinate the arm against resistance (Fig. 5.28).

RATIONALE:

The tendon of the supinator muscle, which supinates the wrist, is attached to the lateral epicondyle. If the condyle itself or the tendon of the supinator that attaches to the condyle is inflamed, resisting supination of the wrist may reproduce irritation to the lateral epicondyle and its attaching tendons. If pain is elicited at the lateral epicondyle, then inflammation of the lateral epicondyle (epicondylitis) is suspect.

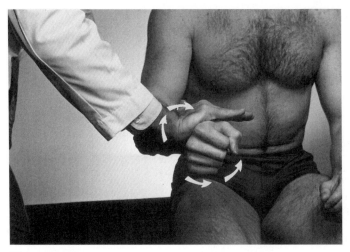

Figure 5.28

MEDIAL EPICONDYLITIS (GOLFER'S ELBOW)

Golfer's Elbow Test (5)

PROCEDURE:

With the patient seated, instruct him to extend the elbow and supinate the hand. Instruct the patient to flex the wrist against resistance (Fig. 5.29).

RATIONALE:

The tendons that flex the wrist are attached to the medial epicondyle (Fig. 5.30). They are the flexor carpi radialis and flexor carpi ulnaris. If the condyle itself or the common flexor tendons that attach to it are inflamed, by resisting wrist flexion, irritation to the medial epicondyle and its attaching tendons may be reproduced. If pain is elicited at the medial epicondyle, then inflammation of the medial epicondyle (epicondylitis) is suspect.

5

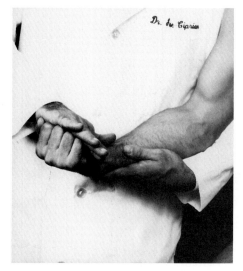

Figure 5.29

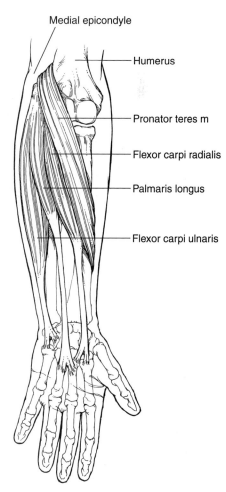

Medial epicondyle

Humerus

Pronator teres m

Flexor carpi radialis

Palmaris longus

Flexor carpi ulnaris

Figure 5.30

LIGAMENTOUS INSTABILITY

Adduction Stress Test (6)

PROCEDURE:

With the patient in the sitting position, stabilize the medial arm and place an adduction pressure on the patient's lateral forearm (Fig. 5.31).

RATIONALE:

By placing an adduction pressure on the lateral forearm, stress is applied to the radial collateral ligament (Fig. 5.32). Gapping and pain are indicative of radial collateral ligament instability.

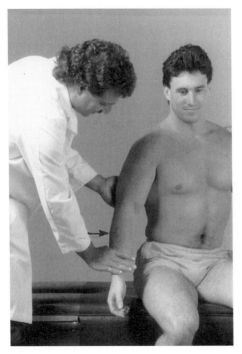

Figure 5.31

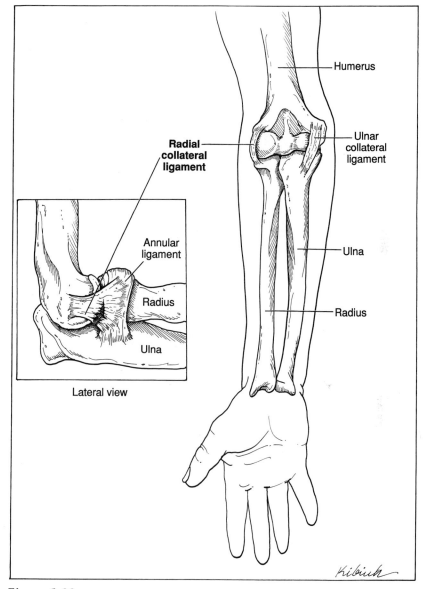

Figure 5.32

Abduction Stress Test (6)

PROCEDURE:

With the patient in the sitting position, stabilize the lateral arm and place an abduction pressure on the medial forearm (Fig. 5.33).

RATIONALE:

By placing an abduction pressure on the medial forearm, stress is applied to the ulnar collateral ligament (Fig. 5.34). Gapping and pain are indicative of ulnar collateral ligament instability.

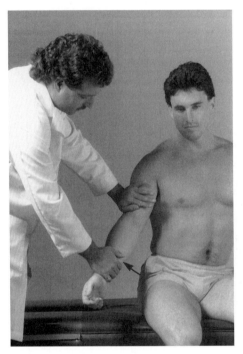

Figure 5.33

5

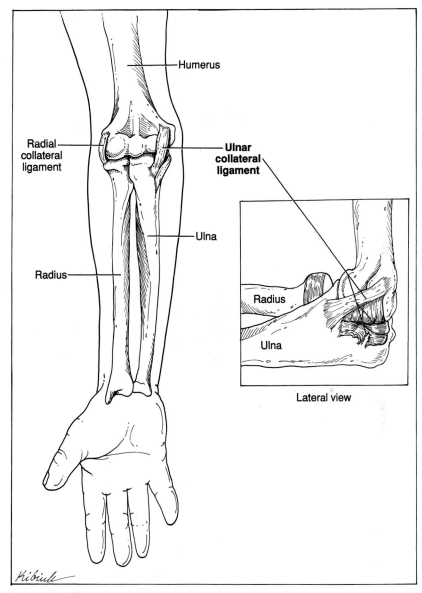

Figure 5.34

NEURITIS/NEUROMA

Tinel's Sign (7)

PROCEDURE:

With the patient seated, tap the groove between the olecranon process and the medial epicondyle with a neurological reflex hammer (Fig. 5.35). The ulnar nerve passes in this groove.

RATIONALE:

This test is designed to elicit pain caused by a neuritis or neuroma of the ulnar nerve. Pain is indicative of a positive test. The nerve can become damaged in the following ways:

1. Excessive use or repetitive injuries or trauma of the elbow
2. Arthritis of the elbow joint
3. Cubital tunnel compression, between the heads of the flexor carpi ulnaris muscle
4. Postural habits that compress the nerve, such as sleeping with elbows flexed and hands under head
5. Recurrent nerve subluxations or dislocations

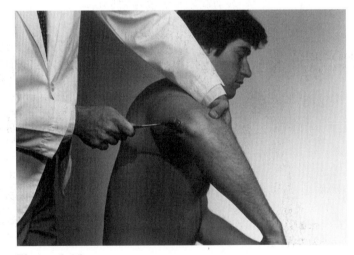

Figure 5.35

Wartenberg's Sign (8)

PROCEDURE:

With the patient sitting, instruct the patient to place his hand on the table. Passively spread the patient's fingers apart (Fig. 5.36). Instruct the patient to bring all the fingers together (Fig. 5.37).

RATIONALE:

The ulnar nerve controls abduction of the fingers. Inability to abduct the little finger to the rest of the hand indicates ulnar nerve neuritis (Fig. 5.38).

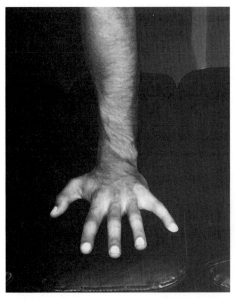

Figure 5.36

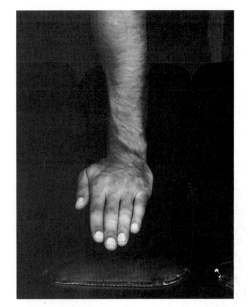

Figure 5.37

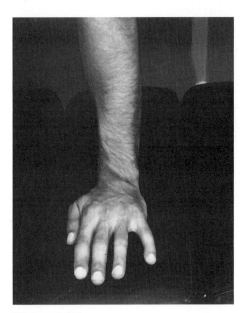

Figure 5.38

Elbow Flexion Test (9)

PROCEDURE:

With the patient in the seated position, instruct the patient to completely flex his elbow for 5 minutes (Fig. 5.39).

RATIONALE:

Flexion of the elbow may compress the ulnar nerve in the cubital tunnel. Paresthesia along the medial aspect of the forearm and hand may indicate compression of the ulnar nerve in the cubital tunnel (cubital tunnel syndrome) (Fig. 5.40). It can also be trapped between the heads of the flexor carpi ulnaris or by scar tissue in the ulnar groove.

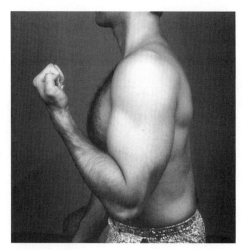

Figure 5.39

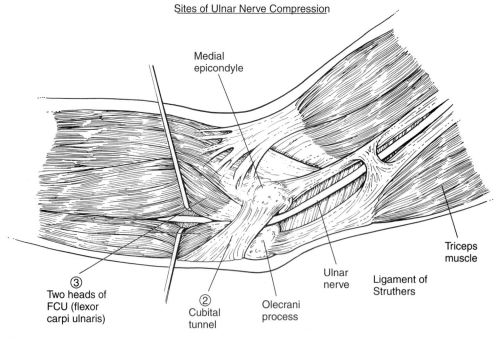

Sites of Ulnar Nerve Compression

Medial
epicondyle

Triceps
muscle

③
Two heads of
FCU (flexor
carpi ulnaris)

②
Cubital
tunnel

Olecrani
process

Ulnar
nerve

Ligament of
Struthers

Figure 5.40

Pinch Grip Test (10)

PROCEDURE:

Instruct the patient to pinch the tips of his index finger and thumb together (Fig. 5.41).

RATIONALE:

Normally, tip to tip pinching should occur. A positive test is when the pulps of the thumb and index finger touch (Fig. 5.42). This result is caused by an injury to the anterior interosseous nerve which is a branch of the median nerve. It may also indicate an entrapment syndrome of the anterior osseous nerve between the two heads of the pronator teres muscle (Fig. 5.43).

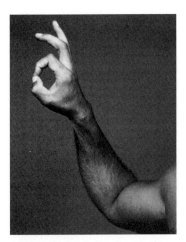

Figure 5.41

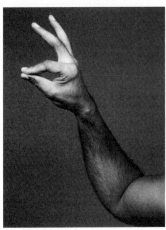

Figure 5.42

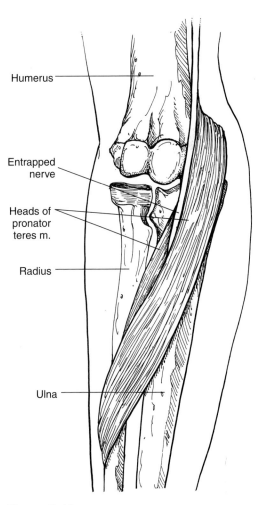

Humerus

Entrapped nerve

Heads of pronator teres m.

Radius

Ulna

Figure 5.43

References

1. American Academy of Orthopaedic Surgeons. The clinical measurement of joint motion. Chicago: American Academy of Orthopaedic Surgeons, 1994.
2. Boone DC, Azen SP. Normal range of motion in male subjects. J Bone Joint Surg 1979;61A:756–759.
3. Lucas GL. Examination of the hand. Springfield, IL: Charles C. Thomas, 1972.
4. Mills GP. The treatment of tennis elbow. Br Med J 1928;1:12–13.
5. McRae R. Clinical orthopedic examination. New York: Churchill Livingstone, 1976;41.
6. Hoppenfeld S. Physical examination of the spine and extremities. New York: Appleton-Century-Crofts, 1976;127.
7. Tinel J. Nerve wounds; symptomatology of peripheral nerve lesions caused by war wounds. Joll CA, ed, Rothwell F, trans. New York: William Wood, 1918.
8. Volz RC, Morrey BF. The physical examination of the elbow. In: Morrey BF, ed. The elbow and its disorder. Philadelphia: WB Saunders, 1985.
9. Magee DJ. Orthopedic physical assessment, 2nd ed. Philadelphia: WB Saunders, 1992.
10. Wiens E, Lane S. The anterior interosseous nerve syndrome. Can J Surg 1978;21:354.

General References

Boyd HB. Tennis elbow. J Bone Joint Surg Am 1973;55:1183–1187.

Cyriax J. Pathology and treatment of tennis elbow. J Bone Joint Surg 1936;18:921.

Cyriax J. Textbook of orthopaedic medicine. Vol. 1. Diagnosis of soft tissue lesions. London: Bailliere Tindall, 1982.

Kapandji IA. The physiology of the joints. Vol. I. Upper limb. New York: Churchill Livingstone, 1970.

McKee GK. Tennis elbow. Br Med J 1937;2:434.

Mennell J McM. Joint pain. Boston: Little, Brown and Co., 1964.

Nagler W, Johnson E, Gardner R. The pain of tennis elbow. Current Concepts Pain Analg, 1985.

Nirschl R, Pettrone F. Tennis elbow. J Bone Joint Surg 1979;61A(6):835.

Post M. Physical examination of the musculoskeletal system. Chicago: Year Book Medical Publishers, 1987.

Roles NC, Maudsley RH. Radial tunnel syndrome: resistant tennis elbow as a nerve entrapment. J Bone Joint Surg Br 1972;54:499.

6

WRIST ORTHOPAEDIC TESTS

6

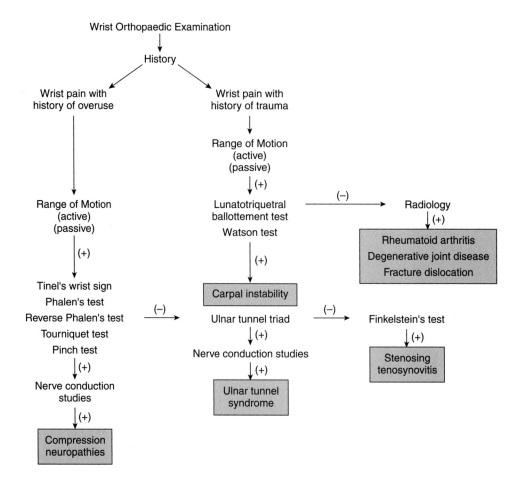

WRIST PALPATION

Anterior Aspect

Flexor Tendons

DESCRIPTIVE ANATOMY:

There are six wrist and digit flexor tendons that cross the wrist. They are as follows:

1. Flexor carpi ulnaris
2. Palmaris longus
3. Flexor digitorum profundus
4. Flexor digitorum superficialis
5. Flexor pollicis longus
6. Flexor carpi radialis
   (Fig. 6.1)

6

PROCEDURE:

Palpate each individual tendon just proximal to the flexor retinaculum, noting any tenderness or calcific deposits (Fig. 6.2). Any noted tenderness may indicate a tenosynovitis of the suspected flexor tendon.

NOTE:

Small pea-like swelling may appear at the anterior or posterior aspect of the wrist. These ganglia are benign tenosynovial tumors and are usually symptom free but may become tender and painful when distended.

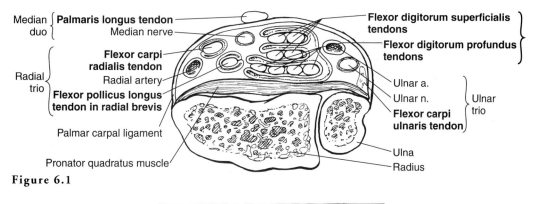

Median duo — **Palmaris longus tendon** — Median nerve

Flexor carpi radialis tendon — Radial artery

Radial trio — **Flexor pollicus longus tendon in radial brevis**

Palmar carpal ligament

Pronator quadratus muscle

Flexor digitorum superficialis tendons

Flexor digitorum profundus tendons

Ulnar a. — Ulnar n. — Ulnar trio — **Flexor carpi ulnaris tendon**

Ulna — Radius

Figure 6.1

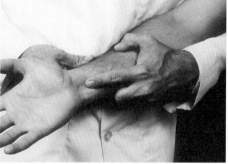

Figure 6.2

Carpal Tunnel

DESCRIPTIVE ANATOMY:

The carpal tunnel is located deep to the palmaris longus at the anterior surface of the wrist. It is bound by the pisiform and the hook of the hamate medially, the tubercle of the scaphoid and tubercle of the trapezium laterally, the flexor retinaculum anteriorly, and the carpal bones posteriorly (Fig. 6.3). Inside the tunnel lie the median nerve and the finger flexor tendons from the forearm to the hand. This tunnel is a very common site for a compression neuropathy.

PROCEDURE:

The actual tunnel and structures within the tunnel are not palpable. The borders of the tunnel should be palpated for deformity and/or tenderness (Fig. 6.4). The area over the tunnel should be palpated for increase in symptoms, such as numbness, tingling, pain, and weakness in the hand. These symptoms may indicate carpal tunnel syndrome.

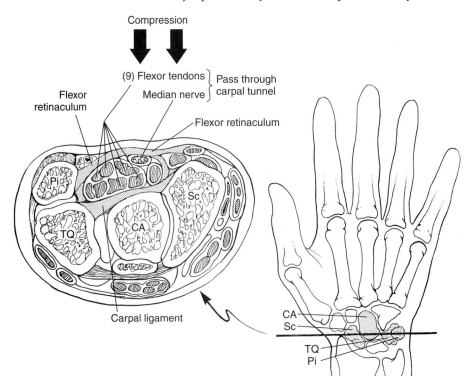

Figure 6.3

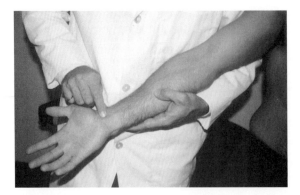

Figure 6.4

Guyon's Canal (Ulnar Tunnel)

DESCRIPTIVE ANATOMY:

The tunnel of Guyon is located between the pisiform and the hook of the hamate. It contains the ulnar nerve and artery (Fig. 6.5). It is also a common site for a compression neuropathy.

PROCEDURE:

The ulnar artery and nerve are not palpable in the tunnel. Palpating over the tunnel may cause increase tenderness to the area and may increase the symptoms to the ulnar distribution of the hand (Fig. 6.6).

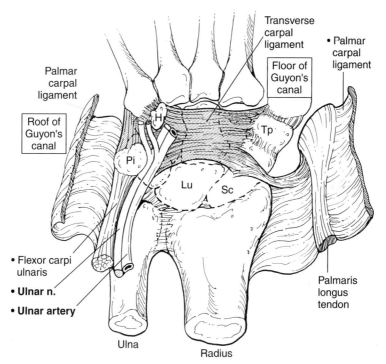

Transverse carpal ligament

• Palmar carpal ligament

Floor of Guyon's canal

Palmar carpal ligament

Roof of Guyon's canal

H

Tp

Pi

Lu

Sc

• Flexor carpi ulnaris

• Ulnar n.

• Ulnar artery

Palmaris longus tendon

Ulna

Radius

Figure 6.5

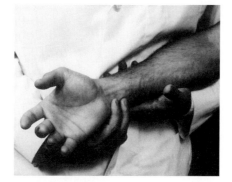

Figure 6.6

Radial and Ulnar Arteries

DESCRIPTIVE ANATOMY:

The radial and ulnar arteries are the two branches of the brachial artery that supply the hand with blood flow. The radial artery is located laterally at the anterior lateral aspect of the wrist, and the ulnar is located at the anterior medial aspect of the wrist (Fig. 6.7).

PROCEDURE:

Palpate each artery one at a time and determine the amplitude of both pulses bilaterally (Figs. 6.8, 6.9). A decrease in amplitude may indicate a compression of the respective artery between the elbow and the wrist if the brachial artery is palpated and not compromised. A common site of compression for the ulnar artery is the tunnel of Guyon.

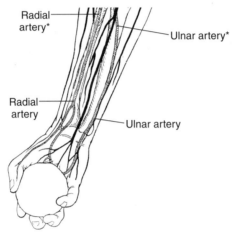

Figure 6.7

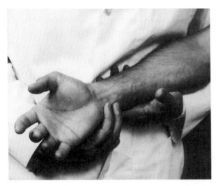

Figure 6.8

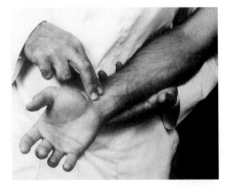

Figure 6.9

Posterior Aspect

Ulnar Styloid Process and Radial Tubercle

DESCRIPTIVE ANATOMY:

The ulnar styloid process is located at the posterior aspect of the wrist proximal to the fifth digit. The radial tubercle is also located at the posterior aspect of the wrist but proximal to the thumb (Fig. 6.10).

PROCEDURE:

Palpate the ulnar styloid process and radial tubercle for tenderness, pain, swelling, or deformity (Figs. 6.11, 6.12). Pain at the radial tubercle secondary to trauma may indicate a fracture, such as a Colles' fracture, which is a fracture of the distal radius with dorsal angulation. Pain at the ulnar styloid may be associated with a distal ulnar fracture. Tenderness, swelling, or deformity at either site may indicate rheumatoid arthritis.

6

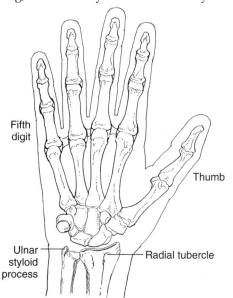

Figure 6.10

Fifth digit

Thumb

Ulnar styloid process

Radial tubercle

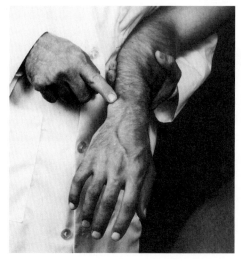

Figure 6.11

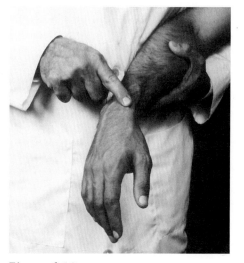

Figure 6.12

Extensor Tendons

DESCRIPTIVE ANATOMY:

There are six fibro-osseous tunnels at the posterior aspect of the wrist. The extensor tendons to the hand pass through these tunnels. These tunnels are bound by the extensor retinaculum superficially and are lined with a synovial sheath. From the thumb laterally, the following are the tunnels and there respective tendons:

1. Tunnel 1: Adductor pollicis longus, extensor pollicis brevis
2. Tunnel 2: Extensor carpi radialis longus and brevis
3. Tunnel 3: Extensor pollicis longus
4. Tunnel 4: Extensor digitorum and extensor indexes
5. Tunnel 5: Extensor digiti minimi
6. Tunnel 6: Extensor carpi ulnaris
   (Fig. 6.13)

PROCEDURE:

Support the patient's hand with your fingers while palpating his wrist with both your thumbs (Fig. 6.14). Note any crepitus or restriction of movement. Crepitus may indicate a tenosynovitis of one of the extensor tendons.

NOTE:

Small pealike swelling may appear at the anterior or posterior aspect of the wrist. These ganglia are benign tenosynovial tumors and are usually symptom free but may become tender and painful when distended.

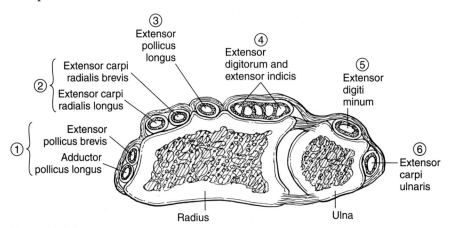

Figure 6.13

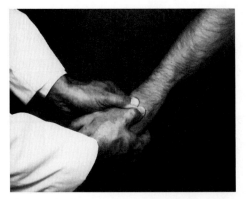

Figure 6.14

146

Wrist Range of Motion

Flexion (1)

With the patient's wrist in the neutral position, place the goniometer in the sagittal plane with the center at the ulnar styloid process (Fig. 6.15). Instruct the patient to flex his wrist downward, and follow the hand with one arm of the goniometer (Fig. 6.16).

NORMAL RANGE:

75 ± 6.6 degrees or greater from the 0 or neutral position (2).

Muscles Involved in Action	*Nerve Supply*
1. Flexor carpi radialis	Median
2. Flexor carpi ulnaris	Ulnar

6

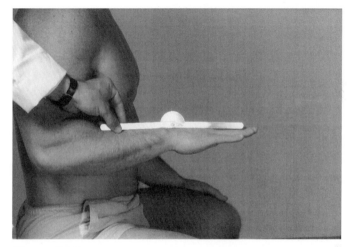

Figure 6.15

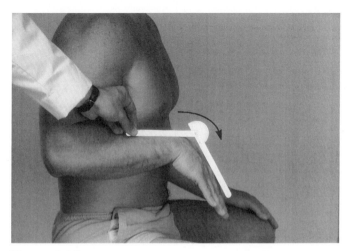

Figure 6.16

Extension (1)

With the patient's wrist in the neutral position, place the goniometer in the sagittal plane with the center at the ulnar styloid process (Fig. 6.17). Instruct the patient to extend his wrist backward while you follow his hand with one arm of the goniometer (Fig. 6.18).

NORMAL RANGE:

74 ± 6.6 degrees or greater from the 0 or neutral position (2).

Muscles Involved in Action	*Nerve Supply*
1. Extensor carpi radialis longus	Radial
2. Extensor carpi radialis brevis	Radial
3. Extensor carpi ulnaris	Radial

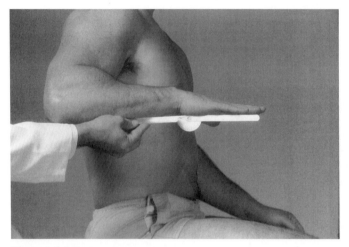

Figure 6.17

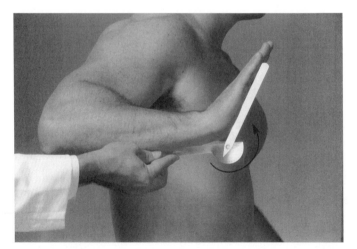

Figure 6.18

Ulnar Deviation (1)

With the patient's wrist in the neutral position and the hand supinated, place the goniometer in the coronal plane with the center at the radial/ulnar junction (Fig. 6.19). Instruct the patient to deviate his wrist medialward, and follow his hand with one arm of the goniometer (Fig. 6.20).

NORMAL RANGE:

35 ± 3.8 degrees or greater from the 0 or neutral position (2).

Muscles Involved in Action	Nerve Supply
1. Flexor carpi ulnaris	Ulnar
2. Extensor carpi ulnaris	Radial

6

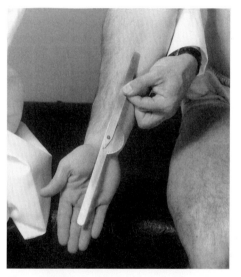

Figure 6.19

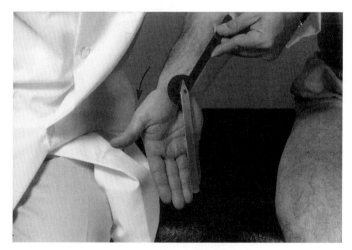

Figure 6.20

Radial Deviation (1)

With the patient's wrist in the neutral position and the hand supinated, place the goniometer in the coronal plane with the center at the radial/ulnar junction (Fig. 6.21). Instruct the patient to deviate his wrist lateralward, and follow his hand with one arm of the goniometer (Fig. 6.22).

NORMAL RANGE:

21 ± 4.0 degrees or greater from the 0 or neutral position (2).

Muscles Involved in Action	Nerve Supply
1. Extensor carpi radialis	Median
2. Extensor carpi radialis longus	Radial
3. Abductor pollicis longus	Radial
4. Extensor pollicis brevis	Radial

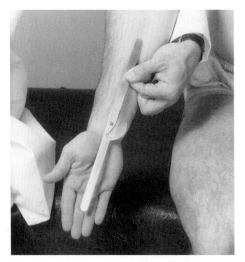

Figure 6.21

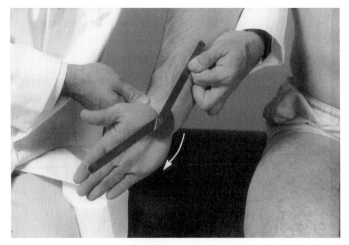

Figure 6.22

CARPAL TUNNEL SYNDROME

Tinel's Wrist Sign (3)

PROCEDURE:

With the patient's hand supinated, stabilize the wrist with one hand. With your opposite hand, tap the palmar surface of the wrist with a neurological reflex hammer (Fig. 6.23).

RATIONALE:

Tingling in the hand along the distribution of the median nerve (thumb, index finger, middle finger, and medial half of the ring finger) is indicative of carpal tunnel syndrome. Carpal tunnel syndrome is a compression of the median nerve either by inflammation of the flexor retinaculum, anterior dislocation of the lunate bone, arthritic changes, or tenosynovitis of the flexor digitorum tendons (see Fig. 6.25).

6

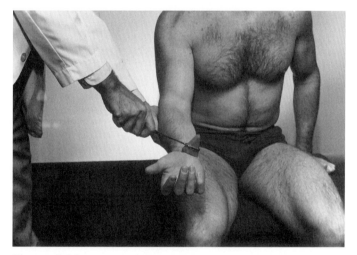

Figure 6.23

Phalen's Test (4,5)

PROCEDURE:

Flex both wrists and approximate them to each other. Hold for 60 seconds (Fig. 6.24).

RATIONALE:

When both wrists are flexed, the flexor retinaculum provides increased compression of the medial nerve in the carpal tunnel. Tingling in the hand after the distribution of the median nerve (thumb, index finger, middle finger, and medial half of the ring finger) is indicative of compression of the median nerve in the carpal tunnel (Fig. 6.25) by either the inflammation of the flexor retinaculum, anterior dislocation of the lunate bone, arthritic changes, or tenosynovitis of the flexor digitorum tendons.

Figure 6.24

Figure 6.25

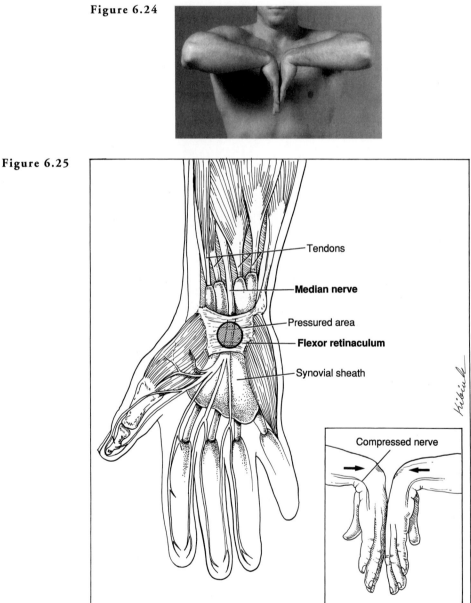

Tendons

Median nerve

Pressured area

Flexor retinaculum

Synovial sheath

Compressed nerve

Test for carpal tunnel syndrome

Reverse Phalens Test (6)

PROCEDURE:

Instruct the patient to extend the affected wrist and have the patient grip your hand. With your opposite thumb, put pressure over the carpal tunnel (Fig. 6.26).

RATIONALE:

Extending the hand and applying pressure to the carpal tunnel further constricts the tunnel. Tingling in the thumb, index finger, and lateral half of the ring finger may indicate a compression of the medial nerve in the carpal tunnel by either the inflammation of the flexor retinaculum, anterior dislocation of the lunate bone, arthritic changes, or tenosynovitis of the flexor digitorum tendons.

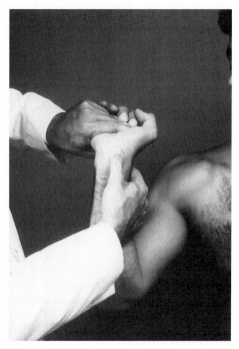

Figure 6.26

Tourniquet Test (7)

PROCEDURE:

Wrap a sphygmomanometer cuff around the affected wrist and inflate it to just above the patient's systolic blood pressure. Hold for 1 to 2 minutes (Fig. 6.27).

RATIONALE:

The inflated sphygmomanometer cuff induces mechanically increased pressure to the median nerve. Tingling in the hand after the distribution of the median nerve (thumb, index finger, middle finger, and medial half of the ring finger), indicates compression of the median nerve in the carpal tunnel by either the inflammation of the flexor retinaculum, anterior dislocation of the lunate bone, arthritic changes, or tenosynovitis of the flexor digitorum tendons.

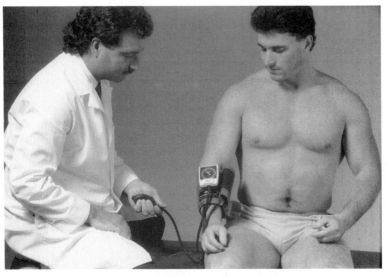

Figure 6.27

Pinch Test (8)

PROCEDURE:

Instruct the patient to pinch a piece of paper between his thumb, index, and middle fingers while you attempt to pull it away (Fig. 6.28).

RATIONALE:

The median nerve innervates the lumbrical muscles, which are used to pinch the piece of paper. With a compression of the median nerve, the patient may experience numbness and/or cramping of the fingers or midpalm region within 1 minute.

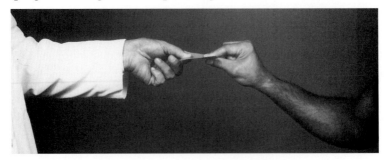

Figure 6.28

ULNAR TUNNEL SYNDROME

Ulnar Tunnel Triad

PROCEDURE:

Inspect and palpate the patient's wrist, looking for tenderness over the ulnar tunnel, clawing of the ring finger, and hypothenar wasting (Fig. 6.29).

RATIONALE:

All three of these signs are indicative of ulnar nerve compression possibly in the tunnel of Guyon.

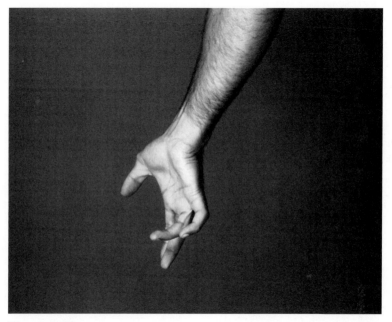

Figure 6.29

6

STENOSING TENOSYNOVITIS

Finkelstein's Test (9)

PROCEDURE:

Instruct the patient to make a fist with the thumb across the palmar surface of the hand (Fig. 6.30). Instruct the patient to stress the wrist medially (Fig. 6.31).

RATIONALE:

Making a fist and stressing it medially stresses the abductor pollicis longus and extensor pollicus brevis tendons. Pain distal to the styloid process of the radius is indicative of stenosing tenosynovitis of the abductor pollicis longus and extensor pollicis brevis tendons (de Quervain's disease).

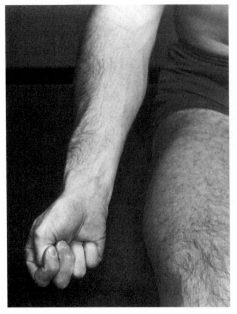

Figure 6.30

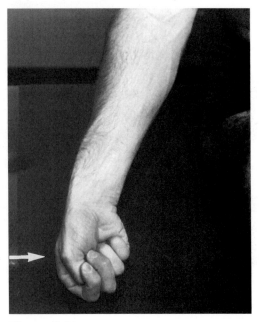

Figure 6.31

CARPAL INSTABILITY

Lunatotriquetral Ballottement Test (10)

PROCEDURE:

With one hand, grasp the triquetrum on the affected side with your thumb and index finger. With your opposite hand, grasp the lunate also with the thumb and index finger (Fig. 6.32). Move the lunate anteriorly and posteriorly, noting any pain, laxity, or crepitus.

RATIONALE:

The lunate and triquetrum are held together by a fibrous articular capsule and by dorsal, palmar, and interosseous ligaments. The lunate is the most commonly dislocated of the carpal bones. Most of the time it dislocates anteriorly and affects the radiolunate and the ligaments between the lunate and the triquetrum. Pain, laxity, or crepitus indicates an instability of the lunatotriquetral articulation, causing a propensity of the lunate to subluxate or dislocate. This instability may lead to carpal tunnel syndrome, medial nerve palsy, flexor tendon constriction, or progressive avascular necrosis of the lunate.

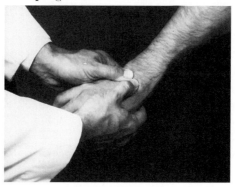

Figure 6.32

Watson Test (10)

PROCEDURE:

With one hand, stabilize the radius and the ulnar. With the opposite hand, grasp the scaphoid, moving it anteriorly and posteriorly (Fig. 6.33).

RATIONALE:

The scaphoid is prone to subluxate or dislocate with hyperextension trauma. Pain, laxity, or crepitus indicates an instability of the scaphoid with propensity to subluxate or dislocate.

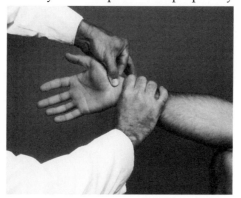

Figure 6.33

References

1. American Academy of Orthopaedic Surgeons. The clinical measurement of joint motion. Chicago: American Academy of Orthopaedic Surgeons, 1994.
2. Boone DC, Azen SP. Normal range of motion in male subjects. J Bone Joint Surg 1979;61A:756–759.
3. Tinel J. Nerve wounds: symptomatology of peripheral nerve lesions caused by war wounds. Joll CA, ed, Rothwell F, trans. New York: William Wood, 1918.
4. Phalen GS. The carpal tunnel syndrome: 17 years experience in diagnosis and treatment of 654 hands. J Bone Joint Surg 1966;48A:211–228.
5. American Society for Surgery of the Hand. The hand examination and diagnosis. Aurora, Colorado, 1978.
6. Post M. Physical examination of the musculoskeletal system. Chicago: Year Book Medical Publishers, 1987.
7. McRae R. Clinical orthopedic examination. New York: Churchill Livingstone, 1976.
8. Ditmars DM, Houin HP. Carpal tunnel syndrome. Hand Clin 1986;2(4):723–736.
9. Finkelstein H. Stenosing tenosynovitis at the radial styloid process. J Bone Joint Surg 1930;12:509.
10. Taleisnik J. Carpal instability. J Bone Joint Surg 1988;70A:1262–1268.

General References

de Quervain F. Clinical surgical diagnosis for students and practitioners. 4th ed. Snowman J, trans. New York: William Wood, 1913.

Ditmars DM, Houin HP. Carpal tunnel syndrome. Hand Clin 1986;2(3):525–532.

Green DP. Carpal dislocations. In: Operative hand surgery. New York: Churchill Livingstone, 1982.

Hoppenfeld S. Physical examination of the spine and extremities. New York: Appleton-Century-Crofts, 1976;127.

Kapandji IA. The physiology of the joints. Vol. I. Upper limb. New York: Churchill Livingstone, 1970.

Stevenson TM. Carpal tunnel syndrome. Proc R Soc Med 1966;59:824.

Thompson WAL, Koppell HP. Peripheral entrapment neuropathies of the upper extremities. N Engl J Med 1959;260:1261.

Wadsworth CT. Wrist and hand examination and interpretation. J Orthop Sports Phys Ther 1983;5:108.

7
HAND ORTHOPAEDIC TESTS

7

HAND PALPATION

Anterior Aspect

Thenar Eminence

DESCRIPTIVE ANATOMY:

The thenar eminence is located at the lateral aspect of the hand with the palm facing out. It is comprised of three muscles that move the thumb: abductor pollicis brevis, opponens pollicis, and flexor pollicis brevis. These muscles are innervated by a branch of the recurrent median nerve (Fig. 7.1). Severe prolonged compression of the median nerve in the carpal tunnel may cause the muscles of the thenar eminence to atrophy.

PROCEDURE:

Palpate the triangular shape of the thenar eminence from the base of the thumb medial to the central aspect of the hand at the base of the carpal bones, then inferior and lateral to the base of the forefinger (Fig. 7.2). Look for hypertrophy or atrophy when compared with the opposite hand. If atrophy or wasting is noted with pain and paresthesia along the medial nerve distribution, then compression of the medial nerve in the carpal tunnel is suspect.

Figure 7.1

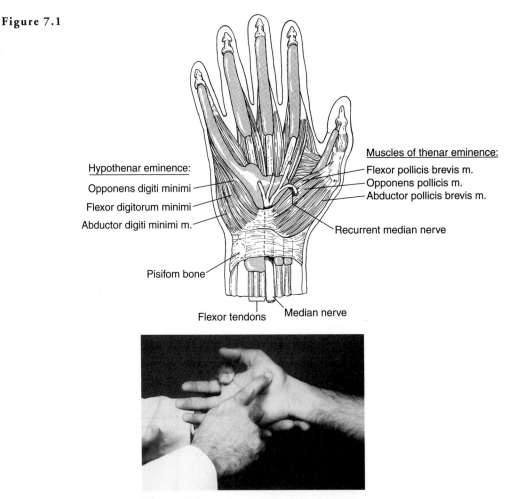

Hypothenar eminence:
Opponens digiti minimi
Flexor digitorum minimi
Abductor digiti minimi m.

Muscles of thenar eminence:
Flexor pollicis brevis m.
Opponens pollicis m.
Abductor pollicis brevis m.

Recurrent median nerve

Pisifom bone

Flexor tendons   Median nerve

Figure 7.2

Hypothenar Eminence

DESCRIPTIVE ANATOMY:

The hypothenar eminence is located at the anterior aspect of the hand from the base of the little finger to the medial aspect of the hand and ends at the pisiform (Fig. 7.1). This eminence contains the abductor digiti minimi, opponens digiti minimi, and flexor digiti minimi. These muscle are supplied by the deep branch of the ulnar nerve. Severe prolonged compression of the nerve either in Guyon's tunnel or, more proximally, in the extremity may cause wasting of the hypothenar eminence.

PROCEDURE:

Palpate the length of the thenar eminence from the base of the little finger to the base of the pisiform (Fig. 7.3). Look for hypertrophy or atrophy when compared with the opposite hand. Wasting of the hypothenar eminence may indicate a compression of the ulnar nerve either in the tunnel of Guyon or, more proximally, in the extremity.

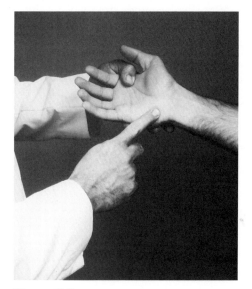

Figure 7.3

7

Posterior Aspect

Extensor Tendons

DESCRIPTIVE ANATOMY:

The posterior aspect of the hand contains an intricate system of ligaments, facial bands, and tendons. This system is called the extensor mechanism. This mechanism provides active extension motion to the fingers and contributes to the stabilization of the hand and digits. The extrinsic extensor tendons run along the entire length of the posterior aspect of the hand to each digit (Fig. 7.4). They can be affected by trauma, which can strain or rupture the tendons. These tendons also can be affected by rheumatoid arthritis and become displaced.

PROCEDURE:

With the patient's fingers and wrists extended, palpate the length of each tendon of the extensor digitorum communis from the base of the wrist to the proximal phalanx (Fig. 7.5). Note any tenderness, cysts, displacement, or loss of continuity of any of the individual tendons. Tenderness and displacement is indicative of rheumatoid arthritis. Loss of continuity secondary to trauma with loss of digit extension may indicate a ruptured extensor tendon. Small pealike cysts may develop between the second and third metacarpal bones and are easily palpable.

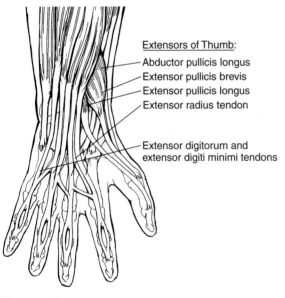

Extensors of Thumb:
— Abductor pullicis longus
— Extensor pullicis brevis
— Extensor pullicis longus
— Extensor radius tendon

— Extensor digitorum and
extensor digiti minimi tendons

Figure 7.4

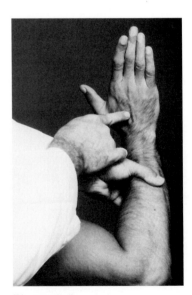

Figure 7.5

Metacarpal and Phalanges

DESCRIPTIVE ANATOMY:

The metacarpal bones and phalanxes are held together by a series of ligaments and joint capsules that supply stability to the joints (Fig. 7.6). The metacarpal and phalangeal bones are easily palpable from the posterior aspect of the hand. They are susceptible to fractures secondary to trauma. The joints may become inflamed and are a common site for rheumatoid arthritis.

PROCEDURE:

Palpate each individual digit and metacarpal bone (Fig. 7.7). Look for tenderness, swelling, temperature differences, and bony nodules. Tenderness and swelling secondary to trauma may indicate a fracture of a suspected bone. Swelling around a joint capsule may indicate an inflammatory process, such as rheumatoid arthritis. Bony nodules (Heberden's nodes) located on the posterior and lateral surfaces of the distal interphalangeal joints may indicate osteoarthritis.

Figure 7.6

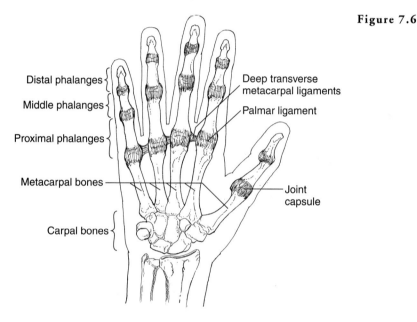

Distal phalanges

Middle phalanges

Proximal phalanges

Deep transverse metacarpal ligaments

Palmar ligament

Metacarpal bones

Joint capsule

Carpal bones

7

Figure 7.7

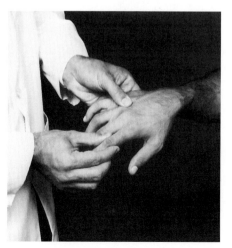

JOINT INSTABILITY

Varus and Valgus Stress Test (1)

PROCEDURES:

With a pinch grip, grasp the suspected joint (either a distal or proximal interphalangeal joint) with one hand. With your opposite hand, pinch grip the adjoining bone and place a varus (Fig. 7.8) and valgus (Fig. 7.9) stress to the joint.

RATIONALE:

These procedures test the integrity of the collateral ligaments and the capsule surrounding the joints. If pain is elicit, then a capsule sprain, subluxation, or dislocation of the joint is suspected. Laxity may indicate a tear to the joint capsule or collateral ligaments of the joint secondary to trauma.

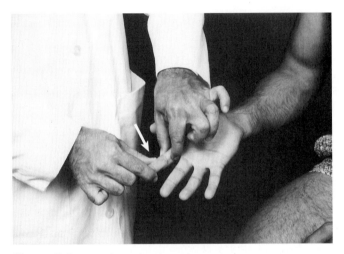

Figure 7.8

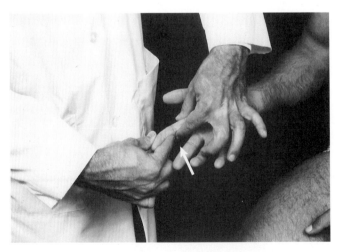

Figure 7.9

Thumb Ulnar Collateral Ligament Laxity Test (2)

PROCEDURE:

With the carpometacarpal joint in extension, stabilize the metacarpal with a pinch grip. With your opposite hand, grasp the proximal phalanx (also with a pinch grip) and push the phalanx radially (Fig. 7.10). Repeat the test with the metacarpophalangeal joint fully flexed (Fig. 7.11).

RATIONALE:

When the thumb is fully extended, 6 degrees of laxity normally results. If laxity is greater than 6 degrees or as much as 30 degrees, then ulnar lateral collateral ligament and volar plate damage exists. If the joint is lax in full flexion, then the ulnar collateral ligament is damaged. If there is no laxity in flexion, then the ligament is intact. If there is no laxity in full flexion and more than 30 degrees of laxity in full extension, then damage exists only to the volar plate.

7

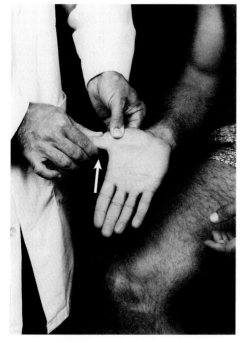

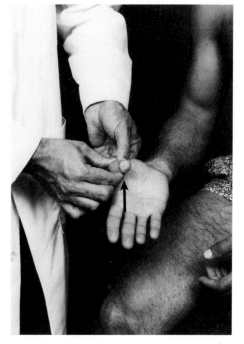

Figure 7.10

Figure 7.11

JOINT CAPSULE AND COLLATERAL LIGAMENT TESTS

Bunnel-Littler Test (3)

PROCEDURE:

Instruct the patient to slightly extend the metacarpophalgeal joint. Then, attempt to move the proximal interphalangeal joint into flexion (Fig. 7.12). Repeat the test with the metacarpophalgeal joint in flexion (Fig. 7.13).

RATIONALE:

If the proximal interphalangeal joint does not flex with the metacarpophalgeal joint in slight extension, then there is a tight intrinsic muscle or a contracture of the joint capsule. If the proximal interphalangeal joint fully flexes with the metacarpophalangeal joint flexed, the intrinsic muscles are tight. A positive test is indicative of an inflammatory process in the fingers, such as osteoarthritis or rheumatoid arthritis.

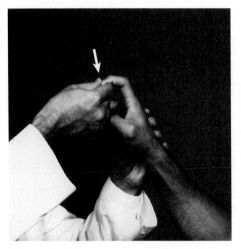

Figure 7.12

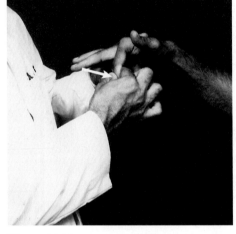

Figure 7.13

Test for Tight Retinacular Ligaments

PROCEDURE:

With the proximal interphalangeal joint in the neutral position, passively attempt to flex the distal interphalangeal joint (Fig. 7.14). Repeat the test with the proximal interphalangeal joint in the flexed position (Fig. 7.15).

RATIONALE:

If the distal interphalangeal joint does not flex with the proximal interphalangeal joint in the neutral position, the collateral ligaments or joint capsule are tight. If the distal interphalangeal joint flexes easily when the proximal interphalangeal joint is flexed, then the collateral ligaments are tight and the capsule is normal.

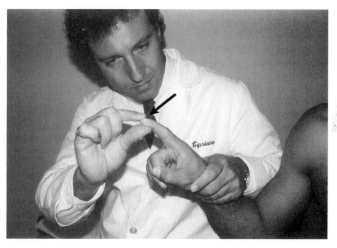

Figure 7.14

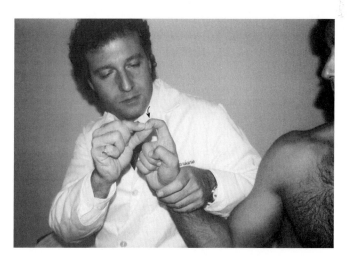

Figure 7.15

TENDON INSTABILITY

Profundus Test (3)

PROCEDURE:

Instruct the patient to flex the suspected distal phalanx while you stabilize the proximal phalanx (Fig. 7.16).

RATIONALE:

Inability to flex the distal phalanx is indicative of a divided flexor digitorum profundus tendon.

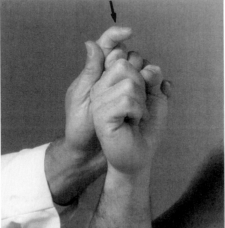

Figure 7.16

Subliminus Test

PROCEDURE:

With the patient's fingers extended, stabilize all except the suspected digit. Instruct the patient to flex the suspected digit at the proximal interphalangeal joint (Fig. 7.17).

RATIONALE:

Inability to flex the joint is indicative of a subliminus tendon injury.

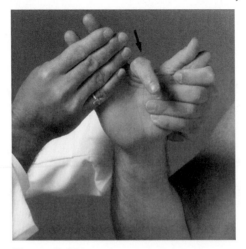

Figure 7.17

Flexor and Extensor Pollicis Longus Test

PROCEDURE:

Stabilize the proximal phalanx of the thumb. Instruct the patient to flex (Fig. 7.18) and extend the distal phalanx (Fig. 7.19).

RATIONALE:

Inability to flex the digit is indicative of an injured flexor pollicis longus tendon. Inability to extend the digit is indicative of an injury to the extensor pollicis longus tendon.

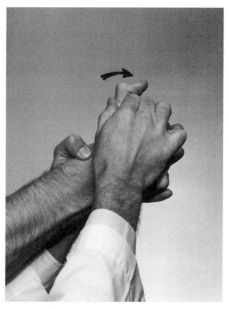

Figure 7.18

7

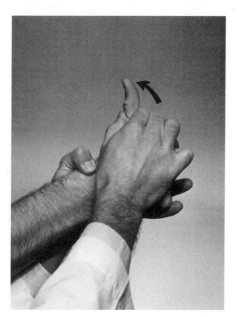

Figure 7.19

Extensor Digitorum Communis Test

PROCEDURE:

With the fingers flexed (Fig. 7.20), instruct the patient to extend his fingers (Fig. 7.21).

RATIONALE:

Inability to extend any of the fingers is indicative of an injury to that particular portion of the extensor digitorum communis tendon (Fig. 7.22).

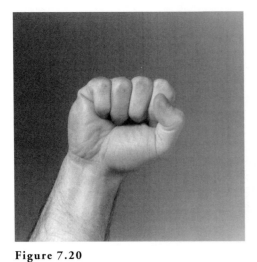

Figure 7.20

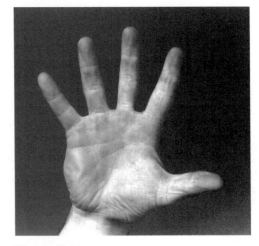

Figure 7.21

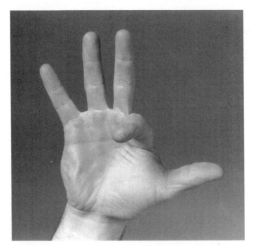

Figure 7.22

References

1. Hartley A. Practical joint assessment. St. Louis: Mosby, 1991.
2. Louis D, et al. Rupture and displacement of the ulnar collateral ligament of the metacarpophalangeal joint of the thumb. J Bone Joint Surg Am 1986;68(9):1320.
3. Hoppenfeld S. Physical examination of the spine and extremities. New York: Appleton-Century-Croft, 1976.
4. Post M. Physical examination of the musculoskeletal system. Chicago: Year Book Medical Publishers, 1987.

General References

Cailliet R. Hand pain and impairment. Philadelphia: Davis, 1971.

Eaton RG. Joint injuries of the hand. Springfield, IL: Charles C. Thomas, 1971.

Maitland GD. The peripheral joints: examination and recording guide. Adelaide, Australia: Virgo Press, 1973.

McRae R. Clinical orthopedic examination. New York: Churchill Livingstone, 1976.

Nicholas JS. The swollen hand. Physiotherapy 1977;63:285.

Wadsworth CT. Wrist and hand examination and interpretation. J Orthop Sports Phys Ther 1983;5:108–120.

7

8
THORACIC ORTHOPAEDIC TESTS

8

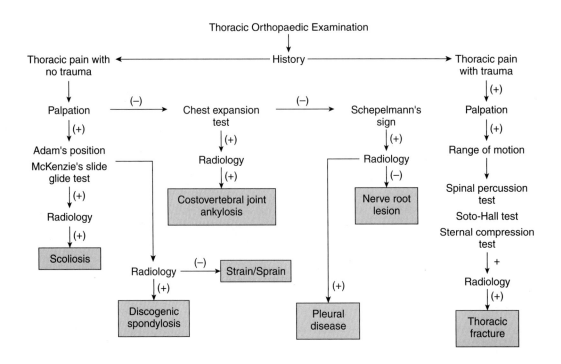

Thoracic Orthopaedic Examination

History

Thoracic pain with no trauma

Thoracic pain with trauma

Palpation

Chest expansion test

Schepelmann's sign

Palpation

Adam's position
McKenzie's slide glide test

Radiology

Radiology

Range of motion

Radiology

Costovertebral joint ankylosis

Nerve root lesion

Spinal percussion test
Soto-Hall test
Sternal compression test

Scoliosis

Radiology

Strain/Sprain

Radiology

Discogenic spondylosis

Pleural disease

Thoracic fracture

PALPATION

Anterior Aspect

Sternum

DESCRIPTIVE ANATOMY:

The sternum is located at the anterior part of the chest wall and it consists of three parts: the manubrium, body, and xiphoid process. It articulates with the costal cartilages on both sides. The manubrium also articulates with the facets of the clavicle on both sides (Fig. 8.1).

PROCEDURE:

Palpate the entire length of the sternum for tenderness or abnormality (Fig. 8.2). Also palpate the costal margins and sternal clavicular articulations for tenderness, pain, and displacement (Fig. 8.3). Pain and tenderness secondary to trauma may indicate a fractured sternum or bruised costal cartilages secondary to trauma. Tender sternocostal or sternoclavicular articulations may indicate a sprain or subluxation of the suspected articulation.

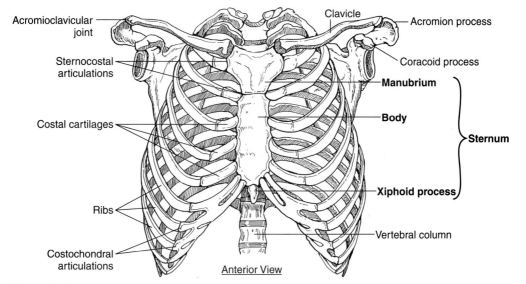

Figure 8.1.

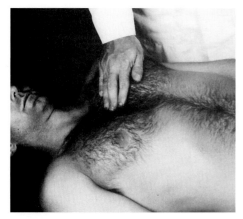

Figure 8.2.

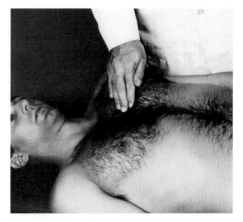

Figure 8.3.

Ribs, Costal Cartilages, and Intercostal Spaces

DESCRIPTIVE ANATOMY:

The ribs at the anterior aspect of the rib cage are attached to the sternum by costal cartilages. The costal cartilages articulate with the ribs, forming the costochondral articulation. They also articulate with the sternum, forming the sternocostal articulations (Fig. 8.4).

PROCEDURE:

Palpate each individual costal cartilage with its associated rib from the lateral aspect of the sternum laterally to the axilla. Then palpate into each intercostal space (Fig. 8.5). Tender costal cartilages may indicate a costochondritis (Tietze syndrome). Tender intercostal spaces may indicate an irritated intercostal nerve or a herpes zoster viral infection. Associated with this infection may be red vesicular eruptions along the course of the intercostal nerve in the intercostal space. Tenderness secondary to trauma may indicate a fractured rib.

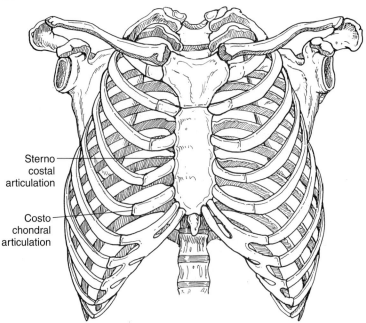

Sterno
costal
articulation

Costo
chondral
articulation

Figure 8.4.

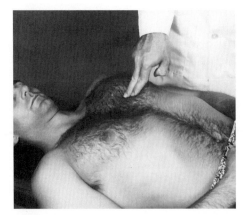

Figure 8.5.

POSTERIOR ASPECT

Scapula

DESCRIPTIVE ANATOMY:

At the posterior aspect of the thorax, the scapula articulates with the posterior aspect of the ribs. It also forms part of the glenoid fossa, which articulates with the head of the humerus. On the anterior aspect, the acromion articulates with the clavicle, forming the acromioclavicular joint. The scapula normally extends from T2 to T7 spinous process. It has three borders: medial, lateral, and superior (Fig. 8.6).

PROCEDURE:

Starting with the medial border, palpate all three borders, noting any tenderness (Figs. 8.7–8.9). Next, palpate the spine of the scapula, noting any tenderness or abnormality (Fig. 8.10). Finally, palpate the posterior surfaces above the spine of the scapula for the supraspinatus muscle (Fig. 8.11) and below the spine for the infraspinatus muscle (Fig. 8.12). Note any tenderness, atrophy, or spasm.

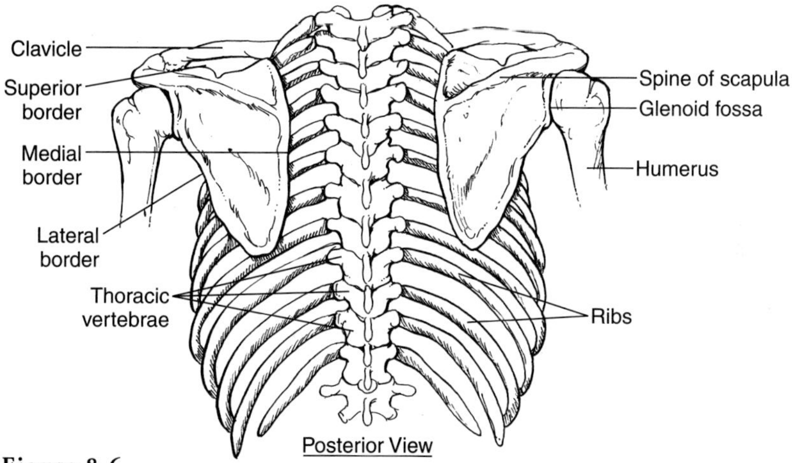

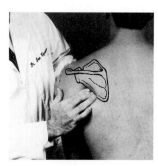

Clavicle

Superior border

Medial border

Lateral border

Thoracic vertebrae

Spine of scapula

Glenoid fossa

Humerus

Ribs

Posterior View

Figure 8.6.

8

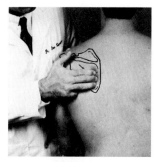

Figure 8.7.

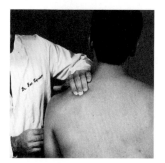

Figure 8.8.

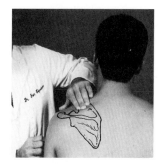

Figure 8.9.

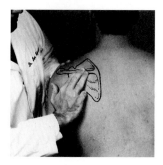

Figure 8.10.

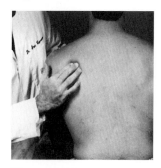

Figure 8.11.

Figure 8.12.

Para-Thoracic Musculature

DESCRIPTIVE ANATOMY:

The thoracic spinal muscles are arranged in three layers: superficial, intermediate, and deep. The superficial layers include the trapezius, latissimus dorsi, levator scapulae, and rhomboid muscles (Fig. 8.13). The intermediate layer contains the serratus posterior, superior, and inferior muscles (Fig. 8.14). The deep muscles of the back are the true back muscles that maintain posture and move the spinal column. These muscles are called are the erector spinae group and consist of the spinalis, longissimus, and iliocostalis (Fig. 8.14).

PROCEDURE:

The superficial layer is palpated by moving the fingers in a transverse fashion over the belly of the muscle, noting any abnormal tone of tenderness (Fig. 8.15). The deep layer is palpated with the fingertips directly adjacent to the spinous processes (Fig. 8.16), also noting any abnormal tone or tenderness. Any abnormal tone or tenderness may be indicative of an inflammatory process in the muscle, such as muscle strain, myofascitis, or fibromyalgia.

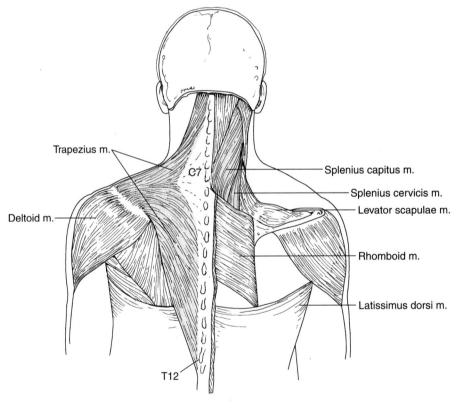

Figure 8.13.

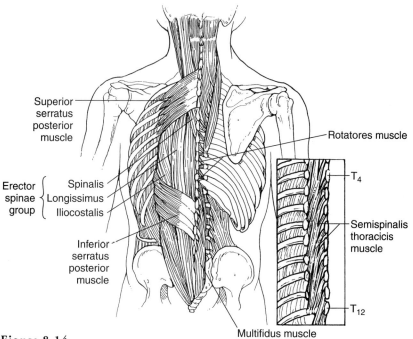

Superior serratus posterior muscle

Rotatores muscle

Erector spinae group { Spinalis, Longissimus, Iliocostalis

T_4

Semispinalis thoracicis muscle

Inferior serratus posterior muscle

T_{12}

Multifidus muscle

Figure 8.14.

8

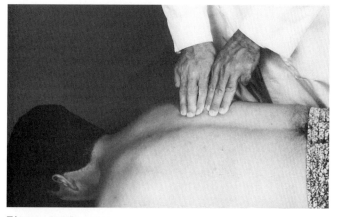

Figure 8.15.

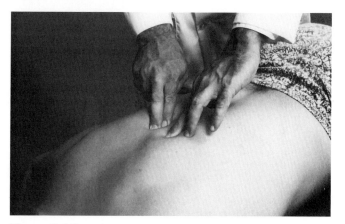

Figure 8.16.

Spinous Processes

DESCRIPTIVE ANATOMY:

The T1 to T12 vertebra have relatively prominent spinous processes that are easily palpable (Fig. 8.17). The tip of each spinous process is located below the transverse process of the same vertebra.

PROCEDURE:

With the patient seated and his thorax slightly flexed, palpate each spinous process with your index and or middle finger. Each spinous should be palpated individually, noting any pain, tenderness, and abnormal alignment (Fig. 8.18). Next, push each spinous process laterally, noting any rotational mobility (Fig. 8.19). Tenderness upon static spinous palpation may indicate subluxation of a thoracic vertebra. Tenderness secondary to flexion/ extension injuries may indicate supraspinous ligament strain, especially in the upper thoracic vertebra. Abnormal gross alignment may indicate scoliosis.

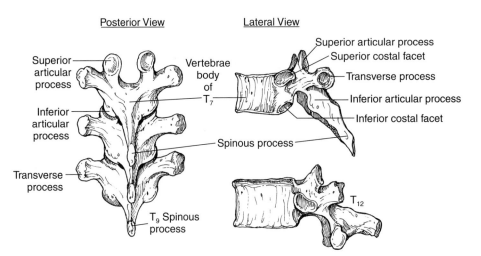

Figure 8.17.

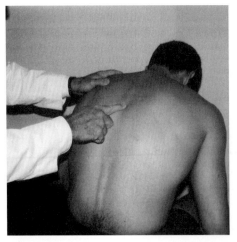

Figure 8.18.

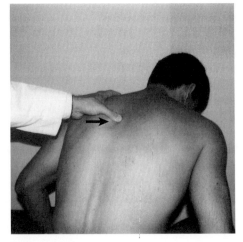

Figure 8.19.

Ribs and Intercostal Spaces

DESCRIPTIVE ANATOMY:

The ribs at the posterior aspect of the rib cage are attached to the vertebral body and transverse process by a capsule and a series of ligaments and muscles (Fig. 8.20). The ribs have an ability to slightly bend under stress but not fracture. Between the ribs in the intercostal spaces are three layers of intercostal muscles and an intercostal nerve. This nerve can become infected with the herpes zoster virus, which invades the spinal ganglia and produces sharp burning pain in the area supplied by the affected intercostal nerve.

PROCEDURE:

Palpate each individual rib from the lateral aspect of the spinal column laterally to the axilla. Then palpate into each intercostal space (Fig. 8.21). Tender or painful ribs secondary to trauma may indicate a fractured rib. Tender intercostal spaces may indicate an irritated intercostal nerve or a herpes zoster viral infection. Associated with this infection may be red vesicular eruptions along the course of the intercostal nerve in the intercostal space.

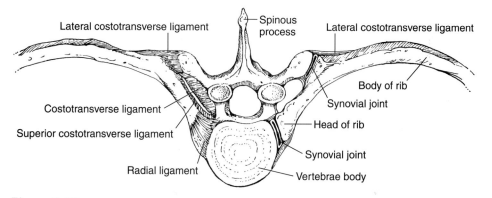

Figure 8.20.

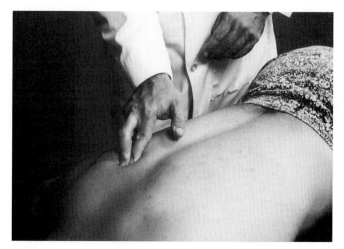

Figure 8.21.

THORACIC RANGE OF MOTION

Flexion (Inclinometer Method) (1)

With the patient in the seated position, place one inclinometer in the sagittal plane at the T1 level and the other inclinometer at the T12 level, also in the sagittal plane (Fig. 8.22). Zero out both inclinometers. Instruct the patient to place his hands on his hips and to flex forward his thoracic spine (Fig. 8.23). Record both inclinations and subtract the T12 from the T1 inclination to arrive at the thoracic flexion angle.

NORMAL RANGE:

50 degrees or greater from the neutral or 0 position.

Muscles Involved in Action	Nerve Supply
1. Rectus abdominous	T6–T12
2. External abdominal oblique	T7–T12
3. Internal abdominal oblique	T7–T12, L1

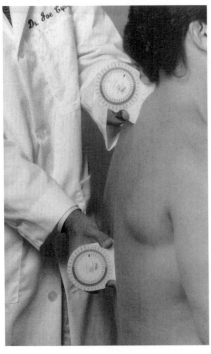

Figure 8.22.

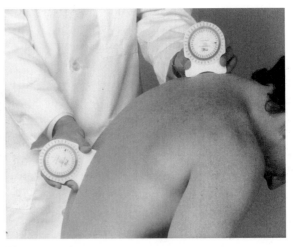

Figure 8.23.

Lateral Flexion (Inclinometer Method) (1)

With the patient standing, place one inclinometer flat against the T1 spinous process and the other flat against the L1 spinous process (Fig. 8.24). Zero out both inclinometers. Instruct the patient to laterally flex the thoracic spine to one side and then the other (Fig. 8.25) and record your finding. Subtract the T1 inclination angle from the T12 inclination angle to arrive at your thoracic lateral flexion angle.

NORMAL RANGE:

20 to 40 degrees from the neutral or 0 position.

Muscles Involved in Action	Nerve Supply
Lateral Flexion to the Same Side	
1. Iliocostalis thoracis	T1–T12
2. Longissimus thoracis	T1–T12
3. Intertransversarii	T1–T12
4. Internal abdominal oblique	T7–T12, L1
5. External abdominal oblique	T7–T12
6. Quadratus lumborum	T7–T12
Lateral Flexion to the Opposite Side	
1. Semispinalis thoracis	T1–T12
2. Multifidus	T1–T12
3. Rotatores	T1–T12
4. External abdominal oblique	T7–T12
5. Transversus abdominis	T7–T12, L1

8

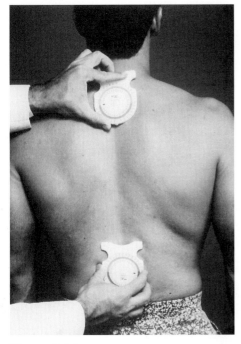

Figure 8.24.

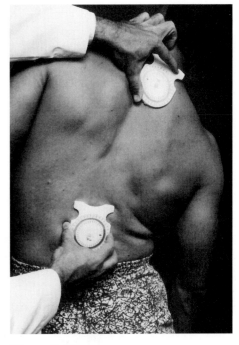

Figure 8.25.

Rotation (Inclinometer Method) (1)

With the patient in the seated position, instruct the patient to flex forward as horizontal as possible, bracing himself with his arms. Place one inclinometer at the T1 level and the other at the T12 level, both in the coronal plane (Fig. 8.26). Zero out both inclinometers. Instruct the patient to rotate his trunk to one side; record both T1 and T12 inclinations (Fig. 8.27). Subtract the T12 from the T1 inclination to arrive at the thoracic rotation angle. Perform this measurement with rotation to the opposite side.

NORMAL RANGE:

30 degrees or greater from the neutral or 0 position.

Muscles Involved in Action	Nerve Supply
Rotation to Same Side	
1. Iliocostalis thoracis	T1–T12
2. Longissimus thoracis	T1–T12
3. Intertransversarii	T1–T12
4. Internal abdominal oblique	T7–T12, L1
Rotation to Opposite Side	
1. Semispinalis thoracis	T1–T12
2. Multifidus	T1–T12
3. Rotatores	T1–T12
4. External abdominal oblique	T7–T12
5. Transversus abdominis	T7–T12, L1

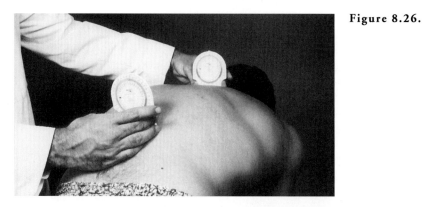

Figure 8.26.

Figure 8.27.

SCOLIOSIS SCREENING

Adam's Position

PROCEDURE:

With the patient standing, stand directly behind the patient and inspect and palpate the entire length of the spine, looking for scoliosis, kyphosis, or kyphoscoliosis (Figs. 8.28, 8.29). Next, instruct the patient to flex forward at the hips. Again, inspect and palpate for scoliosis, kyphosis, or kyphoscoliosis (Fig. 8.30).

RATIONALE:

If scoliosis, kyphosis, or kyphoscoliosis is present in the standing position and the angle reduces upon forward flexion, the scoliosis is a functional adaptation of the spine and surrounding soft tissue structures. It may be caused by poor posture, overdevelopment of unilateral spinal and/or upper extremity musculature, nerve root compromise, leg length deficiency, or hip contracture. This type of scoliosis is usually mild to moderate, measuring less than 25 degrees.

If scoliosis, kyphosis, or kyphoscoliosis is present in the standing position and the angle does not reduce upon forward flexion, then a structural deformity is suspect, such as hemivertebra, compression fracture of a vertebral body, or idiopathic scoliosis.

8

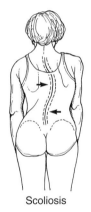 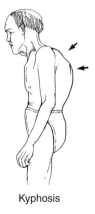

Scoliosis   Kyphosis

Figure 8.28.

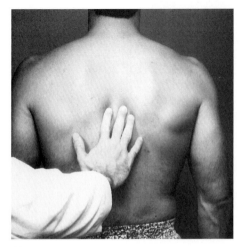

Figure 8.29.

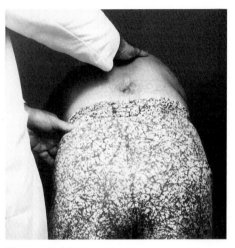

Figure 8.30.

McKenzie's Slide Glide Test (2)

PROCEDURE:

With the patient standing, stand to one side of the patient. With your shoulder, block the thoracic spine. With both hands, grasp the patient's pelvis and pull it toward you; hold this position for 10 to 15 seconds (Fig. 8.31). Repeat this test to the opposite side. If the patient has an evident scoliosis, the side towards which the scoliosis curves should be tested first.

RATIONALE:

This test is performed on patients with a symptomatic scoliosis. By blocking the shoulder and moving the pelvis you are stressing the area of the scoliosis. If the symptoms increase on the affected side, this indicates that the patient's scoliosis is contributing to the patient's symptoms.

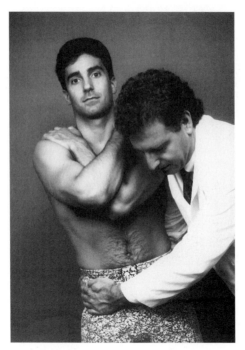

Figure 8.31.

THORACIC FRACTURES

Spinal Percussion Test (3,4)

PROCEDURE:

With the patient sitting and his head slightly flexed, percuss the spinous process (Fig. 8.32) and associated musculature (Fig. 8.33) of each of the thoracic vertebrae with a neurological reflex hammer.

RATIONALE:

Evidence of localized pain indicates a possible fractured vertebra or ligamentous sprain. Evidence of radicular pain indicates a possible disc defect.

NOTE:

Because of the nonspecificity of this test, other conditions will also elicit a positive pain response. A ligamentous sprain will cause a positive sign when percussing the spinous processes. Percussing the paraspinal musculature will elicit a positive sign for muscular strain.

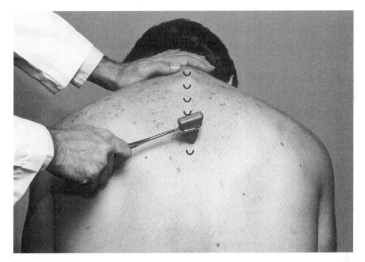

Figure 8.32.

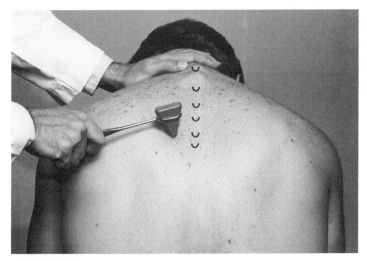

Figure 8.33.

Soto-Hall Test (5)

PROCEDURE:

With the patient in the supine position, assist him in flexing his chin to his chest (Fig. 8.34).

RATIONALE:

Evidence of localized pain indicates osseous, discal, or ligamentous pathology. This test is nonspecific. It merely isolates the cervical and thoracic spine in passive flexion. If this test is found positive, perform tests for strain/sprain, fractures, and space-occupying lesions.

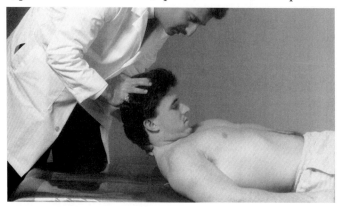

Figure 8.34.

Sternal Compression Test

PROCEDURE:

With the patient in the supine position, exert downward pressure on the sternum (Fig. 8.35).

RATIONALE:

When pressure to the sternum is applied, the lateral borders of the ribs are compressed. If a fracture is sustained at or near the lateral border of the ribs, the pressure you apply to the sternum will cause the fracture to become more pronounced, thus producing or exacerbating pain in the area of the fracture.

NOTE:

Caution must be taken if you suspect a fractured rib, especially if it is displaced. If trauma was induced and you suspect a fractured rib, the area should be radiographed before performing this test.

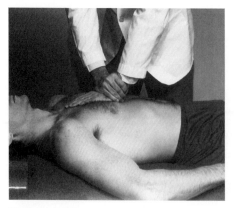

Figure 8.35.

NERVE ROOT LESIONS

Beevor's Sign (6)

PROCEDURE:

With the patient supine, instruct the patient to hook his fingers behind his neck and raise his head toward his feet. This test should mimic a sit-up (Fig. 8.36).

RATIONALE:

In the patient who has no thoracic root lesion, the umbilicus will not move when the patient performs the test because the abdominal muscles are equally innervated and of equal strength. If a root lesion is present, the umbilicus will move in the following manner: If the umbilicus moves in a superior direction, then a bilateral 10 to 12 thoracic nerve root lesion is suspect. If it moves superiorly and laterally, then a unilateral 10 to 12 thoracic nerve root lesion is suspect on the opposite side of the umbilical movement. If the umbilicus moves in an inferior direction, then a bilateral 7 to 10 thoracic nerve root lesion is suspect. If it moves inferiorly and laterally, then a unilateral 7 to 10 thoracic nerve root lesion is suspect on the opposite side of umbilical movement.

8

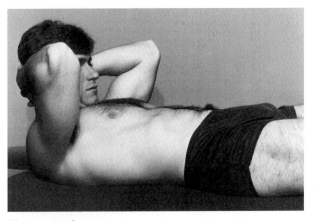

Figure 8.36.

Schepelmann's Sign

PROCEDURE:

With the patient in the seated position, instruct him to flex laterally at the waist to the left side and to the right side (Fig. 8.37).

RATIONALE:

Pain on the side of lateral bending is indicative of intercostal neuritis. Pain on the convex side is indicative of fibrous inflammation of the pleura or intercostal sprain.

When the patient laterally bends, the intercostal nerves on the side of bending are being compressed. If the intercostal nerves are irritated, pain on the side of bending will be elicited.

When the patient bends laterally, the pleura is stretched on the opposite side of bending. If the pleura is inflamed, then pain will be elicited opposite the side of bending. Pain may be also elicited because of injured or spasmed muscles.

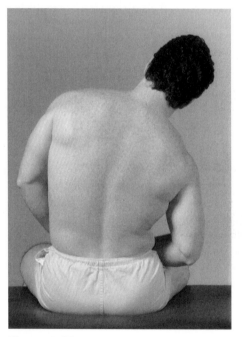

Figure 8.37.

COSTOVERTEBRAL JOINT ANKYLOSIS

Chest Expansion Test (7)

PROCEDURE:

With the patient in the seated position, place a tape measure around the patient's chest at the level of the nipple. Instruct the patient to exhale, and then record the measurement (Fig. 8.38). Next, instruct the patient to inhale maximally; record the measurement (Fig. 8.39).

RATIONALE:

The normal chest expansion for an adult male is 2 inches or more. The normal chest expansion for an adult female is 1 inch or more. A decrease in the normal chest expansion is indicative of an ankylosing condition, such as ankylosing spondylitis at the costotransverse or costovertebral articulations.

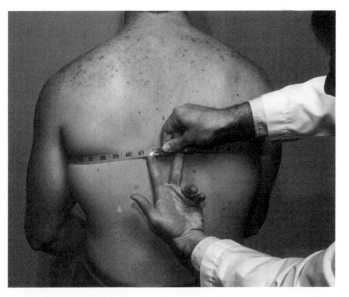

Figure 8.38.

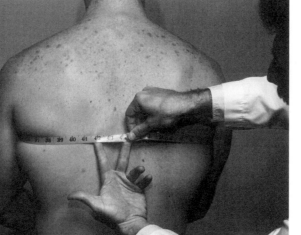

Figure 8.39.

References

1. American Medical Association. Guides to the evaluation of permanent impairment. 3rd ed. Chicago: American Medical Association, 1988.
2. McKenzie RA. The lumbar spine: mechanical diagnosis and therapy. Waikanae, New Zealand: Spinal Publications Ltd., 1981.
3. O'Donoghue D. Treatment of injuries to athletes. 4th ed. Philadelphia: WB Saunders, 1984.
4. Turek SL. Orthopaedics. 3rd ed. Philadelphia: JB Lippincott, 1977.
5. Soto-Hall R, Haldeman K. A useful diagnostic sign in vertebral injuries. Surg Gynecol Obstet: 827–831.
6. Rodnitzky RC. Van Allen's pictorial manual of neurological tests. 3rd ed. Chicago: Year Book Medical Publishers, 1988.
7. Moll JMH, Wright V. An objective clinical study of chest expansion. Ann Rheum Dis 1982;31:1–8.

General References

Boissonault WG. Examination in physical therapy practice. Screening for medical disease. New York: Churchill Livingstone, 1991.

Cyriax JH. Cyriax's illustrated manual of orthopaedic medicine. 2nd ed. London: Butterworth, 1993.

Goodman CC, Snyder TE. Differential diagnosis in physical therapy. Philadelphia: WB Saunders, 1990.

Kapandji IA. The physiology of joints. Vol. 3: the trunk and the vertebral column. New York: Churchill Livingstone, 1974.

Moore Kl. Clinically oriented anatomy. 3rd ed. Baltimore: Williams & Wilkins, 1992.

Post M. Physical examination of the musculoskeletal system. Chicago: Year Book Medical Publishers, 1987.

White AA. Kinematics of the normal spine as related to scoliosis. J Biomech Eng 1971;4:405.

9
LUMBAR ORTHOPAEDIC TESTS

9

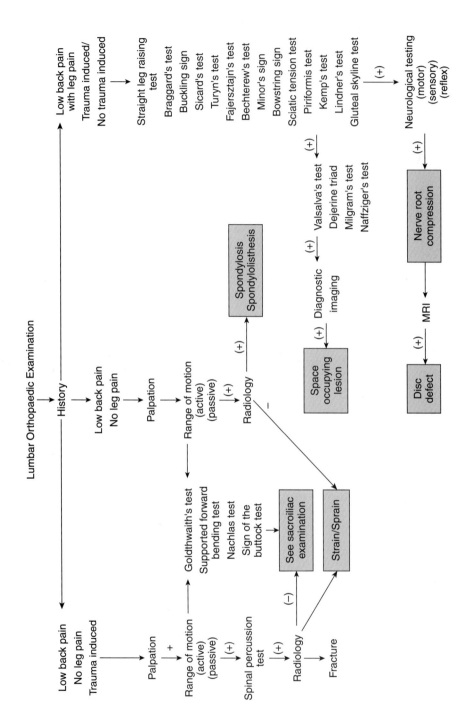

Lumbar Orthopaedic Examination

History

Low back pain with leg pain
Trauma induced/
No trauma induced

→ Straight leg raising test
Braggard's test
Buckling sign
Sicard's test
Turyn's test
Fajersztajn's test
Bechterew's test
Minor's sign
Bowstring sign
Sciatic tension test
Piriformis test
Kemp's test
Lindner's test
Gluteal skyline test

(+) Valsalva's test
Dejerine triad
Milgram's test
Naffziger's test

(+) Diagnostic imaging

(+) Space occupying lesion

(+) Neurological testing (motor) (sensory) (reflex)

(+) Nerve root compression

MRI

(+) Disc defect

Low back pain
No leg pain

Palpation

→ Range of motion (active) (passive)

(+) Radiology

(+) Spondylosis Spondylolisthesis

—

See sacroiliac examination

Strain/Sprain

Low back pain
No leg pain
Trauma induced

Palpation

+

Range of motion (active) (passive)

(+) Spinal percussion test

(+) Radiology

Fracture

Goldthwaith's test
Supported forward bending test
Nachlas test
Sign of the buttock test

(−) See sacroiliac examination

Strain/Sprain

PALPATION

Spinous Processes

DESCRIPTIVE ANATOMY:

The five lumbar spinous processes are large and easily palpable with the spinal column in the flexed position (Fig. 9.1). The fifth lumbar vertebra is the lowest movable segment. In 5% of the population, the fifth lumbar vertebra is congenitally fused to the sacrum: a condition called sacralization. In this condition, the patient will have only four palpable lumbar spinous processes. In other people, the first sacral segment may not be fused to the other segments. This condition is called lumbarization, and six spinous processes may be palpable in the lumbar spine. A common abnormality in the lumbar spinous processes is spina bifida, which is a congenital defect found in 10% of the population. Spina bifida results from a failure of each vertebral arch to grow enough to meet each other and undergo ossification. It is prevalent in the L5 or S1 segments. Another common abnormality in the L4-L5 or L5-S1 interval is spondylolisthesis. This is a fracture of the pars interarticularis that can cause forward slippage of one vertebra on another.

PROCEDURE:

With the patient in the seated position and flexed forward, palpate each spinous process with your index and forefinger (Fig. 9.2). First look for any irregularities, such as spondylolisthesis, spina bifida, lumbarization, or sacralization. Next, place anterior pressure on each process with your thumb (Fig. 9.3). When placing anterior pressure on the spinous processes, note any rigidity or springing. Rigidity may indicate hypomobility and springing may indicate hypermobility.

Figure 9.1

9

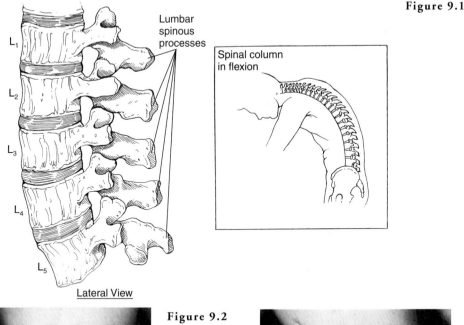

Lumbar spinous processes

Spinal column in flexion

L_1
L_2
L_3
L_4
L_5

Lateral View

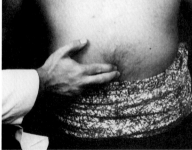

Figure 9.2

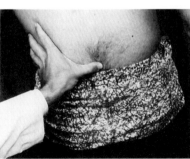

Figure 9.3

Intrinsic Spinal Muscles

DESCRIPTIVE ANATOMY:

The intrinsic spinal muscles in the lumbar spine are the erector spinae group (spinalis, longissimus, and iliocostalis). In the lower spine, these muscles come together to form the sacrospinalis group of muscles (Fig. 9.4).

PROCEDURE:

With the patient in the prone position, palpate the lumbar portions of the erector spine group in a diagonal fashion from medial to lateral (Fig. 9.5). Note any tenderness, inflammation, muscle spasm, or palpable bands. Any of the foregoing findings may indicate muscle strain, myofascitis, fibromyalgia, or active trigger points.

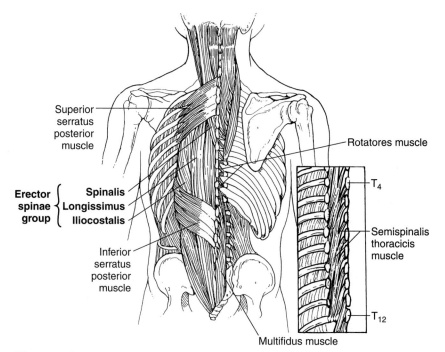

Figure 9.4

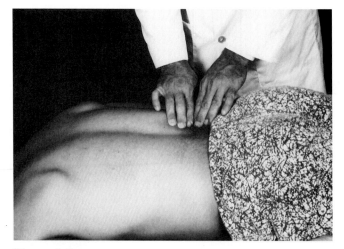

Figure 9.5

Quadratus Lumborum

DESCRIPTIVE ANATOMY:

The quadratus lumborum is located lateral to the thoracolumbar fascia. It is attached to the transverse processes of the lumbar vertebra, the iliac crest and the twelfth rib (Fig. 9.6). It is a common site for myofascial lower back pain.

PROCEDURE:

With the patient in the prone position, palpate the quadratus lumborum from the twelfth rib to the iliac crest (Fig. 9.7). This muscle is located lateral to the erector spinae group. Note any tenderness, inflammation, muscle spasm, or palpable bands. Any of the foregoing findings may indicate a muscle strain, myofascitis, fibromyalgia, or active trigger points.

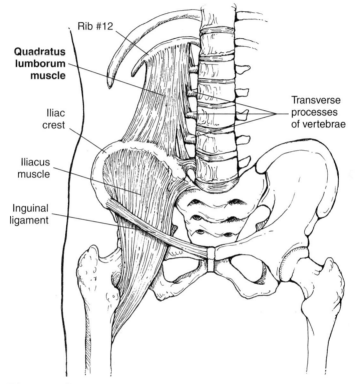

Figure 9.6

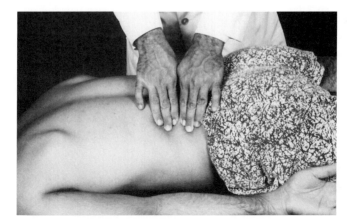

Figure 9.7

197

Gluteal Muscles

DESCRIPTIVE ANATOMY:

The gluteal group of muscles are composed of the gluteus maximus, medius, and minimus. These muscles extend, abduct, and rotate the thigh. They all originate from the ilium and insert into the femur (Fig. 9.8). They can be tender and spastic secondary to trauma. Pain can be referred to the gluteal muscles from a defect in an intervertebral disc, and they can lose muscle tone because of nerve-root involvement. Active myofascial trigger points could be present in the gluteal muscles, which could refer pain into the posterior thigh similar to a sciatic pain pattern from a L5-S1 disc defect with nerve root compression.

PROCEDURE:

With the patient in the prone position, palpate using strong pressure, starting just lateral to the sacrum and moving toward the greater trochanter of the femur (Fig. 9.9). Note any tenderness, spasm, loss of muscle tone, and tender trigger points. Tenderness and spasm secondary to trauma may indicate a muscle strain. A herniated intervertebral disc with nerve root compression may also cause tenderness and spasm to the area. An active myofascial trigger point may cause local tenderness with a referred component to the posterior thigh.

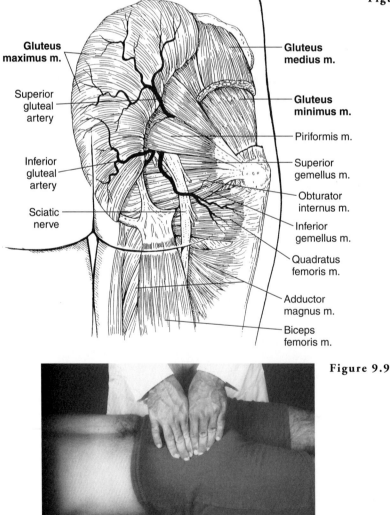

Figure 9.8

Gluteus maximus m.

Gluteus medius m.

Superior gluteal artery

Gluteus minimus m.

Piriformis m.

Inferior gluteal artery

Superior gemellus m.

Obturator internus m.

Sciatic nerve

Inferior gemellus m.

Quadratus femoris m.

Adductor magnus m.

Biceps femoris m.

Figure 9.9

198

Piriformis Muscle

DESCRIPTIVE ANATOMY:

The piriformis muscle is clinically significant because of its proximity to the sciatic nerve (see Fig. 9.8). It may become inflamed and spastic and compress the sciatic nerve, causing pain along the entire course of the nerve. It originates from the sacrum and inserts into the greater trochanter of the femur.

PROCEDURE:

To locate the piriformis, bisect the tip of the coccyx and the posterior superior iliac spine (Fig. 9.10). This will be the inferior border of the piriformis. Palpate the muscle, noting any tenderness or spasm (Fig. 9.11). If the patient presents with lower extremity radicular pain, note if palpation of the piriformis increases that pain. Tenderness and spasm in the piriformis may indicate muscle strain caused by overuse. Because of the proximity of the sciatic nerve to this muscle, a radicular component to the posterior thigh may also be involved. A local tender area may indicate an active myofascial trigger point, which may also cause a radicular pain to the posterior thigh.

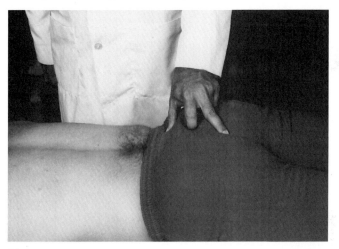

Figure 9.10

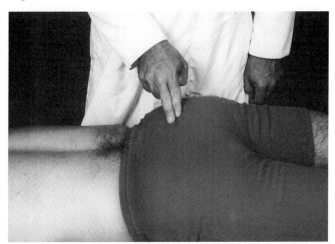

Figure 9.11

Sciatic Nerve

DESCRIPTIVE ANATOMY:

The sciatic nerve is composed of the nerve roots from L4, L5, S1, S2, and S3. The nerve runs through the greater sciatic foramen of the pelvis through the gluteal muscles and below the piriformis (see Fig. 9.9). Once it passes the piriformis, it runs deep to the gluteus maximus midway between the greater trochanter and the ischial tuberosity. In some cases, the sciatic nerve pierces the piriformis muscle rather than passing below it.

PROCEDURE:

Starting midway between the greater trochanter and the ischial tuberosity, palpate the sciatic nerve and follow the nerve as far down the lower extremity as possible (Fig. 9.12). Note any tenderness, burning, or inflammation. If the patient experiences any tenderness, burning, or referred pain into the extremity, then an irritation of the sciatic nerve is suspect.

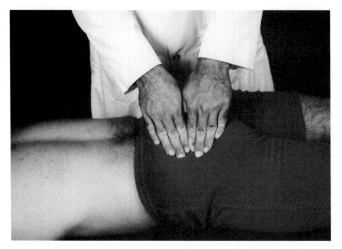

Figure 9.12

LUMBAR RANGE OF MOTION

Flexion (Inclinometer Method) (1)

With the patient standing and the lumbar spine in the neutral position, place one inclinometer over the T12 spinous process in the sagittal plane. Place the second inclinometer at the level of the sacrum, also in the sagittal plane (Fig. 9.13). Zero out both inclinometers. Instruct the patient to flex the trunk forward and record the inclinations of both inclinometers (Fig. 9.14). Subtract the sacral inclination from the T12 inclination to obtain the lumbar flexion angle.

NORMAL RANGE (2):

Male 15–30 years old	66 degrees	Female 15–30 years old	67 degrees
Male 31–60 years old	58 degrees	Female 31–60 years old	60 degrees
Male >61 years old	49 degrees	Female >61 years old	44 degrees

Muscles Involved in Action	Nerve Supply
1. Psoas major	L1–L3
2. Rectus abdominis	T6–T12
3. External abdominal oblique	T7–T12
4. Internal abdominal oblique	T7–T12, L1
5. Transversus abdominis	T7–T12, L1

9

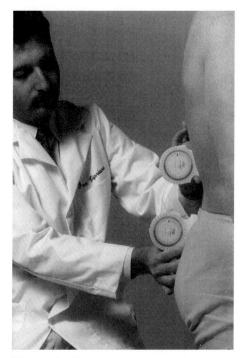

Figure 9.13

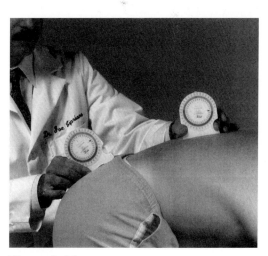

Figure 9.14

Extension (Inclinometer Method) (1)

With the patient standing and the lumbar spine in the neutral position, place one inclinometer slightly lateral to the T12 spinous process in the sagittal plane. Place the second inclinometer at the sacrum, also in the sagittal plane (Fig. 9.15). Zero out both inclinometers. Instruct the patient to extend his trunk backwards and record the inclination of both inclinometers (Fig. 9.16). Subtract the sacral inclination from the T12 inclination to obtain the lumbar extension angle.

NORMAL RANGE (2):

Male 15–30 years old	38 degrees	Female 15–30 years old	42 degrees
Male 31–60 years old	35 degrees	Female 31–60 years old	40 degrees
Male >61 years old	33 degrees	Female >61 years old	36 degrees

Muscles Involved in Action	Nerve Supply
1. Latissimus dorsi	C6–C8
2. Erector spinae	L1–L3
3. Transversospinalis	L1–L5
4. Interspinalis	L1–L5
5. Quadratus lumborum	T12, L1–L4

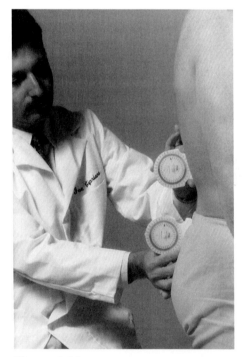

Figure 9.15

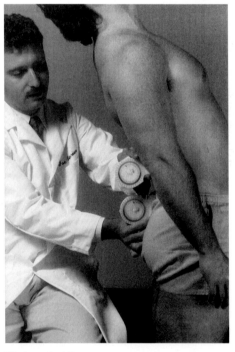

Figure 9.16

Lateral Flexion (Inclinometer Method) (1)

With the patient standing and the lumbar spine in the neutral position, place one inclinometer flat at the T12 spinous process in the coronal plane. Place the second inclinometer at the superior aspect of the sacrum, also in the coronal plane (Fig. 9.17). Zero out both inclinometers. Instruct the patient to flex the trunk to one side, then record the inclination of both inclinometers (Fig. 9.18). Subtract the sacral inclination from the T12 inclination to obtain the lumbar lateral flexion angle. Perform measurements for both right and left lateral flexion.

NORMAL RANGE (3,4):

Male 20–29 years old	38 degrees ± 5.8	Female 15–30 years old	35 degrees ± 6.4
Male 31–60 years old	29 degrees ± 6.5	Female 31–60 years old	30 degrees ± 5.8
Male >61 years old	19 degrees ± 4.8	Female >61 years old	23 degrees ± 5.4

Muscles Involved in Action	Nerve Supply
1. Latissimus dorsi	C6–C8
2. Erector spinae	L1–L3
3. Transversospinalis	L1–L5
4. Intertransversarii	L1–L5
5. Quadratus lumborum	T12, L1–L4
6. Psoas major	L1–L3
7. External abdominal oblique	T7–T12

9

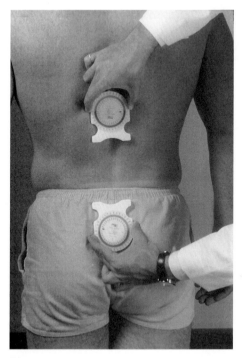

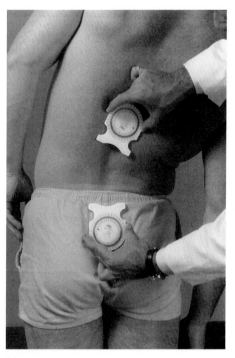

Figure 9.17   **Figure 9.18**

JOINT DYSFUNCTION TESTS

Pheasant Test (5)

PROCEDURE:

With the patient in the prone position, place downward pressure to the lumbar spine (Fig. 9.19). With your other hand, grasp the patient's ankles and passively flex the knees until the heels touch the buttocks (Fig. 9.20).

RATIONALE:

This test is an attempt to hyperextend the spine. If the patient has an unstable lower spinal segment, pain will be elicited in the lower back when the knees are flexed.

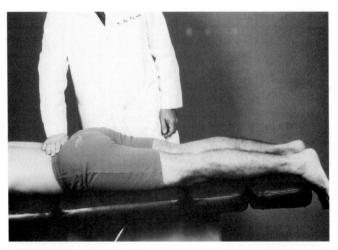

Figure 9.19

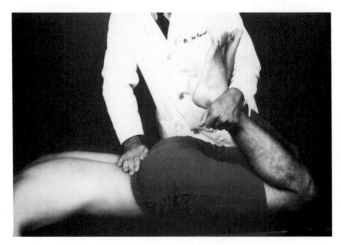

Figure 9.20

Segmental Instability Test (6)

PROCEDURE:

Place the patient in the prone position with the legs over the examination table and the feet resting on the floor. Then apply downward pressure to the lumbar spine (Fig. 9.21). Next, instruct the patient to lift his legs off the floor, and again place downward pressure on the lumbar spine (Fig. 9.22).

RATIONALE:

When the patient lifts his legs off the floor, the lumbar para-vertebral muscle tightens, causing muscle guarding in the lumbar spine. A positive test is when pain is elicited when pressure is applied to the lumbar spine with the feet on the floor, and the pain disappears when the feet are off the floor and the para-vertebral muscle is tightened. By raising the feet off the floor, the mechanical muscle guarding protects the underlying lumbar instability, such as a spondylolisthesis.

Figure 9.21

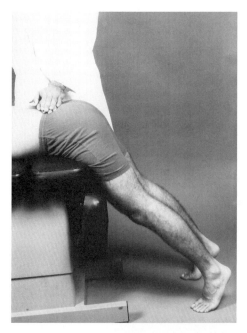

9

Figure 9.22

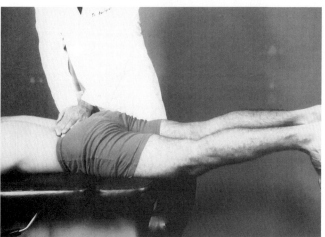

LUMBAR FRACTURES

Spinal Percussion Test (7,8)

PROCEDURE:

With the patient in the sitting position and slightly bent forward, percuss the spinous process (Fig. 9.23) and associated musculature (Fig. 9.24) of each of the lumbar vertebrae with a neurological reflex hammer.

RATIONALE:

Evidence of localized pain indicates a possible fractured vertebra. Evidence of radicular pain indicates a possible disc defect.

NOTE:

Because of the nonspecificity of this test, other conditions will also elicit a positive pain response. A ligamentous sprain will cause a positive sign when percussing the spinous processes. Percussing the paraspinal musculature will elicit a positive sign for muscular strain.

Figure 9.23

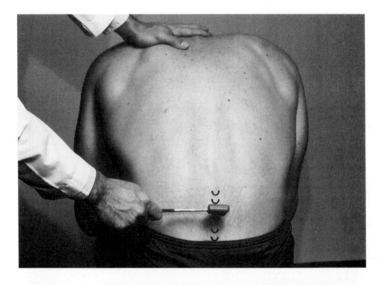

Figure 9.24

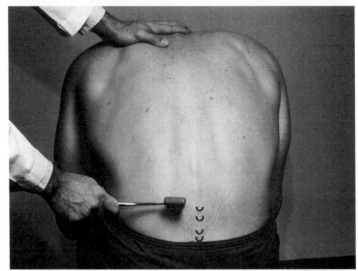

LUMBAR NERVE ROOT AND SCIATIC NERVE IRRITATION/COMPRESSION TESTS

Straight Leg Raising Test (9,10,11,12)

PROCEDURE:

With the patient in the supine position, place an inclinometer at the tibial tuberosity and raise the patient's leg to the point of pain or 90 degrees, whichever comes first (Fig. 9.25).

RATIONALE:

This test primarily stretches the sciatic nerve and spinal nerve roots at the L5, S1, and S2 levels. Between 70 and 90 degrees of hip flexion, these nerve roots are fully stretched. If pain is elicited or is exacerbated after 70 degrees of hip flexion, then lumbar joint pain is suspect. At 35 to 70 degrees of hip flexion, the sciatic nerve roots tense over the intervertebral disc. If radicular pain begins or exacerbates at this level, then sciatic nerve root irritation by intervertebral disc pathology or an intradural lesion is suspect. At 0 to 35 degrees of hip flexion, there is no dural movement, and the sciatic nerve is relatively slack. If pain begins or exacerbates at this level, then extradural sciatic involvement is suspect, i.e., spastic piriformis muscle or sacroiliac joint lesions (Fig. 9.26). If dull posterior thigh pain is elicited, then tight hamstring muscles should be suspect.

If intervertebral disc pathology is suspect, continue with Braggard's and Lasègue's tests and see Chapter 10 to evaluate the suspected neurological level.

Figure 9.25

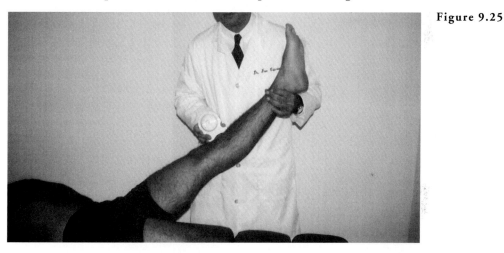

Figure 9.26

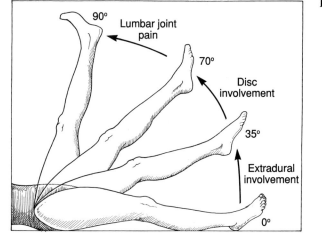

Lasègue's Test (13,14)

PROCEDURE:

With the patient in the supine position, flex the patient's hip with the leg flexed (Fig. 9.27). Keeping the hip flexed, extend the leg (Fig. 9.28).

RATIONALE:

This test is positive for sciatic radiculopathy when: (a) no pain is elicited when the hip is flexed and the leg is flexed; or (b) pain is present when the hip is flexed and the leg is extended.

When both the hip and the leg are flexed, there is no tension on the sciatic nerve. When the hip is flexed and the leg is extended, the sciatic nerve is stretched and, if irritated, will cause pain or will exacerbate existing pain in the leg.

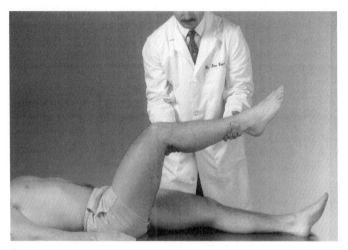

Figure 9.27

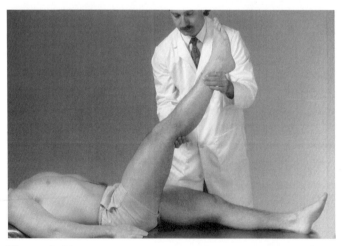

Figure 9.28

Buckling Sign

PROCEDURE:

With the patient in the supine position, perform a straight leg raising test (Fig. 9.29).

RATIONALE:

This test exerts a traction pressure on the sciatic nerve. The patient with severe sciatic radiculopathy will flex the leg at the knee to reduce the traction (Fig. 9.30).

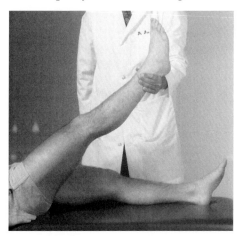 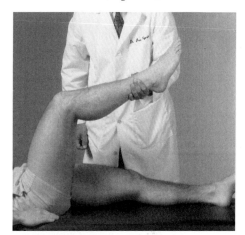

Figure 9.29	Figure 9.30

Femoral Nerve Traction Test (15)

PROCEDURE:

With the patient laying on his side with the affected side up, instruct the patient to slightly flex his unaffected extremity at the hip and knee. Then grasp the affected leg and extend the hip 15 degrees with the knee extended (Fig. 9.31). Next, flex the knee to further stretch the femoral nerve (Fig. 9.32).

RATIONALE:

Extension of the hip and flexion of the knee places a traction pressure on the femoral nerve and nerve roots of L2 to L4. Pain that radiates to the anterior medial thigh indicates an L3 nerve root problem. Pain extending to the mid-tibia is indicative of a L4 nerve root problem. This test may also cause contralateral pain, indicating a nerve root compression/irritation on the opposite side.

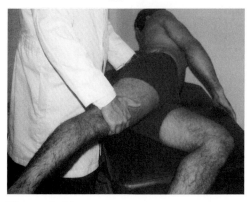 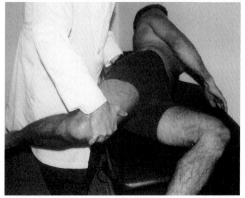

Figure 9.31	Figure 9.32

Braggard's Test (10)

PROCEDURE:

With the patient in the supine position, raise his leg to the point of leg pain. Lower the leg 5 degrees and dorsiflex the foot (Fig. 9.33).

RATIONALE:

The raising of the leg and dorsiflexion of the foot places a traction pressure on the sciatic nerve. If the dorsiflexion produces pain in the 0 to 35 degree range, then extradural sciatic nerve irritation is suspect. If pain occurs with dorsiflexion of the foot at 35 to 70 degrees, then irritation of the sciatic nerve roots from a intradural problem is suspect, usually from an intervertebral disc lesion (see Straight Leg Raising Test). Dull posterior thigh pain is indicative of tight hamstring muscles. If intervertebral disc pathology is suspect, see Chapter 10 to evaluate which neurological level is affected.

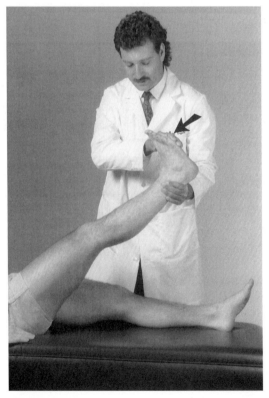

Figure 9.33

Sicard's Test

PROCEDURE:

With the patient in the supine position, raise his leg to the point of pain. Lower the leg 5 degrees and dorsiflex the big toe (Fig. 9.34).

RATIONALE:

The raising of the leg and dorsiflexion of the big toe places a traction pressure on the sciatic nerve. If the dorsiflexion produces pain in the 0 to 35 degree range, then extradural sciatic nerve irritation is suspect. If pain occurs with dorsiflexion of the foot at 35 to 70 degrees, then irritation of the sciatic nerve roots from an intradural problem is suspect, usually from an intervertebral disc lesion (see straight leg raising test). Dull posterior thigh pain is indicative of tight hamstring muscles. If intervertebral disc pathology is suspect, see chapter 10 to evaluate which neurological level is affected.

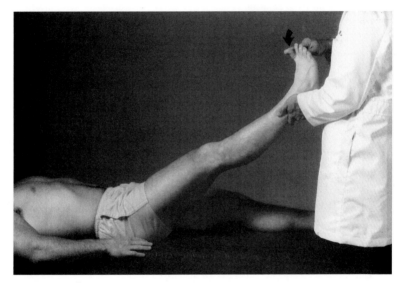

Figure 9.34

9

Turyn's Test

PROCEDURE:

With the patient in the supine position, dorsiflex the patient's big toe (Fig. 9.35).

RATIONALE:

Dorsiflexion of the big toe stretches the sciatic nerve. Pain in the gluteal region and/or radiating pain indicates sciatic nerve root irritation, either intradurally or extradurally.

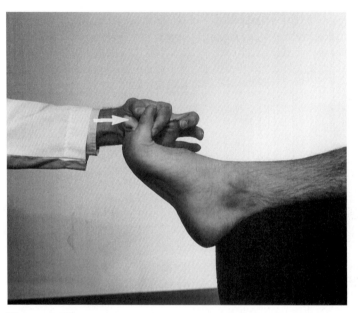

Figure 9.35

Fajersztajn's Test (16,17)

PROCEDURE:

With the patient supine, raise the unaffected leg to 75 degrees or to the point of leg pain, and dorsiflex the foot (Fig. 9.36).

RATIONALE:

This test causes ipsilateral and contralateral stretching of the nerve roots (Fig. 9.37), pulling laterally on the dural sac. A positive sign is elicited if an increase in leg pain or pain is reproduced on the affected leg side. This pain is indicative of a disc protrusion usually medial to the nerve root.

When the well leg is raised, the nerve root on that side is stretched, causing the nerve root on the opposite side to slide down and toward the midline (Fig. 9.38). If a medial disc protrusion is present, this movement will increase tension on the nerve root opposite the side of hip flexion, thus increasing the patient's pain on the affected leg side. If pain decreases on the affected leg side when the well leg is raised, then a lateral disc protrusion is suspect because the nerve root is being pulled away from the disc (Fig. 9.39).

If this test is positive, see Chapter 10 to evaluate the neurological level affected.

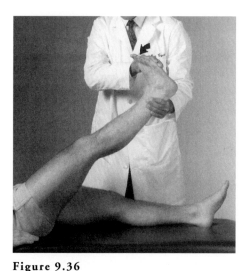

Figure 9.36

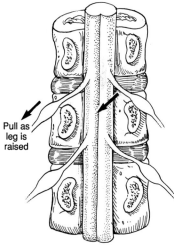

Pull as leg is raised

Figure 9.37

9

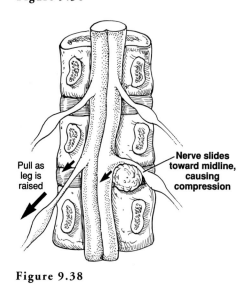

Pull as leg is raised

Nerve slides toward midline, causing compression

Figure 9.38

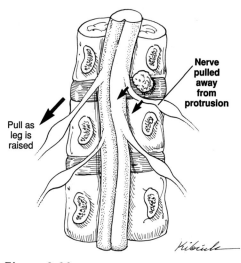

Nerve pulled away from protrusion

Pull as leg is raised

Figure 9.39

Bechterew's Test

PROCEDURE:

Place the patient in the seated position with the legs hanging over the examination table. Instruct the patient to extend one knee at a time alternately (Fig. 9.40).

If a positive response is not elicited, instruct the patient to raise both legs together (Fig. 9.41).

RATIONALE:

With the patient seated and the leg flexed, the sciatic nerve is relatively slack. When the leg is extended, a traction pressure is placed on the sciatic nerve. If the patient is unable to perform this test because of radicular pain or if the patient performs the test but leans back, then compression to the sciatic nerve or lumbar nerve roots, either intradurally or extradurally, is indicated. This test is usually positive in disc protrusion cases.

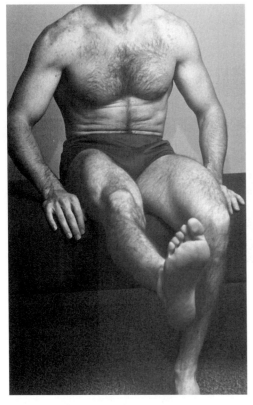

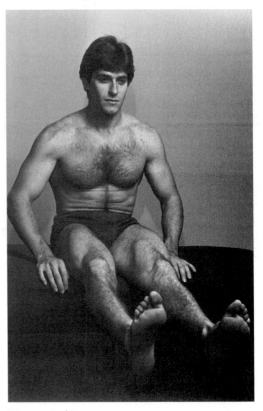

Figure 9.40   **Figure 9.41**

Minor's Sign

PROCEDURE:

With the patient in the seated position, instruct the patient to stand (Fig. 9.42).

RATIONALE:

The patient with sciatic radiculopathy will support himself on the healthy side and keep the affected leg flexed. By flexing the affected leg, the patient decreases the tension on the sciatic nerve, thus relieving pain. The patient in Figure 9.42 is demonstrating sciatic radiculopathy down the left lower extremity.

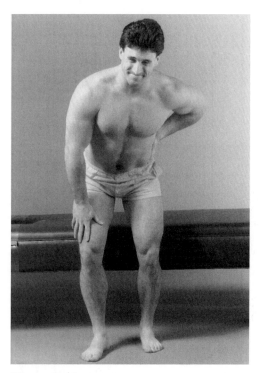

Figure 9.42

9

Bowstring Sign (18)

PROCEDURE:

With the patient in the supine position, place the patient's leg atop your shoulder. At this point, firm pressure should be exerted on the hamstring muscles (Fig. 9.43). If pain is not elicited, apply pressure to the popliteal fossa (Fig. 9.44).

RATIONALE:

Pain in the lumbar region or radiculopathy is a positive sign for sciatic nerve compression, either intradurally or extradurally. By applying pressure to the hamstring muscles or popliteal fossa, tension on the sciatic nerve is increased, thus eliciting or exacerbating the patient's pain.

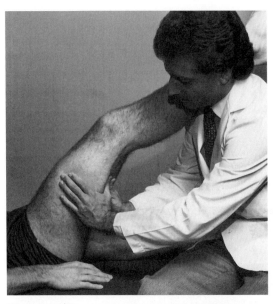

Figure 9.43

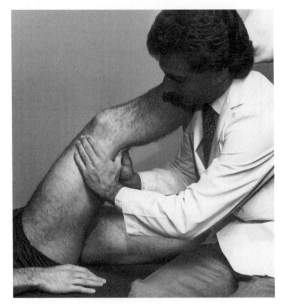

Figure 9.44

Sciatic Tension Test (19)

PROCEDURE:

With the patient in the seated position, passively extend the affected limb to the point of pain (Fig. 9.45). Lower the limb below the point of pain and grasp the leg between your knees. With both your hands, place posterior to anterior pressure in the popliteal space (Fig. 9.46).

RATIONALE:

The action of flexing the leg places a traction pressure of the sciatic nerve. By lowering the leg, the traction is reduced; if the sciatic nerve is irritated, the pain will reduce. By placing an additional pressure in the popliteal space with your fingers, the traction pressure of the sciatic nerve is increased, causing radicular pain if the sciatic nerve is irritated. An increase in pain is indicative of an irritation to the sciatic nerve, either intradurally or extradurally.

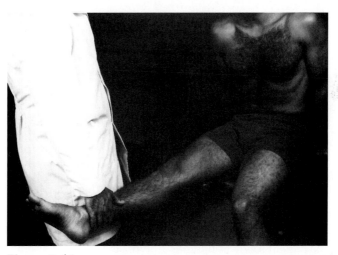

Figure 9.45

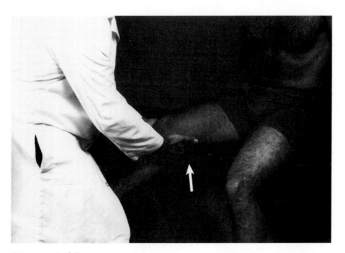

Figure 9.46

Piriformis Test (20)

PROCEDURE:

Instruct the patient to lay on his or her side close to the edge of the examination table. Have the patient flex the hip and knee to 90 degrees. Place your hand on the patient's pelvis for stabilization, and with your opposite hand place downward pressure on the patient's knee (Fig. 9.47).

RATIONALE:

This test stresses the external rotators and piriformis muscle. If the sciatic nerve passes through the piriformis or if the piriformis is in spasm, either situation may be impinging the sciatic nerve and may reproduce the pain in the buttock or radicular pain into the extremity.

Figure 9.47

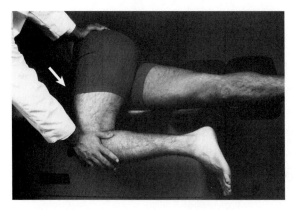

Gluteal Skyline Test (21)

PROCEDURE:

Instruct the patient to lay on the examination table in the prone position, the head straight and the arms by the patient's side or hanging down. Stand at the patient's feet and observe the height of the buttock. Instruct the patient to contract each gluteal muscle (Fig. 9.48).

RATIONALE:

The L5, S1, S2, and inferior gluteal nerve innervate the gluteal muscles. If the affected gluteal muscle is flat and shows less contraction than the nonaffected side, then damage to the L5, S1, S2, and inferior gluteal nerve is suspect.

Figure 9.48

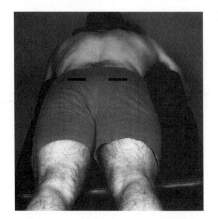

Kemp's Test

PROCEDURE:

With the patient either sitting or standing, stabilize the posterior superior iliac spine with one hand. With your other hand, reach around the front of the patient and grasp his shoulder. Passively bend the dorsolumbar spine obliquely backward (Fig. 9.49).

RATIONALE:

When the patient bends obliquely backward, the dural sac on the side of bending moves laterally. If a lateral disc lesion is present, this movement will increase the nerve root tension over that disc lesion, producing pain in the lower back—usually with a radicular component on the same side of oblique bending (Fig. 9.50). On the opposite side of oblique bending, the dural sac moves medially. If a medial disc lesion is present, this movement will increase the tension over that disc lesion, producing pain in the lower back—usually with a radicular component on the opposite side of oblique bending (Fig. 9.51). If the test is positive, see Chapter 10 to evaluate the affected neurological level. If the patient presents with localized lower back pain with no radicular component, then lumbar muscle spasm or facet capsulitis may be suspect.

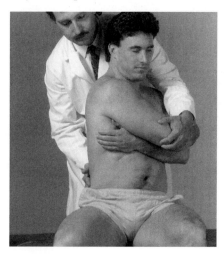

Figure 9.49

9

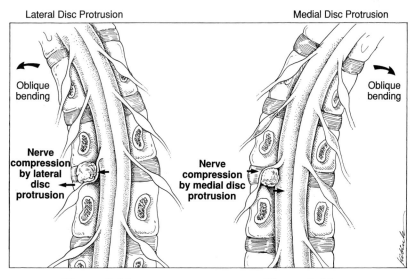

Figure 9.50   **Figure 9.51**

Lindner's Sign

PROCEDURE:

With the patient in the supine position, passively flex the patient's head (Fig. 9.52).

RATIONALE:

Passive flexion of the patient's head stretches the dural sac. Reproduction of the patient's pain indicates a disc lesion at the level of pain. Sharp, diffuse pain or involuntary hip flexion may be indicative of meningeal irritation (see Brudzinski's test). If disc pathology is suspect, see Chapter 10 to evaluate the affected level.

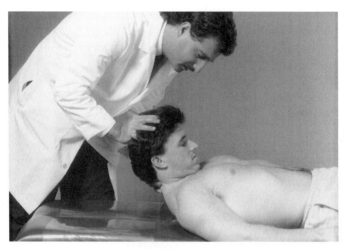

Figure 9.52

SPACE-OCCUPYING LESIONS

Valsalva's Maneuver (22)

PROCEDURE:

With the patient in the seated position, instruct him to bear down as if straining at stool but concentrating the bulk of the stress at the lumbar region (Fig. 9.53). Ask the patient if he feels any increased pain; if so, ask him to point to its location. This test is very subjective and requires an accurate response from the patient.

RATIONALE:

This test increases intrathecal pressure. Localized pain secondary to the increased pressure may indicate a space-occupying lesion (e.g., disk defect, mass, osteophyte) in the lumbar canal or foramen.

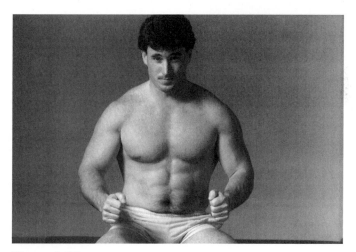

Figure 9.53

Dejerine's Triad

PROCEDURE:

With the patient seated, instruct him to cough, sneeze, and bear down as if straining at stool (Valsalva's maneuver).

RATIONALE:

Pain localized in the lumbar region after any of the previous actions is indicative of increased intrathecal pressure, most likely induced by a space-occupying lesion (e.g., disc defect, mass, osteophyte).

NOTE:

If the patient is unable to sneeze, give the patient a dash of pepper to inhale (Lewin Snuff Test).

Milgram's Test (23)

PROCEDURE:

With the patient in the supine position, instruct him to raise his legs until they are 2 or 3 inches above the table (Fig. 9.54).

RATIONALE:

The patient should be able to perform this test for at least 30 seconds without low back pain. If pain is present, a space-occupying lesion inside or out of the spinal canal is suspected. A positive test is usually present in disc protrusion cases.

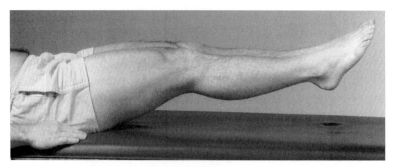

Figure 9.54

Naffziger's Test (24)

PROCEDURE:

With the patient in the seated position, compress the jugular veins. The veins are located approximately 1 inch lateral to the tracheal cartilage (Fig. 9.55). Hold the compression for 1 minute.

RATIONALE:

By compressing the jugular veins, an increase in the intrathecal pressure is induced. Localized pain in the lumbar region indicates a space-occupying lesion, usually a disc protrusion or prolapse. Radicular pain may indicate nerve root involvement.

The theca is the covering of the spinal cord, which consists of the pia mater, arachnoid mater, and dura mater.

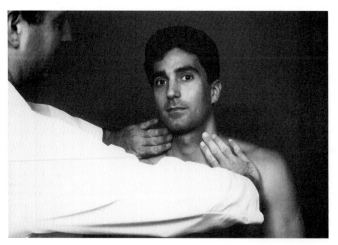

Figure 9.55

DIFFERENTIAL DIAGNOSIS: LUMBAR INVOLVEMENT VERSUS SACROILIAC INVOLVEMENT

Goldthwaith's Test

PROCEDURE:

With the patient in the supine position, place one hand under the lumbar spine with each finger under an interspinous space. With the other hand, perform a straight leg raising test. Note whether pain is elicited before, during, or after the spinous processes fan out (Fig. 9.56).

RATIONALE:

Radicular pain before fanning out of the lumbar vertebrae indicates an extradural lesion, such as a sacroiliac joint disorder (0 to 35 degrees). Radicular pain during lumbar fanning indicates an intradural lesion, such as an intrathecal space occupying lesion (e.g., disc defect osteophyte, mass) (35 to 70 degrees). Localized pain after lumbar fanning indicates a posterior lumbar joint disorder (after 70 degrees) (see Straight Leg Raising Test).

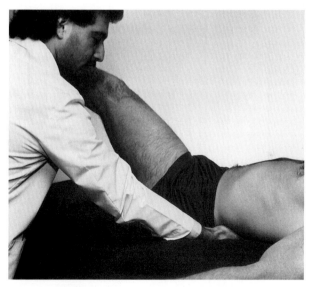

Figure 9.56

9

Supported Forward Bending Test

PROCEDURE:

With the patient in the standing position, instruct the patient to bend forward, keeping the knees straight (Fig. 9.57). Repeat the test, but support the ilia with your hands while bracing the patient's sacrum with your hip (Fig. 9.58).

RATIONALE:

By stabilizing the ilia, the sacroiliac joints are immobilized; thus, when bending is performed, a lumbar lesion will elicit pain in both instances because the lumbar vertebrae are not immobilized either time. If a sacroiliac joint lesion is present, pain will be elicited only when the ilia are not immobilized.

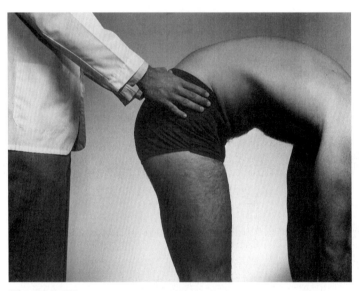

Figure 9.57

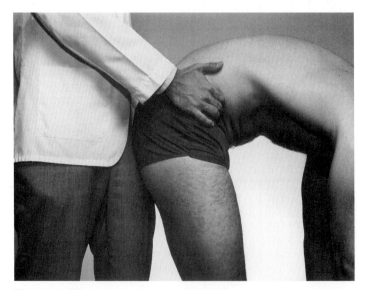

Figure 9.58

Nachlas Test (25)

PROCEDURE:

With the patient in the prone position, approximate the patient's heel to his buttock on the same side (Fig. 9.59).

RATIONALE:

Flexing the leg to the buttock stretches the quadriceps muscles and the femoral nerve, which is the largest branch of the lumbar plexus (L2,L3,L4). Radicular pain into the anterior thigh may indicate a compression or irritation of the L2, L3, and L4 nerve roots by an intradural lesion (e.g., disc defect, spur, mass), a lumbar plexus, or femoral nerve compression or irritation by an extradural lesion (piriformis muscle hypertrophy). Stretching the quadriceps muscles causes the sacroiliac joint and the lumbosacral joints to move inferiorly. Pain in the buttock may indicate a sacroiliac joint lesion. Pain in the lumbosacral joint may indicate a lumbosacral lesion.

NOTE:

Local pain at the anterior thigh and inability to completely approximate the heel to the buttock may indicate a quadriceps muscle contracture.

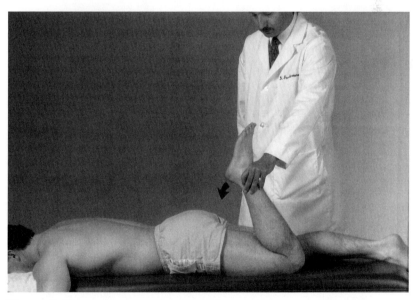

Figure 9.59

9

Sign of the Buttock Test (26)

PROCEDURE:

With the patient in the supine position, perform a passive straight leg raising test (Fig. 9.60). If restriction is found, flex the patient's knee and see if hip flexion increases (Fig. 9.61).

RATIONALE:

If hip flexion increases and the patient's pain is exacerbated, then the problem is in the lumbar spine because there is full movement in the sacroiliac joint when the knee is flexed. This result indicates a negative sign. If hip flexion does not increase when the knee is flexed, then dysfunction in the sacroiliac joint is present. This dysfunction indicates a pathology of the sacroiliac joint or buttocks, such as an inflammatory process, bursitis, mass, or an abscess. This result is a positive sign.

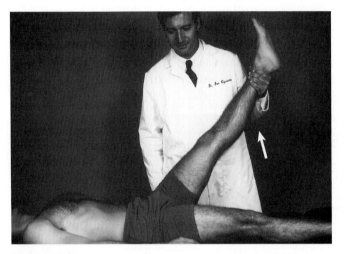

Figure 9.60

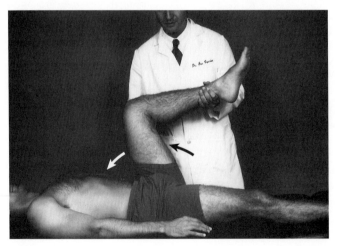

Figure 9.61

References

1. American Academy of Orthopaedic Surgeons. The clinical measurement of joint motion. Chicago: American Academy of Orthopaedic Surgeons, 1994.
2. Loebl WY. Measurement of spinal posture and range of spinal movements. Ann Phys Med 1967;9:103–110.
3. Fitzgerald GK, Wynveen KJ, Rheault W, et al. Objective assessment with establishment of normal values for lumbar spinal range of motion. Phys Ther 1983;63:1776–1781.
4. Einkauf DK, Gohdes ML, Jensen GM, et al. Objective assessment with establishment of normal values for lumbar spinal range of motion. Phys Ther 1987;67:370–375.
5. Kirkaldy-Willis WH. Managing low back pain. Edinburgh: Churchill Livingstone, 1983.
6. Wadsworth CT. Manual examination and treatment of the spine and extremities. Baltimore: Williams & Wilkins, 1988.
7. O'Donoghue D. Treatment of injuries to athletes. 4th ed. Philadelphia: WB Saunders, 1984.
8. Turek SL. Orthopaedics. 3rd ed. Philadelphia: JB Lippincott, 1977.
9. Breig A, Troup JDG. Biomechanical considerations in straight-leg-raising test: cadaveric and clinical studies of the effects of medial hip rotation. Spine 1979;4:242.
10. Fahrni WH. Observations on straight-leg-raising with special reference to nerve root adhesions. Can J Surg 1966;9:44.
11. Hoppenfeld S. Physical examination of the spine and extremities. New York: Appleton-Century-Crofts, 1976:127.
12. Urban LM. The straight-leg-raising test: a review. J Orthop Sports Phys Ther 1981;2:117.
13. Lasègue C. Considerations sur la sciatique. Arch Gen de Meil 1864;24:558.
14. Wilkins RH, Brody IA. Lasègue's sign. Arch Neurol 1969;21:219.
15. Dyck P. The femoral nerve traction test with lumbar disc protrusion. Surg Neurol 1976;6:163.
16. Hudgins WR. The crossed-straight-leg-raising test. N Engl J Med 1977;297:1127.
17. Woodhall R, Hayes GJ. The well-leg-raising test of Fajersztajn in the diagnosis of ruptured lumbar intervertebral disc. J Bone Joint Surg 1950;32A:786.
18. Cram RH. Sign of sciatic nerve root pressure. J Bone Joint Surg 1953;35B:192.
19. Magee JM. Orthopaedic physical assessment. 2nd ed. Philadelphia: WB Saunders, 1992.
20. Hartley A. Practical joint assessment. St. Louis: Mosby, 1991.
21. Katznelson A, Nerubay J, Level A. Gluteal skyline: a search for an objective sign in the diagnosis of disc lesions of the lower lumbar spine. Spine 1982;7:74.
22. DeGowin EL, DeGowin RL. Bedside diagnostic examination. 2nd ed. London: MacMillan, 1969.
23. Scham SM, Taylor TKF. Tension signs in lumbar disc prolapse. Clin Orthop Relat Res 1971;75:195.
24. Arid RB, Naffziger HC. Prolonged jugular compression: a new diagnostic test of neurologic value. Trans Am Neural Assoc 1941;66:45–48.
25. Criax J. Textbook of orthopaedic medicine. 4th ed. Vol. I. London: Bailliere Tindall, 1975.

General References

American Medical Association. Guides to the evaluation of permanent impairment. 3rd ed. Chicago: American Medical Association, 1988.

Bogduk N, Twomey LT. Clinical anatomy of the lumbar spine. New York: Churchill Livingstone, 1987.

Chadwick PR. Examination, assessment and treatment of the lumbar spine. Physiotherapy 1984;70:2.

Charnley J. Orthopaedic signs in the diagnosis of disc protrusion with special reference to the straight-leg-raising test. Lancet 1951;1:156.

Cyriax J. Textbook of orthopaedic medicine. Vol. 1. Diagnosis of soft tissue lesions. London: Bailliere Tindall, 1982.

D'Ambrosia RD. Musculoskeletal disorders: regional examination and differential diagnosis. 2nd ed. Philadelphia: JB Lippincott, 1986.

Derosa C, Portefielf J. Review for advanced orthopaedic competencies: the low back and sacroiliac joint and hip. Chicago: 1989.

Edgar MA, Park WM. Induced pain patterns on passive straight-leg-raising in lower lumbar disc protrusion. J Bone Joint Surg 1974; 56B:658.

Farfan HF. Mechanical disorders of the low back. Philadelphia: Lea & Febiger, 1973.

Farfan HF, Cossette JW, Robertson GW, et al. Effects of torsion on lumbar intervertebral joints: the role of torsion in the production of disc degeneration. J Bone Joint Surg 1970; 52A:468.

Finneson BE. Low back pain. 2nd ed. Philadelphia: JB Lippincott, 1981.

Fisk JW. The painful neck and back. Chicago: Charles C. Thomas, 1977

9

Goddard BS, Reid JD. Movements induced by straight-leg-raising in the lumbo-sacral roots, nerves, and plexus and in the intrapelvic section of the sciatic nerve. J Neurol Neurosurg Psychiatry 1965;28:12.

Gracovetsky S, Farfan HF, Lamy C. The mechanism of the lumbar spine. Spine 1981;6: 249–262.

Grieve GP. Common vertebral joint problems. 2nd ed. New York: Churchill Livingstone, 1988.

Helfet AJ, Lee DM. Disorders of the lumbar spine. Philadelphia: JB Lippincott, 1978.

Kapandji IA. The physiology of joints, Vol. 3. The trunk and the vertebral column. New York: Churchill Livingstone, 1974.

Loeser JD. Pain due to nerve injury. Spine 1985;10:232.

Macnab I. Backache. Baltimore: Williams & Wilkins, 1977.

Mayer TG, Tencer AF, Kristoferson S, et al. Use of non-invasive techniques for quantification of spinal range-of-motion in normal subjects and chronic low back dysfunction patients. Spine 1984;9:588–595.

McKenzie RA. The lumbar spine: mechanical diagnosis and therapy. Waikanae, New Zealand: Spinal Publications Ltd., 1981.

McRae R. Clinical orthopaedic examination. New York: Churchill Livingstone, 1976.

Nachemson A. Towards a better understanding of low back pain: a review of the mechanics of the lumbar disc. Rheumatol Rehabil 1975; 14:129.

Panjabi M, Krag M, Chung T. Effects of disc injury on mechanical behavior of the human spine. Spine 1984;9(7):707.

Post M. Physical examination of the musculoskeletal system. Chicago: Year Book Medical Publishers, 1987.

Ruge D, Wiltse LL. Spinal disorder diagnosis and treatment. Philadelphia: Lea & Febiger, 1977.

Travell JG, Simmons DG. Myofascial pain and dysfunction: the trigger point manual. Vol. 2. The lower extremities. Baltimore: Williams & Wilkins, 1992.

White AA, Panjabi MM. Clinical biomechanics of the spine. Toronto: JB Lippincott, 1978.

Wooden MJ. Preseason screening of the lumbar spine. J Orthop Sports Phys Ther 1981;3:6.

10
LUMBAR NERVE ROOT LESIONS

10

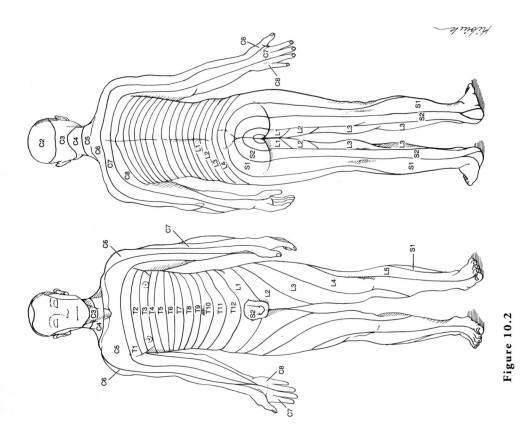

Figure 10.2

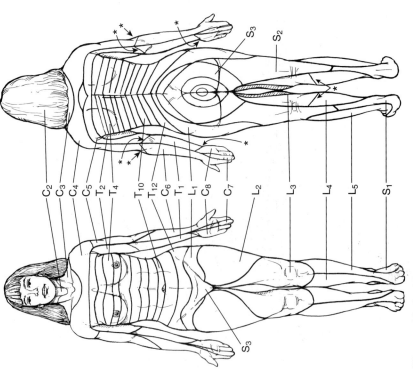

Figure 10.1

If a lumbar nerve root lesion is suspect, you must evaluate three important clinical aspects of the neurological examination: sensory dysfunction, motor dysfunction, and reflex dysfunction.

The sensory deficit evaluation attempts to test the segmental cutaneous innervation to the skin. It is tested with a sterile or disposable neurotip or pinwheel in specific dermatomal patterns. Two dermatomal maps are provided here. Figure 10.1 indicates the body areas of intact sensation when roots above and below an isolated root are interrupted, sensation loss when one or more continuous roots are interrupted, or the pattern of herpetic rash and hypersensitivity in isolated root involvement. Figure 10.2 presents the hyposensitivity to pin scratch in various root lesions and is consistent with electrical skin resistance studies showing axial dermatomes extending to the distal extremities. This pattern is useful in evaluating paresthesias and hyperesthesias secondary to root irritation. This is the pattern that will be delineated to evaluate sensory root dysfunction. Remember that a fair amount of segmental overlap exists; therefore, a single unilateral lesion may affect more than one dermatomal level. Motor function will be tested by evaluating the muscle strength of specific muscles innervated by a particular nerve root or roots using the muscle grading chart adopted by the American Academy of Orthopaedic Surgeons (Fig. 10.3). The reflex arc will be tested by evaluating the superficial stretch reflex associated with the particular nerve root. These reflexes are graded by the Wexler scale (Fig. 10.4).

5	Complete range of motion against gravity with full resistance.
4	Complete range of motion against gravity with some resistance.
3	Complete range of motion against gravity.
2	Complete range of motion with gravity eliminated.
1	Evidence of slight contractility. No joint motion.
0	No evidence of contractility.

Figure 10.3   Muscle Grading Chart

10

0	No response
+1	Hyporeflexia
+2	Normal
+3	Hyperreflexia
+4	Hyperreflexia with transient clonus
+5	Hyperreflexia with sustained clonus

Figure 10.4   Wexler Scale

The clinical presentation of nerve root lesions depends on two important factors: the **location** and the **severity** of the injury or pathology. The combination of these two factors determines the lesion's clinical presentation. The possibilities are endless and can range from no clinical presentations or slight clinical manifestation, such as slight loss of sensation and pain, to total denervation with loss of total function to the structures innervated by suspected nerve root (motor, sensory, and reflex).

Each nerve root will have its own sensory distribution, muscle test or tests, and a stretch reflex, which will be grouped together to facilitate the identification of the suspected level.

Remember that the clinical evaluation is not made solely on one aspect of the "Neurological Package" but is instead determined by the combination of history, inspection, palpation, the three individual tests (motor, reflex, and sensory), and appropriate diagnostic imaging and/or functional neurological testing, such as EMG. We must also realize that the injury or pathology we are attempting to evaluate may not necessarily be affecting a nerve root, but it may be affecting the lumbar plexus, a trunk of that plexus, or a named nerve. Depending on the severity and location of the injury or pathology, various combinations of neurological dysfunction may be elicited.

ANATOMIC NOTE

The nerve roots in the lower thoracic and lumbar spine gradually exit the intervertebral foramen at the upper aspect of the intervertebral foramen. This causes the nerve root in these areas to be affected by the intervertebral disc above the exiting nerve root (Fig. 10.5). The lower thoracic area and upper lumbar area (T12-L2) are transitions to this anatomic consideration and in this area may be affected either by the intervertebral disc at the same interval or the intervertebral disc at the level above the exiting nerve root. This situation may depend on the laterality of the disc defect. The L3, L4, and L5 nerve roots exit the intervertebral foramen at the upper end of the foramen 80% of the time, and they are usually affected by the intervertebral disc above the exiting nerve root. Because of its anatomic position, the S1 nerve root is usually affected by the L5-S1 intervertebral disc.

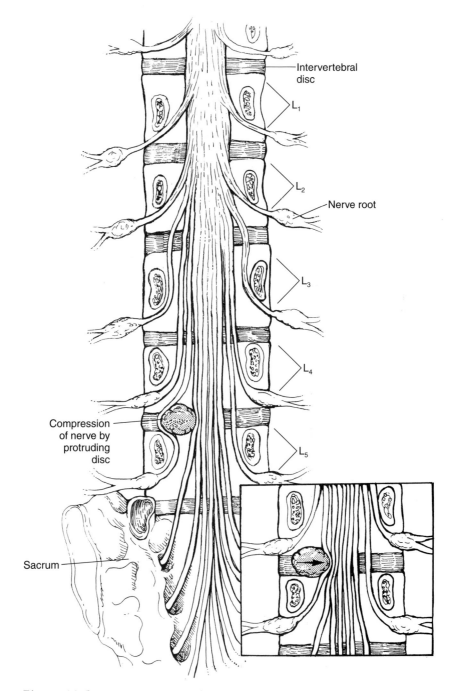

Figure 10.5

T12, L1, L2, L3

The T12, L1, L2, and L3 nerve roots exit the spinal canal at their respective levels. The T12 and L1 nerve roots can be affected by the intervertebral disc at their respective levels or levels above them, depending on the size and laterality of the disc defect (Fig. 10.6).

Figure 10.6

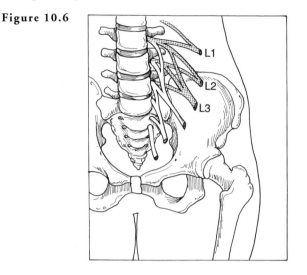

Motor

Iliopsoas (T12, L1, L2, L3 Nerve Root Innervation)

PROCEDURE:

With the patient sitting at the edge of the examination table, instruct the patient to raise his thigh off the table. Place your hand on the patient's knee and instruct the patient to continue to raise his thigh against your resistance (Fig. 10.7). Perform the test on the opposite thigh. Grade according to the muscle grading chart and evaluate bilaterally.

RATIONALE:

A grade 0 to 4 unilaterally may indicate a neurological deficit of the T12, L1, L2, or L3 nerve roots. A weak or strained iliopsoas muscle may be suspected if the sensory portion of the T12, L1, L2, or L3 "Neurological Packages" is intact.

Figure 10.7

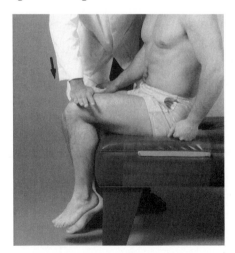

Reflex

None

Sensory

PROCEDURE:

With a pin, stroke the dermatomal area corresponding to each nerve root (Fig. 10.8) and evaluate bilaterally.

RATIONALE:

Unilateral hypoesthesia may indicate a neurological deficit of the corresponding T12, L1, L2, or L3 nerve root or the femoral nerve.

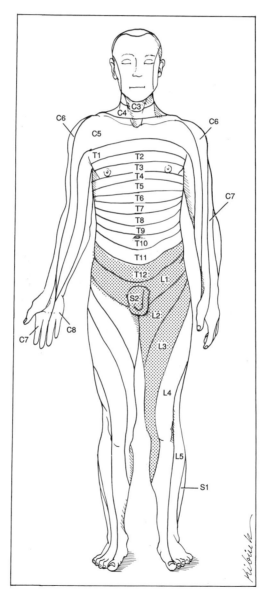

Figure 10.8

L2, L3, L4

The L2, L3, and L4 nerve roots exit the spinal canal at their respective levels and can be affected by the intervertebral disc at their respective levels or levels above them, depending on the size and laterality of the disc defect (Fig. 10.9).

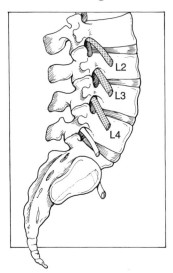

Figure 10.9

Motor

Quadriceps Muscle (L3, L4-Femoral Nerve Innervation)

PROCEDURE:

With the patient sitting at the edge of the examination table, instruct the patient to extend his knee. Place one hand on the patient's thigh for stabilization and place the other hand on his leg. Exert pressure on the leg while instructing the patient to resist flexion (Fig. 10.10). Grade according to the muscle grading chart and evaluate bilaterally.

RATIONALE:

A grade 0 to 4 unilaterally may indicate a neurological deficit of the L2, L3, or L4 nerve roots or femoral nerve. A weak or strained quadriceps muscle may be suspected if the sensory portion of the L2, L3, or L4 "Neurological Packages" is intact.

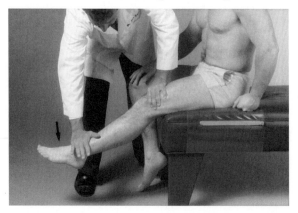

Figure 10.10

Reflex

Patella Reflex

The patella reflex is primarily an L4 reflex and is tested with the L4 neurological level.

Sensory

PROCEDURE:

With a pin, stroke the dermatomal area corresponding to each nerve root (Fig. 10.11) and evaluate bilaterally.

RATIONALE:

Unilateral hypoesthesia may indicate a neurological deficit of the corresponding L2, L3, or L4 nerve roots or the femoral nerve.

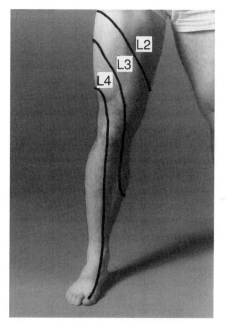

10

Figure 10.11

L4

The L4 nerve root exits the spinal canal between the L4 and L5 vertebrae and is usually affected by the L3-L4 intervertebral disc (Fig. 10.12).

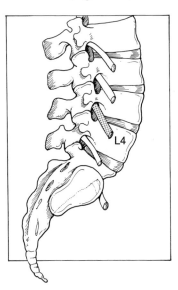

Figure 10.12

Motor

Tibialis Anterior (L4, L5-Deep Peroneal Nerve Innervation)

PROCEDURE:

With the patient seated at the edge of the examination table, instruct the patient to dorsiflex and invert the foot. Grasp the patient's ankle with one hand, grasp his foot with your other hand, and attempt to force his foot into plantar flexion and eversion against patient resistance (Fig. 10.13). Grade according to the muscle grading chart and evaluate bilaterally.

RATIONALE:

A grade 0 to 4 unilaterally may indicate a neurological deficit of the L4 nerve root or the deep peroneal nerve. A weak or strained tibialis anterior muscle may be suspected if the sensory and reflex portions of the L4 "Neurological Packages" are intact.

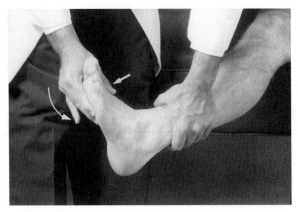

Figure 10.13

Reflex

Patella Reflex

PROCEDURE:

With the patient seated at the edge of the examination table, tap the infrapatellar tendon with the neurological reflex hammer (Fig. 10.14).

RATIONALE:

Unilateral hyporeflexia may indicate a nerve root deficit. Loss of reflex unilaterally may indicate an interruption of the reflex arc (lower motor neuron lesion). Unilateral hyperreflexia may indicate an upper motor neuron lesion.

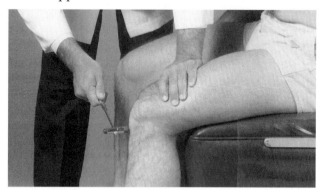

Figure 10.14

Sensory

PROCEDURE:

With a pin, stroke the medial aspect of the leg and foot (Fig. 10.15) and evaluate bilaterally.

RATIONALE:

Unilateral hypoesthesia may indicate a neurological deficit of the L4 nerve root.

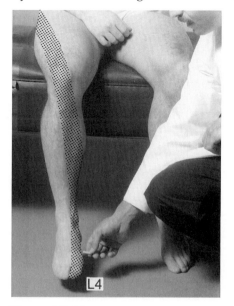

Figure 10.15

L5

The L5 nerve root exits the spinal canal between the L5 vertebrae and the first sacral segment and is usually affected by the L4-L5 intervertebral disc (Fig. 10.16).

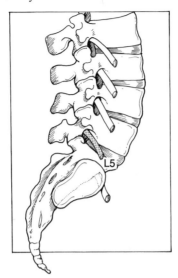

Figure 10.16

Motor

Extensor Hallucis Longus (L5, S1-Deep Peroneal Nerve Innervation)

PROCEDURE:

With the patient seated at the edge of the examination table, grasp the patient's calcaneus with one hand for stabilization. With your opposite hand, pinch the great toe and instruct the patient to dorsiflex it against your resistance (Fig. 10.17). Grade according to the muscle grading chart and compare bilaterally.

RATIONALE:

A grade 0 to 4 unilaterally may indicate a neurological deficit of the L5 nerve root or the deep peroneal nerve. A weak or strained extensor hallucis longus muscle may be suspected if the sensory and reflex portions of the L5 "Neurological Package" are intact.

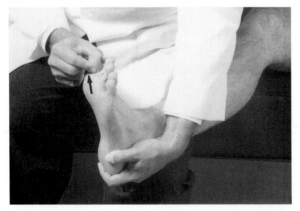

Figure 10.17

Gluteus Medius (L5, S1-Superior Gluteal Nerve Innervation)

PROCEDURE:

With the patient lying on his side on the examination table, instruct the patient to abduct his superior leg (Fig. 10.18). Place your hand on the lateral aspect of the patient's knee and attempt to push the knee into adduction against patient resistance (Fig. 10.19). Grade according to the muscle grading chart and evaluate bilaterally.

RATIONALE:

A grade 0 to 4 unilaterally may indicate a neurological deficit of the L5 nerve root or the superior gluteal nerve. A weak or strained gluteus medius muscle may be suspected if the sensory and reflex portions of the L5 "Neurological Package" are intact.

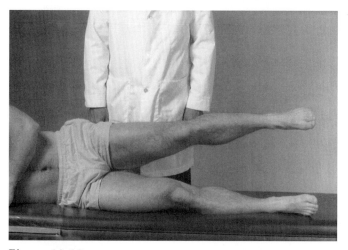

Figure 10.18

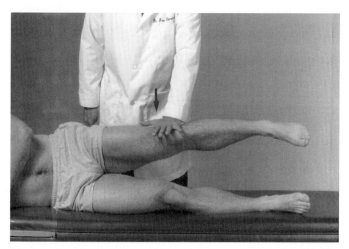

Figure 10.19

10

Extensor Digitorum Longus and Brevis (L5, S1-Deep Peroneal Nerve Innervation)

PROCEDURE:

With the patient sitting at the edge of the examination table, grasp the calcaneus to stabilize the foot. With your opposite hand, grasp the patient's second through fifth toes and instruct the patient to dorsiflex his toes against your resistance (Fig. 10.20).

RATIONALE:

A grade 0 to 4 unilaterally may indicate a neurological deficit of the L5 nerve root or the superficial peroneal nerve. A weak or strained extensor digitorum longus and/or brevis muscle may be suspected if the sensory and reflex portions of the L5 "Neurological Package" are intact.

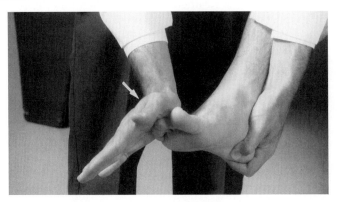

Figure 10.20

Reflex

Medial Hamstring Reflex

PROCEDURE:

With the patient in the prone position, slightly flex the patient's knee and place your thumb on the medial hamstring tendon. With a neurological reflex hammer, tap the medial hamstring tendon (Fig. 10.21). The patient should exhibit a slight flexion of the knee.

RATIONALE:

Unilateral hyporeflexia may indicate a nerve root deficit. Loss of reflex unilaterally may indicate an interruption of the reflex arc (lower motor neuron lesion). Unilateral hyper-reflexia may indicate an upper motor neuron lesion.

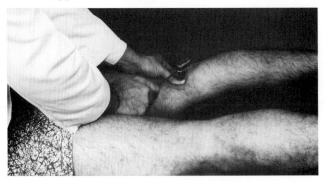

Figure 10.21

Sensory

PROCEDURE:

With a pin, stroke the lateral leg and dorsum of the foot (Fig. 10.22). Evaluate bilaterally.

RATIONALE:

Unilateral hypoesthesia may indicate a neurological deficit of the L5 nerve root.

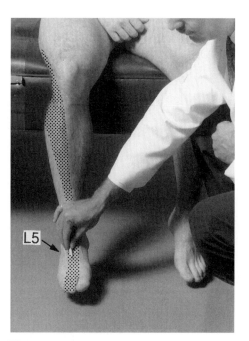

Figure 10.22

S1

The S1 nerve root exits the spinal canal through the first sacral foramen and is usually affected by the L5-S1 intervertebral disc (Fig. 10.23).

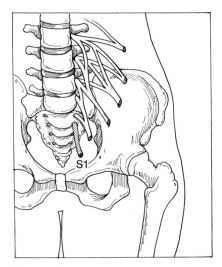

Figure 10.23

Motor

Peroneus Longus and Brevis (L5, S1-Superficial Peroneal Nerve Innervation)

PROCEDURE:

With the patient sitting at the edge of the examination table, stabilize the calcaneus with one hand and grasp the lateral aspect of his foot with your opposite hand. Instruct the patient to plantar flex, and evert his foot against your resistance (Fig. 10.24). Grade according to the muscle grading chart and evaluate bilaterally.

RATIONALE:

A grade 0 to 4 unilaterally may indicate a neurological deficit of the S1 nerve root or the superficial peroneal nerve. A weak or strained peroneus longus and/or brevis muscle may be suspected if the sensory and reflex portions of the S1 "Neurological Package" are intact.

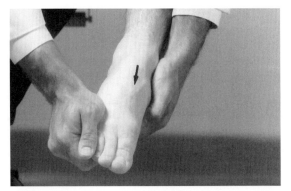

Figure 10.24

Reflex

Achilles Reflex

PROCEDURE:

With the patient seated at the edge of the examination table, place slight dorsiflexion on the foot. With a neurological reflex hammer, tap the Achilles tendon (Fig. 10.25). The patient should exhibit a slight plantar flexion of the foot.

RATIONALE:

Unilateral hyporeflexia may indicate a nerve root deficit. Loss of reflex unilaterally may indicate an interruption of the reflex arc (lower motor neuron lesion). Unilateral hyper-reflexia may indicate an upper motor neuron lesion.

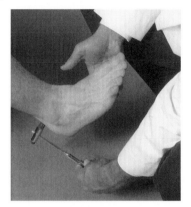

Figure 10.25

Sensory

PROCEDURE:

With a pin, stroke the lateral aspect of the foot (Fig. 10.26).

RATIONALE:

Unilateral hypoesthesia may indicate a neurological deficit of the S1 nerve root.

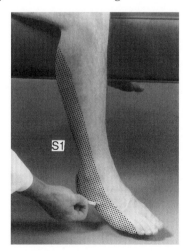

Figure 10.26

General References

Barrows HS. Guide to neurological assessment. Philadelphia: JP Lippincott, 1980.

Bronisch FW. The clinically important reflexes. New York: Grune & Stratton, 1952.

Chusid JG. Correlative neuroanatomy and functional neurology. 16th ed. Los Altos, CA: Lange Medical Publishers, 1976.

DeJong RN. The neurologic examination. 4th ed. Hagerstown, MD: Harper & Row, 1979.

Devinsky O, Feldmann E. Examination of the cranial and peripheral nerves. New York: Churchill Livingstone, 1988.

Geenberg DA, Aminoff MJ, Simon RP. Clinical neurology. 2nd ed. East Norwalk: Appleton & Lange, 1993.

Hoppenfeld S. Physical examination of the spine and extremities. New York: Appleton-Century-Croft, 1976;127.

Kendall FP, McCreary EK, Provance PG. Muscles: testing and function. 4th ed. Baltimore: Williams & Wilkins, 1993.

Mancall E. Essentials of the neurologic examination. 2nd ed. Philadelphia: FA Davis, 1981.

Parsons N. Color atlas of clinical neurology. Chicago: Year Book Medical Publishers, 1989.

VanAllen MW, Rodnitzky RL. Pictorial manual of neurologic tests. 2nd ed. Chicago: Year Book Medical Publishers, 1981.

11
SACROILIAC ORTHOPAEDIC TESTS

11

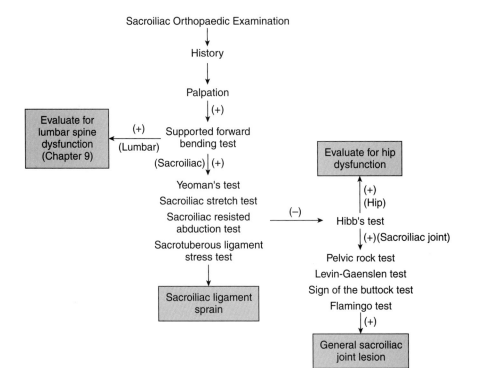

PALPATION

Posterior Superior Iliac Spine and Iliac Crest

DESCRIPTIVE ANATOMY:

The iliac crest and posterior superior iliac spine are important bony landmarks used to assess postural deviations and leg length deficiencies. The iliac crest extends through the inferior margin of the flank and is easily palpable. The posterior superior iliac spine is located inferior to the iliac crest, lateral to the S2 sacral segment (Fig. 11.1).

PROCEDURE:

With the patient standing, palpate the iliac crest for tenderness (Fig. 11.2). Tenderness may be caused by contusions, periosteitis, and avulsion fractures. Next, place your forefingers on each iliac crest and your thumbs on the posterior superior iliac spines of each ilium (Fig. 11.3). Note any difference in longitudinal position. A difference in longitudinal position may indicate a leg length deficiency, scoliosis, sacroiliac joint subluxation, or hip joint dislocation.

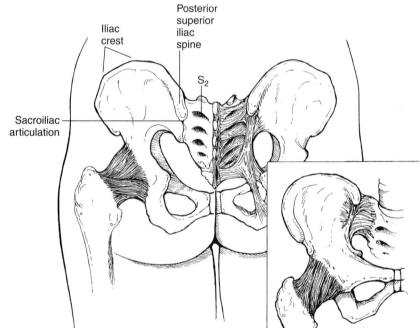

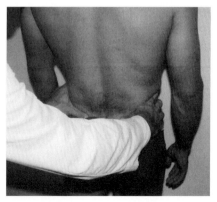

Figure 11.1

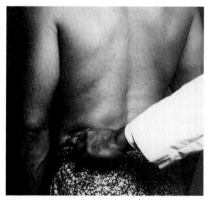

Figure 11.2

Figure 11.3

Sacroiliac Articulations

DESCRIPTIVE ANATOMY:

The sacroiliac articulations are located inferiorly and medially to the posterior superior iliac spine (Fig. 11.1). The articulations are synovial and are held together by interosseous ligaments, dorsal sacroiliac ligaments, and ventral sacroiliac ligaments. The movement of the sacroiliac joints is limited to slight gliding and rotation. These joints are primarily weight bearing. They transfer the weight of the trunk to the hip joints.

PROCEDURE:

Place the patient in the prone position, flex the patient's knee to 90 degrees, and externally rotate the hip. With your opposite hand, palpate the sacroiliac joint from just below the posterior superior iliac spine to the sacral notch (Fig. 11.4). Note any pain or tenderness that may indicate an inflammatory process in the sacroiliac joint.

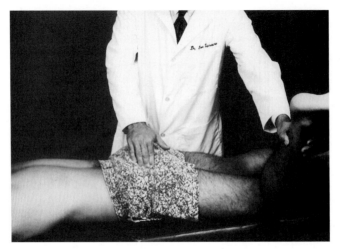

Figure 11.4

Ischial Tuberosity

DESCRIPTIVE ANATOMY:

The ischial tuberosity is located just below the gluteal fold (Fig. 11.1) and can be palpated easily with the hip flexed. The hamstring muscles originate from the tuberosity and may be injured by direct trauma or trauma to the hamstring muscles.

PROCEDURE:

Have the patient lay on one side and instruct him to flex his thigh by bringing his knee to his chest. Palpate the ischial tuberosity, noting any pain or tenderness (Fig. 11.5). Pain may indicate a contusion secondary to trauma, an avulsion fracture caused by severe hamstring pull, or ischial tuberosity bursitis.

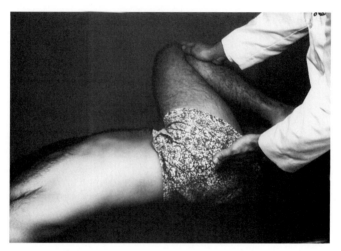

Figure 11.5

11

Gluteal Muscles

See lumbar spine chapter.

Piriformis Muscle

See lumbar spine chapter.

SACROILIAC SPRAIN

Yeoman's Test (1)

PROCEDURE:

With the patient prone, flex the patient's leg and extend the thigh (Fig. 11.6).

RATIONALE:

Extension of the thigh stresses the sacroiliac joint and anterior sacroiliac joint ligaments on the side of thigh extension. If pain is elicited on the ipsilateral side, then a sprain of the anterior sacroiliac joint ligaments is suspect, i.e., iliofemoral or ischiofemoral ligaments (Fig. 11.7). Pain may also indicate an inflammatory process or abscess in the sacroiliac joint.

NOTE:

This test also stresses the lower lumbar vertebra by slightly extending the lumbar spine. Lumbar pain, either localized or radiating, may indicate lumbar involvement. See Chapter 9 for evaluation.

Figure 11.6

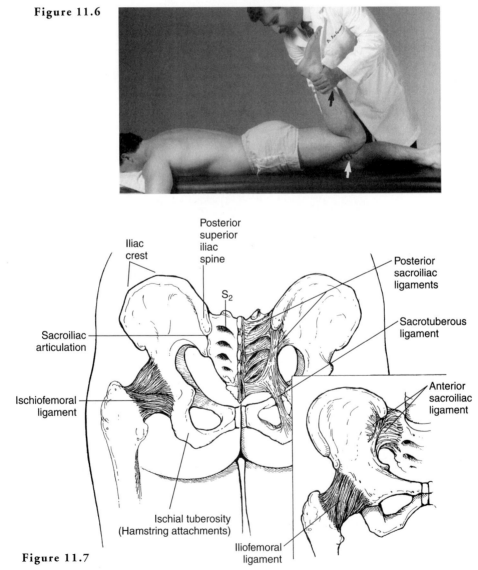

Figure 11.7

252

Sacroiliac Stretch Test

PROCEDURE:

With the patient in the supine position, cross the patient's arms and apply downward and lateral pressure to the anterior superior iliac spine of each ilium (Fig. 11.8).

RATIONALE:

Pressure on both anterior and superior iliac spines compresses both sacroiliac joint surfaces and stretches the anterior sacroiliac ligaments simultaneously. If pain is elicited in one or both joints, then a strain of the anterior sacroiliac ligaments is suspect, i.e., iliofemoral or ischiofemoral ligaments (See Fig. 11.6); an inflammatory process in the affected sacroiliac joint is also suspect.

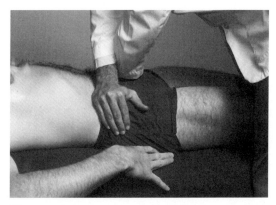

Figure 11.8

Sacroiliac Resisted Abduction Test

PROCEDURE:

Instruct the patient to lie on one side with his inferior limb slightly flexed. His superior leg should be straight out and abducted. Place pressure on the abducted limb against patient resistance (Fig. 11.9).

11

RATIONALE:

Resisting abduction of the thigh stresses the sacroiliac joint and abductor muscles of the thigh. Pain in the sacroiliac joint indicates a sprain of the sacroiliac joint ligaments on the ipsilateral side. Pain in the buttock or lateral thigh indicates a strain of the abductor muscles of the thigh (tensor fasciae latae and gluteus group).

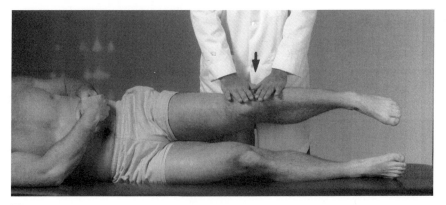

Figure 11.9

Sacrotuberous Ligament Stress Test (2)

PROCEDURE:

Place the patient in the supine position. Fully flex the patient's knee and hip and adduct and internally rotate the hip. With your opposite hand, palpate the sacrotuberous ligament, which runs from the posterior aspect of the sacrum to the ischial tuberosity (Fig. 11.10).

RATIONALE:

The sacrotuberous ligament anchors the sacrum to the ischial tuberosity. The action of hip adduction and medial hip rotation stresses the sacrotuberous ligament. Pain in the area of the sacrotuberous ligament may indicate sacrotuberous ligament sprain.

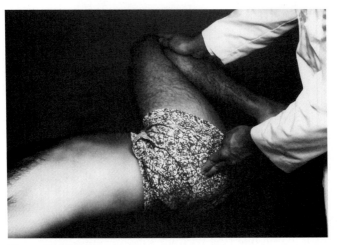

Figure 11.10

GENERAL SACROILIAC JOINT LESIONS

Hibb's Test

PROCEDURE:

With the patient in the prone position, flex the patient's leg to his buttock and move the leg outward, internally rotating the hip (Fig. 11.11).

RATIONALE:

This procedure causes a stressed internal rotation of the femoral head into the acetabular cavity and causes a slight distraction on the sacroiliac joint. This test is mainly a hip joint test but, because of the sacroiliac joint distraction, it may help evaluate sacroiliac joint lesions. Pain in the sacroiliac joint indicates a sacroiliac joint lesion, such as an inflammatory process or abscess in the sacroiliac joint or a sprain of the sacroiliac ligaments. Pain in the hip joint indicates a hip joint lesion (See Hibb's test in Chapter 12).

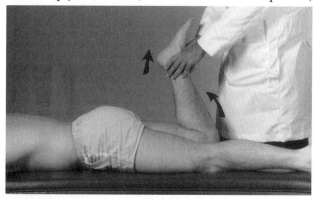

Figure 11.11

Pelvic Rock Test (Iliac Compression Test) (3)

PROCEDURE:

With the patient lying on his side, exert a strong downward pressure on the ilium. Perform this test bilaterally (Fig. 11.12).

RATIONALE:

Placing a downward pressure on the ilium transfers a compression pressure to the joint surfaces of the sacroiliac joints. Pain in either sacroiliac joint indicates a sacroiliac joint lesion, such as an inflammatory process in the joint surfaces on the affected side.

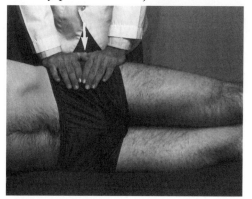

Figure 11.12

Lewin-Gaenslen Test

PROCEDURE:

With the patient lying on his unaffected side, instruct him to flex his inferior leg (Fig. 11.13). Take the superior leg and extend it while you stabilize the lumbosacral joint. (Fig. 11.14).

RATIONALE:

Extension of the leg stresses the sacroiliac joint and anterior sacroiliac joint ligaments on the side of leg extension. Pain on that side indicates a general sacroiliac joint lesion, i.e., anterior sacroiliac ligament sprain (iliofemoral, ischiofemoral ligaments), or inflammatory process in the sacroiliac joint.

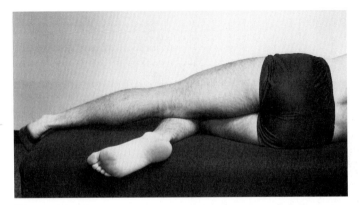

Figure 11.13

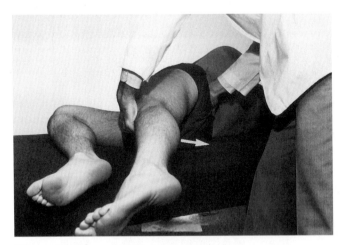

Figure 11.14

Gaenslen's Test (4)

Procedure:

With the patient in the supine position and with the affected side toward the edge of the table, instruct the patient to approximate the knee to his chest on the unaffected side (Fig. 11.15). Then place downward pressure on the affected thigh until it is lower than the edge of the table (Fig. 11.16).

Rationale:

Extension of the leg stresses the sacroiliac joint and anterior sacroiliac joint ligaments on the side of leg extension. Pain on that side indicates a general sacroiliac lesion, i.e., anterior sacroiliac ligament sprain (iliofemoral, ischiofemoral), or inflammatory process in the sacroiliac joint.

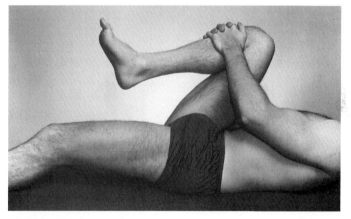

Figure 11.15

11

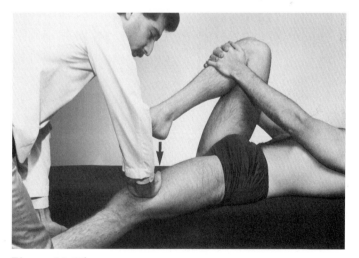

Figure 11.16

Sign of the Buttock Test (5)

PROCEDURE:

With the patient in the supine position, perform a passive straight leg raising test (Fig. 11.17). If restriction is found, flex the patient's knee and see if hip flexion increases (Fig. 11.18).

RATIONALE:

If hip flexion increases and the patient's pain is exacerbated, then the problem is in the lumbar spine because there is full movement in the sacroiliac joint when the knee is flexed. This indicates a negative sign. If hip flexion does not increase when the knee is flexed, then there is a dysfunction in the sacroiliac joint. This indicates a pathology of the sacroiliac joint or buttocks, such as an inflammatory process, bursitis, mass, or an abscess. This is a positive sign.

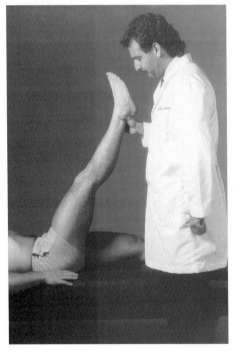

Figure 11.17

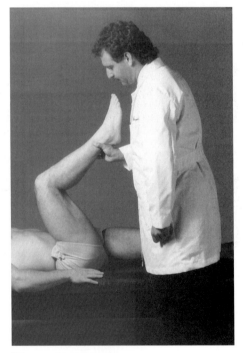

Figure 11.18

Flamingo Test (6)

PROCEDURE:

With the patient standing, instruct him to stand on one leg at a time (Fig. 11.19). Instruct the patient to hop, which increases stress on the joint (Fig. 11.20).

RATIONALE:

This test increases the pressure in the hip, sacroiliac articulation, and symphysis pubis articulation. Increased pain in any of these joints may indicate an inflammatory process on the standing leg side. Pain secondary to trauma may indicate a fracture into the suspected joint. Pain in the hip joint may also indicate a trochanteric bursitis.

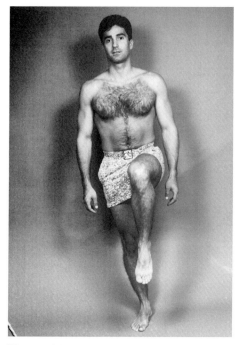

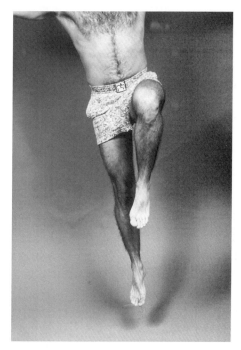

Figure 11.19

Figure 11.20

11

References

1. Yeoman W. The relation of arthritis of the sacro-iliac joint to sciatica. Lancet 1928;2:1119–1122.
2. Lee D. The pelvic girdle. Edinburgh: Churchill Livingstone, 1989.
3. Hoppenfeld S. Physical examination of the spine and extremities. New York: Appleton-Century-Crofts, 1976:127.
4. Gaenslen FJ. Sacroiliac arthrodesis. JAMA 1927;89:2031–2035.
5. Cyriax J. Textbook of orthopaedic medicine. 4th ed. Vol. I. London: Bailliere Tindall, 1975:541.
6. Magee DJ. Orthopedic physical assessment. 2nd ed. Philadelphia: WB Saunders, 1992.

General References

Alderink GJ. The sacroiliac joint: review of anatomy, mechanics, and function. J Orthop Sports Phys Therap 1991;13:71.

DeGowin EL, DeGowin RL. Bedside diagnostic examination. 3rd ed. New York: MacMillan, 1976.

Gray H. Sacro-iliac joint pain: the finer anatomy. New Internat Clin 1938;2:54.

Hartley A. Practical joint assessment. St. Louis: Mosby, 1991.

McRae R. Clinical orthopedic examination. New York: Churchill Livingstone, 1976.

Norkin C, Levangie P. Joint structure and function: a comprehensive analysis. Philadelphia: FA Davis, 1987.

Post M. Physical examination of the musculo-skeletal system. Chicago: Year Book Medical Publishers, 1987.

Wells PE. The examination of the pelvic joints. In: Grieve GP, ed. Modern manual therapy of the vertebral column. Edinburgh: Churchill Livingstone, 1986.

12

Hip Joint Orthopaedic Tests

12

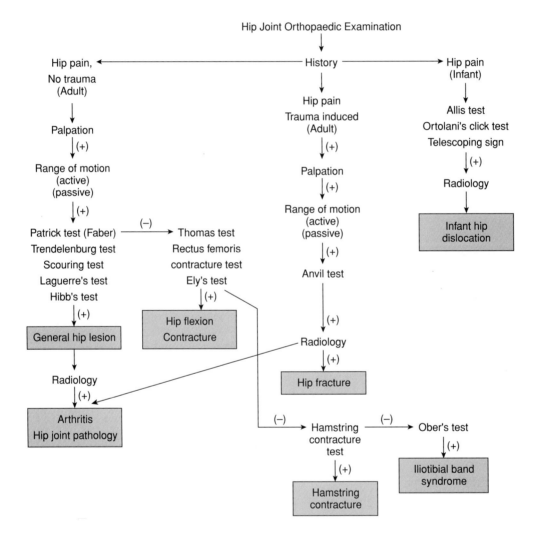

Hip Joint Orthopaedic Examination

History

Hip pain,
No trauma
(Adult)

Hip pain
Trauma induced
(Adult)

Hip pain
(Infant)

Palpation
(+)

Allis test
Ortolani's click test
Telescoping sign
(+)

Range of motion
(active)
(passive)
(+)

Palpation
(+)

Radiology

Patrick test (Faber)   (−)   Thomas test
Trendelenburg test   Rectus femoris
Scouring test   contracture test
Laguerre's test   Ely's test
Hibb's test   (+)
(+)

Range of motion
(active)
(passive)
(+)

Infant hip
dislocation

General hip lesion

Hip flexion
Contracture

Anvil test

Radiology
(+)

Radiology
(+)

Hip fracture

Arthritis
Hip joint pathology

(−)   Hamstring
       contracture
       test
       (+)

(−)   Ober's test
       (+)

Iliotibial band
syndrome

Hamstring
contracture

PALPATION

Iliac Crest, Anterior, Superior, and Inferior Iliac Spine

DESCRIPTIVE ANATOMY:

The iliac crest is located at the inferior margin of the flank from the anterior; from the posterior, its highest point is at the level of the L4 spinous process (Fig. 12.1). The iliacus, external oblique, and tensor fasciae latae muscles originate from the iliac crest. At the anterior terminal end of the iliac crest lies the anterior superior iliac spine (Fig. 12.1). It is the attachment of the sartorius muscle and is easily palpable.

The anterior inferior iliac spine is located just below the anterior superior iliac spine. The rectus femoris muscle and iliofemoral ligament are attached to it (Fig. 12.1).

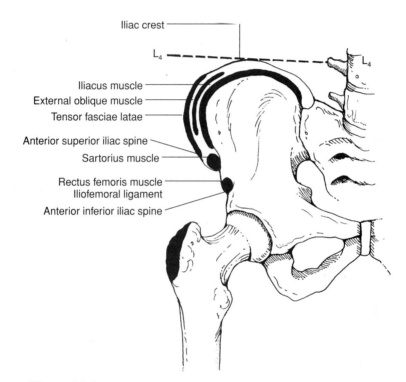

Figure 12.1

12

PROCEDURE:

With the patient supine, palpate the iliac crests for point tenderness and swelling (Fig. 12.2). This may indicate periostitis, strain or avulsion of the iliacus, external oblique, or tensor fasciae latae muscles. Contusion to the iliac crest secondary to trauma is common in the athlete. Palpate the iliac crests with the patient standing as well, checking for unevenness of the crests (Fig. 12.3). Unevenness may be a sign of scoliosis, anatomical short leg, or contracture deformity. The anterior superior iliac spine should be palpated next (Fig. 12.4). Look for point tenderness and swelling, which may indicate a sartorius muscle strain or avulsion fracture. Just below the anterior superior iliac spine is the anterior inferior iliac spine (Fig. 12.5). With your thumb or forefinger, palpate this area and note any point tenderness or swelling. It may indicate a sprained or avulsed rectus femoris muscle or strained iliofemoral ligament.

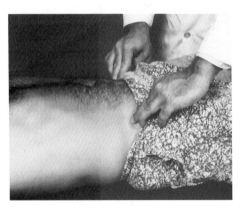

Figure 12.2

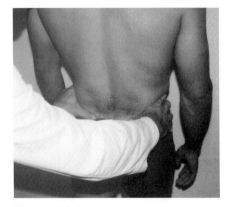

Figure 12.3

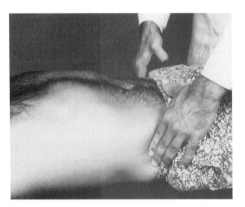

Figure 12.4

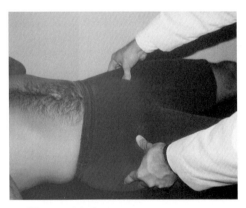

Figure 12.5

Greater Trochanter

DESCRIPTIVE ANATOMY:

The greater trochanter is located approximately 10 cm inferior and lateral to the anterior superior iliac spine (Fig. 12.6). The greater trochanter is the attachment of the gluteus medius, gluteus minimus, and vastus lateralis muscles. The trochanteric bursa also lies under these muscles.

PROCEDURE:

With the patient in the supine position, slightly abduct the thigh and palpate the greater trochanter (Fig. 12.7). Note any point tenderness or swelling. This may indicate a strain of the gluteus medius, gluteus minimus, or vastus lateralis muscles. An increase in the temperature differential associated with tenderness and swelling is an indication of trochanteric bursitis.

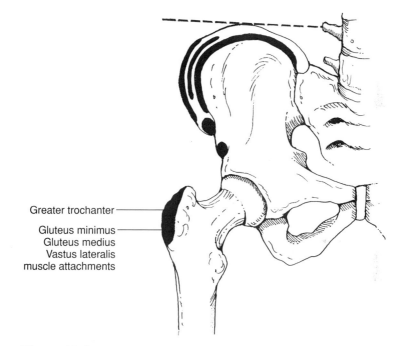

Greater trochanter —————
Gluteus minimus —————
Gluteus medius
Vastus lateralis
muscle attachments

12

Figure 12.6

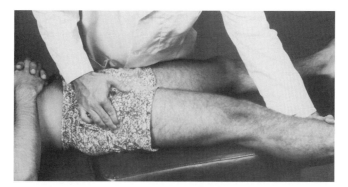

Figure 12.7

Hip Joint

DESCRIPTIVE ANATOMY:

The hip joint is a ball and socket synovial joint, and the femur head is held in place by the iliofemoral, pubofemoral, and ischiofemoral ligaments (Fig. 12.8). The iliofemoral ligament is the largest and strongest of these ligaments that hold the femur into the acetabular cavity.

The hip joint is difficult at best to palpate because it lies deep in the body. Unless the joint is severely traumatized to the point of fracture or dislocation, palpation of the actual joint will reveal little clinical information. The palpation of the surrounding tissue may be a better indicator of hip joint pathology.

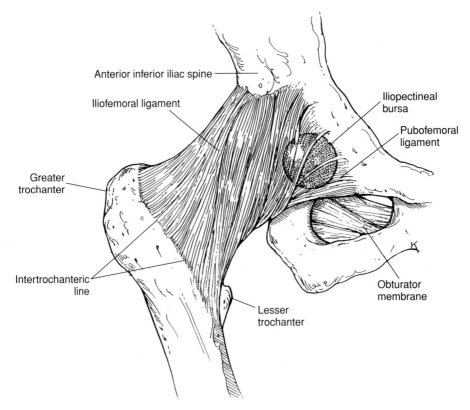

Anterior inferior iliac spine

Iliofemoral ligament

Iliopectineal bursa

Pubofemoral ligament

Greater trochanter

Intertrochanteric line

Lesser trochanter

Obturator membrane

Figure 12.8

Tensor Fasciae Latae Muscle

DESCRIPTIVE ANATOMY:

The tensor fasciae latae muscle is located on the anterior lateral side of the thigh. It originates from the anterior outer lip of the iliac crest and inserts into the iliotibial band that attaches to the lateral epicondyle of the tibia (Fig. 12.9).

PROCEDURE:

With the patient laying on the unaffected side, palpate the tensor fasciae latae muscle from just below the anterior superior iliac spine down over the greater trochanter to the lateral aspect of the knee (Fig. 12.10). Note any tenderness, spasm, increase in skin temperature, or inflammation. These may indicate a strain of the muscle. If point tenderness is present, then an active trigger point that may refer pain to the upper half of the medial thigh is suspect. If the muscle becomes strained through microtrauma as it moves over the greater trochanter of the femur, it can cause greater trochanteric bursitis.

Figure 12.9

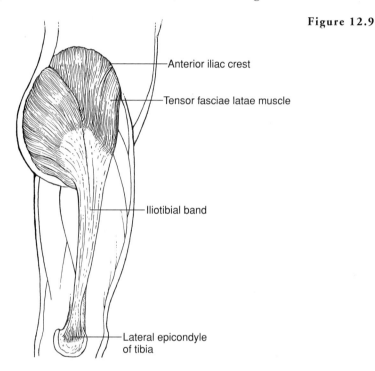

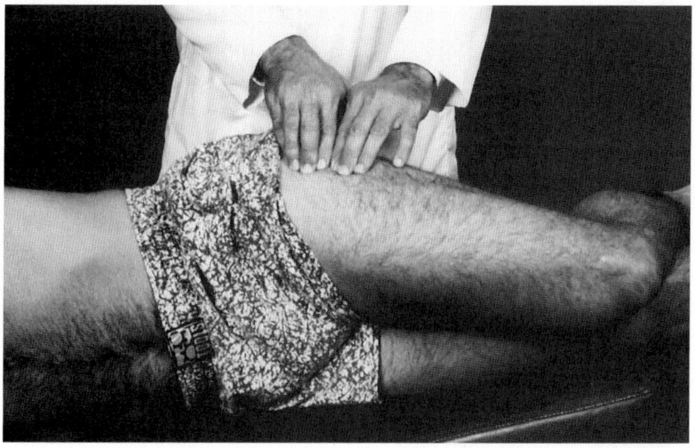

Anterior iliac crest

Tensor fasciae latae muscle

Iliotibial band

Lateral epicondyle of tibia

12

Figure 12.10

Femoral Triangle

DESCRIPTIVE ANATOMY:

The femoral triangle is a clinically important region. It is bound superiorly by the inguinal ligament, medially by the adductor longus muscle, and laterally by the sartorius muscle (Fig. 12.11). The triangle contains the femoral artery and vein, lymph nodes, and the femoral nerve.

PROCEDURE:

With the patient supine, palpate the inguinal ligament, which extends from the anterior superior iliac spine to the pubic tubercle. Note any tenderness, which may indicate a sprain. Next, palpate the adductor longus and sartorius muscle, again noting any tenderness or inflammation. This may indicate a strain or active trigger points in the affected muscle. Once the borders are palpated, palpate the interior of the triangle for inflamed lymph nodes, which may indicate a lower extremity or systemic infection (Fig. 12.12). Palpate the femoral artery for amplitude. A decrease in the amplitude indicates a compromise to the vascular supply to the lower extremity.

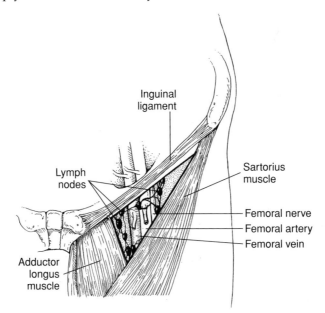

Figure 12.11

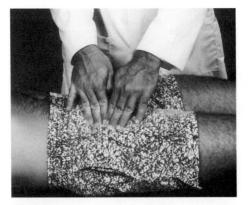

Figure 12.12

HIP RANGE OF MOTION

Flexion (1)

With the patient in the supine position, place the goniometer in the sagittal plane at the level of the hip (Fig. 12.13). Instruct the patient to flex his hip, and follow his thigh with one arm of the goniometer (Fig. 12.14).

NORMAL RANGE (2):

121 ± 6.4 degrees or greater from the 0 or neutral position.

Muscles Involved in Action	*Nerve Supply*
1. Psoas	L1–L3
2. Iliacus	Femoral nerve
3. Rectus femoris	Femoral nerve
4. Sartorius	Femoral nerve
5. Pectineus	Femoral nerve
6. Adductor longus and brevis	Obturator nerve
7. Gracilis	Obturator nerve

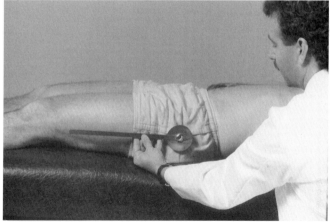

Figure 12.13

12

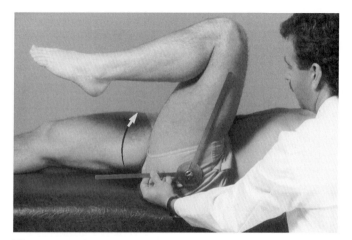

Figure 12.14

Extension (1)

With the patient in the prone position, place the goniometer in the sagittal plane at the level of the hip joint (Fig. 12.15). Instruct the patient to raise his thigh off the table as far as possible, and follow his thigh with one arm of the goniometer (Fig. 12.16).

NORMAL RANGE (2):

12 ± 5.4 degrees or greater from the 0 or neutral position.

Muscles Involved in Action	*Nerve Supply*
1. Biceps femoris	Sciatic
2. Semimembranosus	Sciatic
3. Semitendinosus	Sciatic
4. Gluteus maximus	Inferior gluteal
5. Gluteus medius	Superior gluteal
6. Adductor magnus	Sciatic

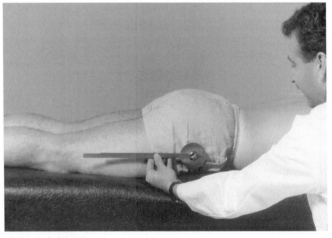

Figure 12.15

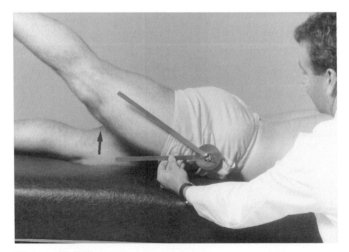

Figure 12.16

Abduction (1)

With the patient in the supine position, place the goniometer in the coronal plane with the center at the level of the hip (Fig. 12.17). Instruct the patient to move his thigh lateralward while following his thigh with one arm of the goniometer (Fig. 12.18).

NORMAL RANGE (2):

41 ± 6.0 degrees or greater from the 0 or neutral position.

Muscles Involved in Action	*Nerve Supply*
1. Tensor fasciae latae	Superior gluteal
2. Gluteus minimus	Superior gluteal
3. Gluteus medius	Superior gluteal
4. Gluteus maximus	Inferior gluteal
5. Sartorius	Femoral

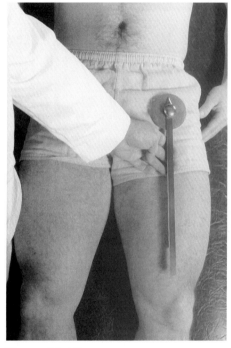

Figure 12.17

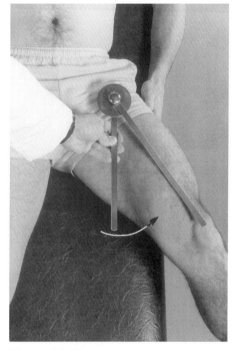

Figure 12.18

12

Adduction (1)

With the patient in the supine position and the opposite hip flexed, place the goniometer in the coronal plane with the center at the level of the hip (Fig. 12.19). Instruct the patient to move his thigh medialward while following the thigh with one arm of the goniometer (Fig. 12.20).

NORMAL RANGE (2):

27 ± 3.6 degrees or greater from the 0 or neutral position.

Muscles Involved in Action	*Nerve Supply*
1. Adductor longus, brevis, magnus	Obturator
2. Gracilis	Obturator
3. Pectineus	Femoral

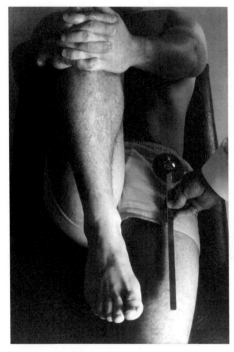

Figure 12.19

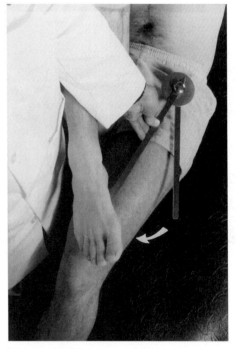

Figure 12.20

Internal Rotation (1)

With the patient in the seated position, place the goniometer in front of the patella (Fig. 12.21). Instruct the patient to rotate his leg outward while following the leg with one arm of the goniometer (Fig. 12.22). This movement internally rotates the hip.

NORMAL RANGE (2):

44 ± 4.3 degrees or greater from the 0 or neutral position.

Muscles Involved in Action	*Nerve Supply*
1. Adductor longus, brevis, magnus	Obturator
2. Gluteus minimus, medius	Superior gluteal
3. Tensor fasciae latae	Superior gluteal
4. Pectineus	Femoral
5. Gracilis	Obturator

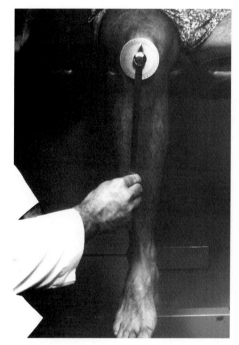

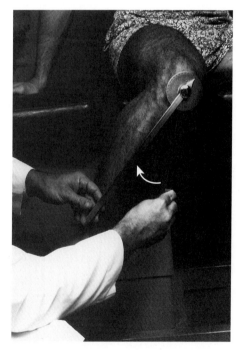

Figure 12.21   **Figure 12.22**

12

External Rotation (1)

With the patient in the seated position, place the goniometer in front of the patella (Fig. 12.23). Instruct the patient to rotate his thigh medialward while following the leg with one arm of the goniometer (Fig. 12.24).

NORMAL RANGE (2):

44 ± 4.8 degrees or greater from the 0 or neutral position.

Muscles Involved in Action	*Nerve Supply*
1. Gluteus maximus	Inferior gluteal
2. Obturator internus, externus	Obturator
3. Quadratus femoris	N. to quadratus femoris
4. Piriformis	L5, S1, S2
5. Gemellus superior, inferior	N. to obturator internus
6. Sartorius	Femoral
7. Gluteus medius	Superior gluteal

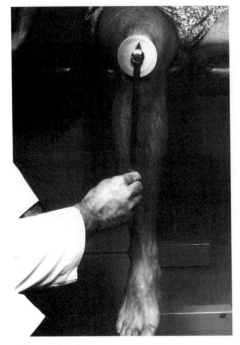

Figure 12.23

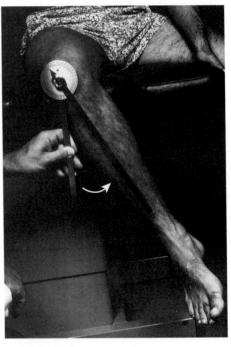

Figure 12.24

PEDIATRIC HIP DISLOCATION

Allis Test (3)

PROCEDURE:

With the infant in the supine position, flex the knees. The patient's feet should approximate each other bilaterally on the table (Fig. 12.25).

RATIONALE:

A difference in the height of the knees is indicative of a positive test. If the knee is short on the affected side, a posterior displacement of the femoral head or decreased tibial length is indicated. If the knee is long on the affected side, an anterior displacement of the femoral head or an increase in tibial length is indicated.

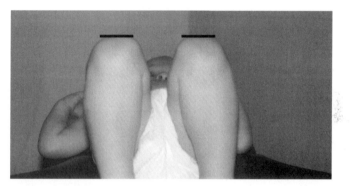

Figure 12.25

Ortolani's Click Test (4)

PROCEDURE:

With the infant in the supine position, grasp both thighs with your thumbs on the lesser trochanters. Then flex and abduct the thighs bilaterally (Fig. 12.26).

RATIONALE:

A palpable and/or audible click are the signs of a positive test. The click signifies a displacement of the femoral head in or out of the acetabular cavity.

12

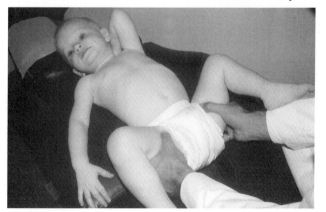

Figure 12.26

Barlow's Test (4)

PROCEDURE:

With the infant in the supine position, grasp the thigh with your middle finger behind the greater trochanter and your thumb on the medial aspect of the thigh. Flex the infant's hip to 90 degrees and fully flex the thigh. With your middle finger, put anterior pressure on the greater trochanter, attempting to dislocate the hip forward (Fig. 12.27). Then apply pressure backward and outward with your thumb in an attempt to reduce the dislocation (Fig. 12.28).

RATIONALE:

This test is similar to Ortolani's click test only that you are now attempting to reduce the dislocation with your thumbs. This is indicative of a unstable hip, which can be dislocated.

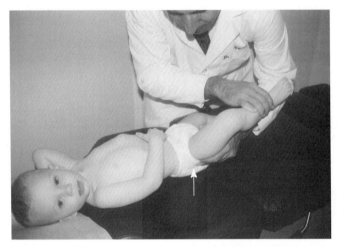

Figure 12.27

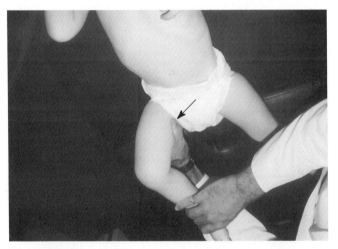

Figure 12.28

Telescoping Sign (5)

Procedure:

With the child in the supine position, flex the suspected hip and knee to 90 degrees. Next, grasp the thigh and push it down towards the table (Fig. 12.29) and then pull it up away from the table (Fig. 12.30).

Rationale:

If the child has a dislocated hip or a hip that could dislocate, excessive movement or a click will occur with this action. Normally, little movement occurs when this function is performed. This excessive movement is called telescoping.

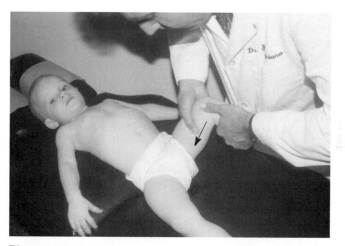

Figure 12.29

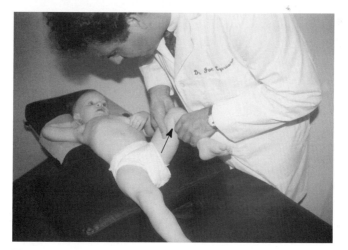

Figure 12.30

12

HIP FRACTURES

Anvil Test

PROCEDURE:

With the patient in the supine position, tap the inferior calcaneus with your fist (Fig. 12.31).

RATIONALE:

Tapping the inferior calcanous transfers quick sharp compression-type blows to the hip joint. Localized pain in the hip joint secondary to trauma may indicate a femoral head fracture or joint pathology.

NOTE:

Localized pain in the thigh or leg secondary to trauma may indicate a femoral, tibial, or fibula fracture. Pain localized to the calcaneus may indicate a calcaneal fracture.

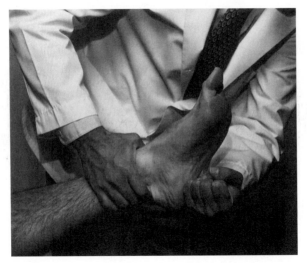

Figure 12.31

HIP CONTRACTURE TESTS

Thomas Test (6)

PROCEDURE:

With the patient supine, instruct him to approximate each knee to his chest one at a time. Palpate the quadriceps muscles on the unflexed leg (Fig. 12.32).

RATIONALE:

If the patient significantly flexes the opposite knee and tightness is palpated on the side of the involuntary flexed knee, a hip flexion contracture is indicated (Fig. 12.33). If no tightness in the rectus femoris muscle exists, then the probable cause of restriction is at the hip joint structure or joint capsule.

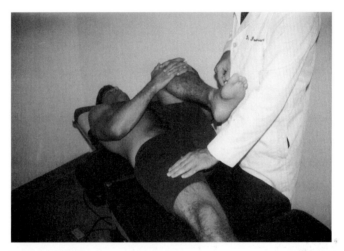

Figure 12.32

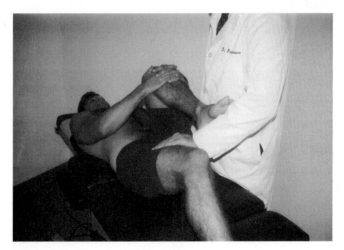

Figure 12.33

12

Rectus Femoris Contracture Test (5)

PROCEDURE:

Instruct the patient to lay supine on the examination table with the leg off the table and flexed to 90 degrees. Instruct the patient to flex the opposite knee to his or her chest and hold it. Palpate the quadriceps muscles of the leg that is flexed off the table for tightness (Fig. 12.34).

RATIONALE:

If the patient involuntarily extends the knee of the leg that is flexed off the table and tightness is palpated in that thigh (Fig. 12.35), a hip flexion contracture is indicated. If there is no tightness in the rectus femoris muscle, then the probable cause of restriction is at the hip joint structure or joint capsule.

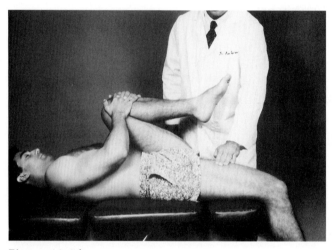

Figure 12.34

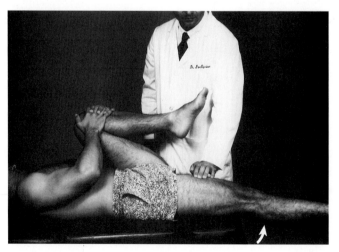

Figure 12.35

Ely's Test (7)

PROCEDURE:

Instruct the patient to lay prone on the examination table. Then grasp the patient's leg and passively flex it (Fig. 12.36).

RATIONALE:

If the patient has a tight rectus femoris muscle or hip flexion contracture, then the hip on the same side will flex (Fig. 12.37), raising the buttock off the table. This spontaneous flexion of the hip reduces the traction pressure on the rectus femoris muscle induced by the passive leg flexion.

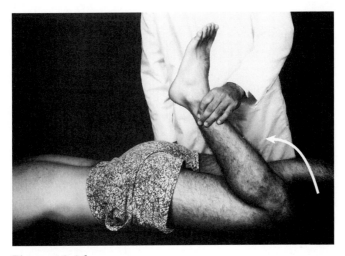

Figure 12.36

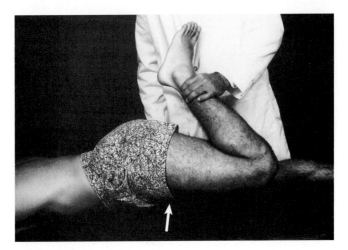

Figure 12.37

12

Ober's Test (8)

PROCEDURE:

With the patient lying on his side, abduct the patient's leg (Fig. 12.38) and then release it (Fig. 12.39). Perform this test bilaterally.

RATIONALE:

The tensor fasciae latae and iliotibial band abduct the hip. If the leg fails to descend smoothly, contracture of the tensor fasciae latae muscle or iliotibial band is suspected.

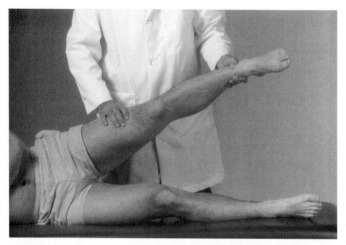

Figure 12.38

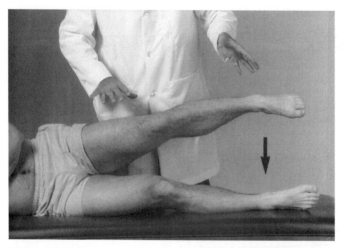

Figure 12.39

Hamstring Contracture Test (5)

PROCEDURE:

Instruct the patient to sit on the examination table with one hip abducted and the knee flexed and the other knee extended (Fig. 12.40). Next, instruct the patient to flex his trunk and touch his toes with his fingers on the extended leg side (Fig. 12.41). Repeat the test with the opposite side flexed and compare bilaterally.

RATIONALE:

If the patient is unable to touch his toes, then the test is positive for a tight hamstring muscle group on the side of the extended leg.

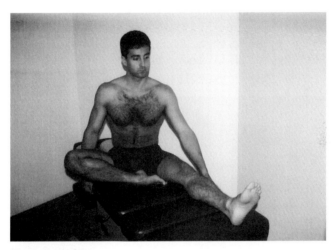

Figure 12.40

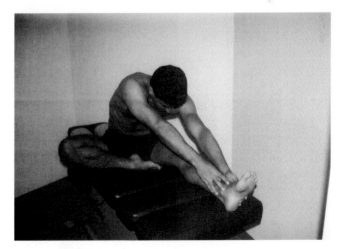

Figure 12.41

12

GENERAL HIP JOINT LESIONS

Patrick Test (Faber) (9)

PROCEDURE:

With the patient in the supine position, flex his leg and place the foot flat on the table. Grasp the femur and press it into the acetabular cavity (Fig. 12.42). Next, cross the patient's leg to the opposite knee. Stabilize the opposite anterior superior iliac spine and press down on the knee that is being tested (Fig. 12.43).

RATIONALE:

This test forces the femoral head into the acetabular cavity, giving maximal congruence to the articular surfaces. Pain in the hip indicates an inflammatory process present in the hip joint. Pain secondary to trauma may indicate a fracture in the acetabular cavity, rim of the acetabular cavity, or femoral neck. Pain may also be indicative of avascular necrosis of the femoral head. Faber stands for flexion, abduction, and external rotation. This is the position of the hip when the test begins.

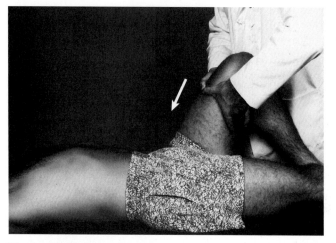

Figure 12.42

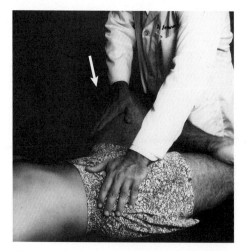

Figure 12.43

Trendelenburg Test (10)

PROCEDURE:

With the patient standing, grasp the patient's waist and place your thumbs on the posterior superior iliac spine of each ilium. Next, instruct the patient to flex one leg at a time (Fig. 12.44).

RATIONALE:

When the patient is standing with one leg flexed, the patient is supported by an intact hip joint with its associated ligaments and muscles on that side. If the patient is unable to stand on one leg because of pain and/or because the opposite pelvis falls or fails to raise, this is considered a positive test. This result may indicate a weak gluteus medius muscle opposite the side of hip flexion, and it tests the integrity of the hip joint and associated musculature and ligaments on the opposite side of hip flexion. This test is often positive secondary to hip joint pathology.

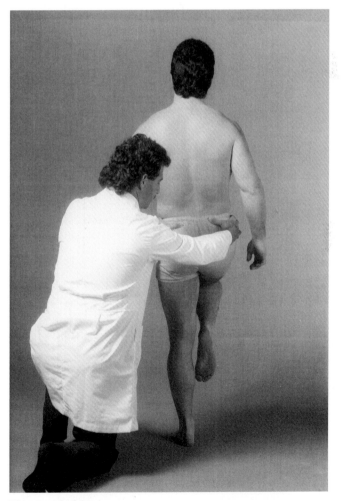

12

Figure 12.44

Scouring Test (11)

PROCEDURE:

With the patient in the supine position, flex the patient's hip to 90 degrees, fully flex the knee, and internally rotate the hip (Fig. 12.45). Grasp the knee (assuming the patient has no injury or pathology to the knee) and apply a downward and lateral pressure on the knee (Fig. 12.46).

RATIONALE:

This test is similar to the Patrick test. In this test, we are stressing the anteromedial and posterolateral aspect of the joint capsule. Pain and/or a grating sensation is indicative of a positive test. This result may indicate an inflammatory process in the acetabular joint, such as osteoarthritis. Pain secondary to trauma may indicate a fracture of the acetabular cavity or rim.

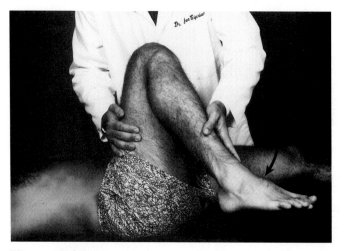

Figure 12.45

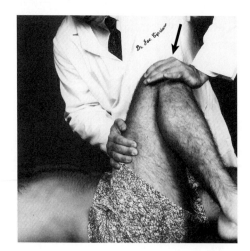

Figure 12.46

Laguerre's Test

PROCEDURE:

With the patient in the supine position, flex the hip and knee to 90 degrees. Rotate the thigh outward and rotate the knee medially. With one hand, press down on the knee, and pull up on the ankle with the other hand (Fig. 12.47).

RATIONALE:

This test externally forces the head of the femur into the acetabular cavity, stressing the anterior aspect of the joint capsule. This test may be indicative of an inflammatory process in the acetabular joint, such as osteoarthritis. Pain secondary to trauma may indicate a fracture of the acetabular cavity or rim.

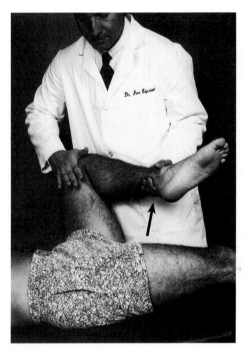

Figure 12.47

Hibb's Test

See general sacroiliac joint lesions.

TUBERCULOSIS OF THE HIP

Gauvain's Test (13,14)

PROCEDURE:

With the patient lying on his nonaffected side, grasp the ankle of the patient's affected leg and abduct the leg while rotating it externally (Fig. 12.48) and internally (Fig. 12.49). Place your superior hand on the patient's abdomen.

RATIONALE:

When you rotate the patient's foot, a reflex spasm with tightening of the abdominal musculature may be indicative of tuberculosis of the hip.

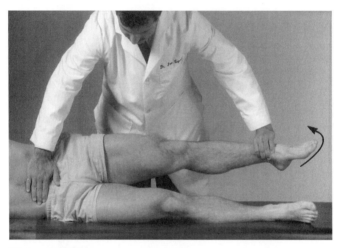

Figure 12.48

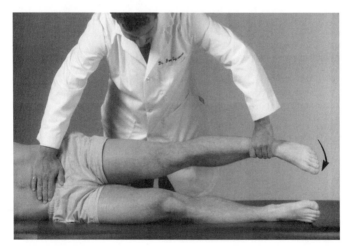

Figure 12.49

References

1. American Academy Of Orthopaedic Surgeons. The clinical measurement of joint motion. Chicago: American Academy of Orthopaedic Surgeons, 1994.
2. Boone DC, Azen SP. Normal range of motion of joints in male subjects. J Bone Joint Surg Am 1979;61:756–759.
3. Hensinger RN. Congenital dislocation of the hip. Summit, New Jersey: CIBA Clinical Symposia 1979;31(1).
4. Tachdjian MO. Pediatric orthopedics. Philadelphia: WB Saunders, 1972.
5. Magee DJ. Orthopedic physical assessment. 2nd ed. Philadelphia: WB Saunders, 1992.
6. Hoppenfeld S. Physical examination of the spine and extremities. New York: Appleton-Century-Crofts, 1976:127.
7. GrueBel-Lee DM. Disorders of the hip. Philadelphia: JB Lippincott, 1983.
8. Ober FB. The role of the iliotibial and fascia lata as a factor in the causation of low-back disabilities and sciatica. J Bone Joint Surg 1936;18:105.
9. Kenna C, Murtagh J. Patrick or Faber test. Aust Fam Physician 1989;18:375.
10. Trendelenburg F. Dtsch. Med. Wschr 21, 21-4 (R.S.M. Translation) 1895.
11. Maitland GD. The peripheral joints: examination and recording guide. Adelaide, Australia: Vergo Press, 1973.
12. Lee D. The pelvic girdle. Edinburgh: Churchill Livingstone, 1989.
13. Gauvain HJ. Tuberculosis disease of hip joint: a sign of pathological activity. Lancet 1918;2:666.
14. Gauvain HJ. The treatment and training of cases of surgical tuberculosis. J State Med 1918;26:44–50.

General References

Alderink GJ. The sacroiliac joint: review of anatomy, mechanics and function. J Orthop Sports Phys Ther 1991;13:71.

Beetham WP, Polley HF, Slocumb CH, et al. Physical examination of the joints. Philadelphia: WB Saunders, 1965.

Chung SMK. Hip disorders in infants and children. Philadelphia: Lea & Febiger, 1981.

Cyriax J. Textbook of orthopaedic medicine, 2nd ed, Vol 1. London: Bailliere Tindal, 1982.

Kapandji LA. The physiology of the joints. Vol. 2. Lower limb. New York: Churchill Livingstone, 1970.

McRae R. Clinical orthopedic examination. New York: Churchill Livingstone, 1976.

Moore KL. Clinically oriented anatomy. 2nd ed. Baltimore: Williams & Wilkins, 1992.

Noble HB, Hajek MR, Porter M. Diagnosis and treatment of iliotibial band tightness in runners. Physician Sports Med 1984;10:67.

Phillips EK. Evaluation of the hip. Phys Ther 1975;55:975–981.

Post M. Physical examination of the musculoskeletal system. Chicago: Year Book Medical Publishers, 1987.

Rydell N. Biomechanics of the hip joint. Clin Orthop 1973;92:6.

Singleton MC. The hip joint: clinical oriented anatomy—a review. Common disorders of the hip. New York: Haworth, 1986.

Wells PE. The examination of the pelvic joints. In: Grieve GP, ed. Modern manual therapy of the vertebral column. Edinburgh: Churchill Livingstone, 1986.

12

13
KNEE ORTHOPAEDIC TESTS

13

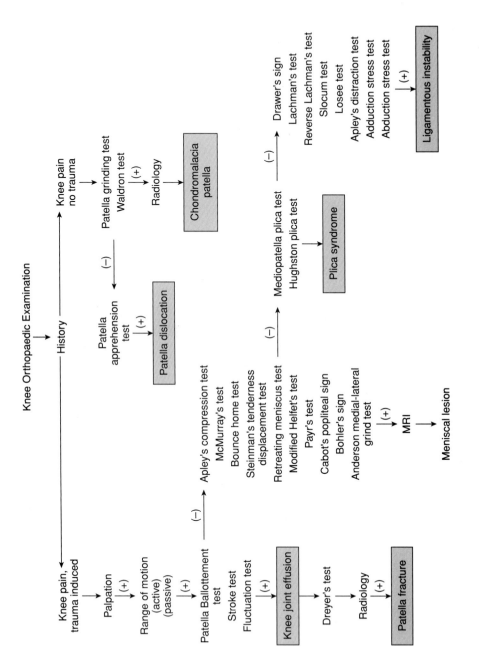

Knee Orthopaedic Examination

History

Knee pain no trauma

Patella grinding test
Waldron test

(+)

Radiology

Chondromalacia patella

(−)

Patella apprehension test

(+)

Patella dislocation

Apley's compression test
McMurray's test
Bounce home test
Steinman's tenderness displacement test
Retreating meniscus test
Modified Helfet's test
Payr's test
Cabot's popliteal sign
Bohler's sign
Anderson medial-lateral grind test

(+)

MRI

Meniscal lesion

(−)

Mediopatella plica test
Hughston plica test

Plica syndrome

(−)

Drawer's sign
Lachman's test
Reverse Lachman's test
Slocum test
Losee test
Apley's distraction test
Adduction stress test
Abduction stress test

(+)

Ligamentous instability

Knee pain, trauma induced

Palpation

(+)

Range of motion (active) (passive)

(+)

Patella Ballottement test
Stroke test
Fluctuation test

(+)

Knee joint effusion

Dreyer's test

Radiology

(+)

Patella fracture

(−)

PALPATION

Anterior Aspect

Patella, Quadriceps Femoris Tendon, and Patella Ligament

DESCRIPTIVE ANATOMY:

The patella is anchored to the anterior aspect of the knee superiorly by the suprapatellar tendon. This tendon is an extension of the quadriceps muscle and it is continued inferiorly by the patella ligament (Fig. 13.1). The patella ligament is a thick and strong ligament that is continuous with the fibrous capsule of the knee joint, and it attaches to the tibial tuberosity. These structures function as a lever to extend the leg when the quadriceps muscle contracts. These structures are located superficially and are easily palpable.

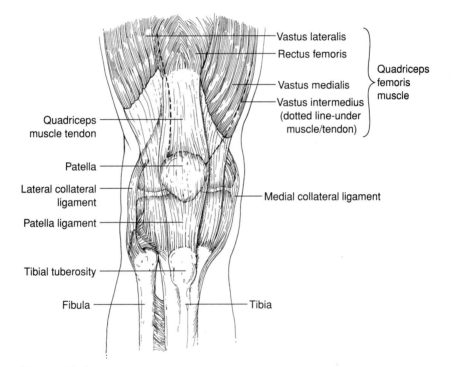

Figure 13.1

13

PROCEDURE:

With the patient supine and the knee extended, palpate the patella and its margins (Fig. 13.2). Note any tenderness, inflammation, temperature differences, and/or roughness. Tenderness and pain from direct trauma may result in a periosteal contusion or fracture of the patella. Swelling and increase in temperature may suggest a prepatellar bursitis. Roughness at the margins of the patella may indicate chondromalacia patella, which is a degeneration of the undersurface of the patella.

Next, palpate the quadriceps femoris tendon (Fig. 13.3). Tenderness may indicate tendinitis caused by overuse or strain resulting from overstress. Continue palpation inferior to the patella, which is the patella ligament. Palpate from the apex of the patella, which is the inferior margin of the patella, down to the tibial tubercle, which is the attachment of the patella ligament (Fig. 13.4). Note any pain, tenderness, swelling, or temperature differences. Any of these findings may indicate ligament strain. If symptoms are localized to the tibia tuberosity, then Osgood-Schlatter disease may be suspect in the adolescent. Osgood-Schlatter disease is an enlargement of the tibial tuberosity, which is common in young adults.

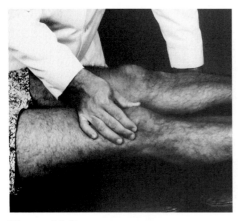

Figure 13.2

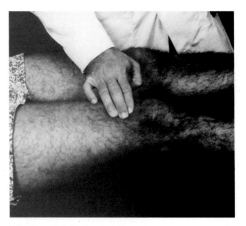

Figure 13.3

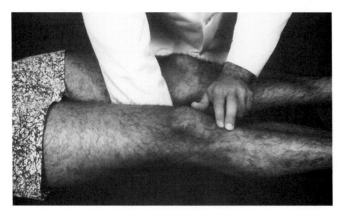

Figure 13.4

Anterior Knee Bursa

DESCRIPTIVE ANATOMY:

There are several clinically important bursa in the anterior aspect of the knee. They are: suprapatella bursa, prepatella bursa, superficial infrapatella bursa, and deep infrapatella bursa (Fig. 13.5). The suprapatella bursa is an extension of the synovial capsule and is located between the femur and the quadriceps femoris tendons. It allows for movement of the quadriceps tendon over the distal end of the femur. The prepatella bursa is located superficial to the patella between the skin and anterior surface of the patella. It allows movement of the skin over the underlying patella. The superficial infrapatella bursa is located between the tibial tuberosity and the skin. It allows for movement of the skin over the tibial tuberosity. The deep infrapatella bursa lies between the patella ligament and the tibia. This allows for movement of the patella ligament over the tibia.

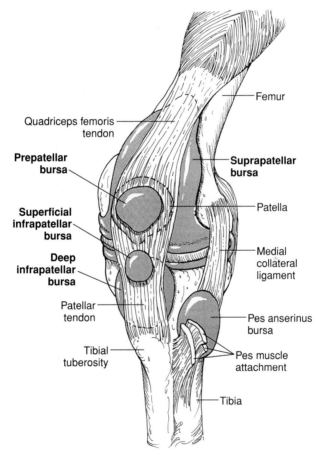

Figure 13.5

13

PROCEDURE:

Palpate the suprapatella bursa above the patella (Fig. 13.6). Note any thickening, tenderness, or temperature differences. These signs may indicate a bursitis to the suprapatella bursa or pathology to the quadriceps femoris tendon. Next, palpate the prepatella bursa, which is located superficial to the patella (Fig. 13.7). Note any thickening, swelling, tenderness, or temperature differences. These signs may indicate prepatella bursitis (Housemaid's knee). Continue palpating the superficial and deep infrapatella bursa (Fig. 13.8). Note any thickening, swelling, tenderness, or temperature differences.

Any of the following may indicate infrapatella bursitis or patella ligament pathology.

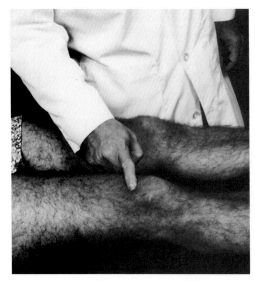

Figure 13.6

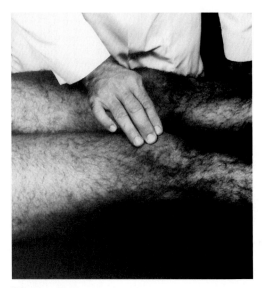

Figure 13.7

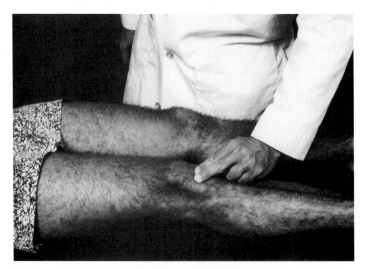

Figure 13.8

Quadriceps Femoris Muscle

DESCRIPTIVE ANATOMY:

The quadriceps femoris muscle consists of four muscles: rectus femoris, vastus lateralis, medialis, and intermedius (Fig. 13.9). The primary action of these muscles is to extend the leg at the knee joint. They all unite to form the quadriceps tendon, which inserts into the patella.

PROCEDURE:

Palpate the entire length of the quadriceps muscle, noting any swelling, tenderness, temperature differences, or masses (Fig. 13.10). Tenderness and/or swelling may indicate a muscle strain or hematoma. Point tenderness at the upper aspect of the muscle may be indicative of active trigger points and may refer pain to the knee. A hard mass secondary to trauma may indicate myositis ossificans, which is an ossification of muscle tissue.

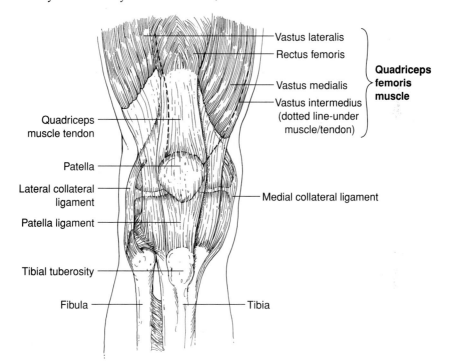

Figure 13.9

13

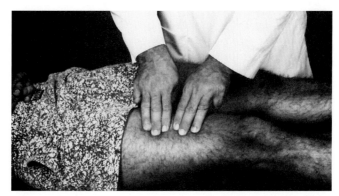

Figure 13.10

Medial Aspect

Medial Femoral Condyle, Tibial Plateau, and Joint Line

DESCRIPTIVE ANATOMY:

The medial femoral condyle is a bony prominence on the medial aspect of the distal femur, which is the attachment of the medial collateral ligament. The medial tibial plateau and joint line are important palpable landmarks of the medial aspect of the knee joint. The medial aspect of the meniscus is in the joint line, and the coronary ligament attaches the meniscus to the tibial plateau (Fig. 13.11).

PROCEDURE:

With the knee in 90 degrees of flexion, palpate the medial femoral condyle with your index and middle finger (Fig. 13.12). Note any tenderness or pain. These signs may indicate a strain, avulsion, or calcification (Pellegrini-Stieda disease) of the medial collateral ligament. Next, palpate the tibial plateau and medial joint line. Note any tenderness or pain. These signs may indicate a tear of the medial meniscus or strain of the coronary ligament.

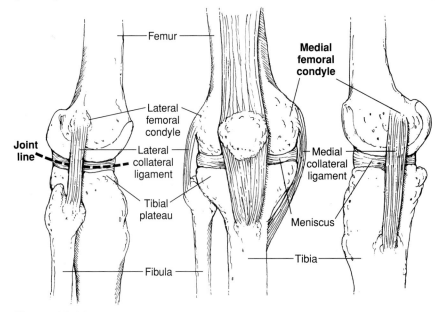

Figure 13.11

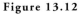
Figure 13.12

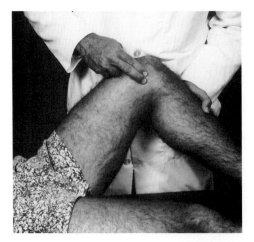

Medial Collateral Ligament

DESCRIPTIVE ANATOMY:

The medial collateral or tibial collateral ligament is a strong, broad, flat band that extends from the medial epicondyle of the femur to the medial condyle and upper medial aspect of the tibia (Fig. 13.13). It contributes to the medial stability of the knee. Its fibers are attached to the medial meniscus and the fibrous capsule of the knee.

PROCEDURE:

With the patient supine and the leg extended, palpate the medial collateral ligament from the medial epicondyle of the femur to the medial condyle of the tibia with your index and middle fingers (Fig. 13.14). Note any pain, tenderness, or defect in the ligament. Pain and tenderness may indicate a sprain of the ligament. A deficit secondary to trauma may indicate a tear of the ligament, which is usually associated with capsular and meniscal damage. A defect either at the medial femoral epicondyle or medial tibial condyle may suggest an avulsion fracture at either attachment secondary to trauma.

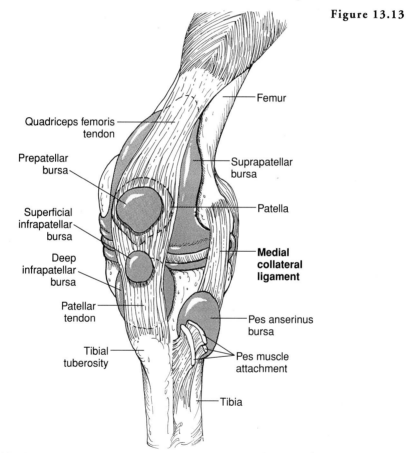

Figure 13.13

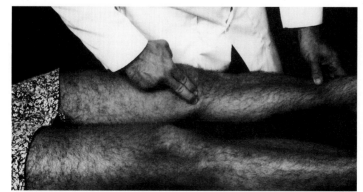

Figure 13.14

Lateral Aspect

Lateral Femoral Condyle and Joint Line

Descriptive Anatomy:

The lateral femoral condyle is a bony prominence on the lateral aspect of the distal femur, which is the attachment of the lateral collateral ligament and iliotibial band. This structure is important for the lateral stability of the knee. The lateral joint line is an important palpable landmark of the lateral aspect of the knee joint. The lateral aspect of the meniscus and the coronary ligament, which attaches the meniscus to the tibia, are in the joint line (Fig. 13.15).

Procedure:

With the knee in 90 degrees of flexion, palpate the lateral femoral condyle with your index and middle finger (Fig. 13.16). Note any tenderness or pain. These signs may indicate an strain, avulsion, or calcification of the lateral collateral ligament. Next, palpate the lateral joint line. Note any tenderness or pain. These signs may indicate a tear of the lateral meniscus or strain of the coronary ligament.

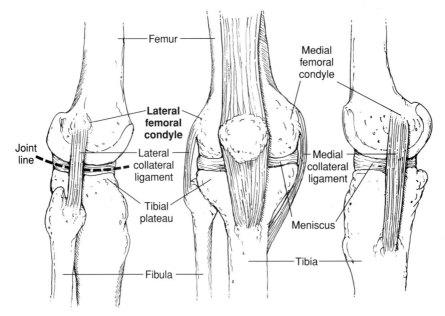

Figure 13.15

Figure 13.16

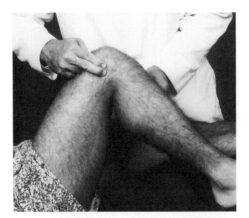

Lateral Collateral Ligament and Iliotibial Band

DESCRIPTIVE ANATOMY:

The lateral collateral ligament is a round cord that extends from the lateral epicondyle of the femur to the head of the fibula (see Fig. 13.15). This structure is important for the lateral stability of the knee. As opposed to the medial collateral ligament, the fibers are not attached to the meniscus. The tendon of the popliteus muscle passes deep to the ligament, separating it from the meniscus of the knee. The iliotibial band is a continuation of the tensor fasciae latae muscle, and it attaches to the lateral condyle of the tibia (Fig. 13.17). This band helps keep the knee extended while erect and it is important for lateral stability of the knee.

PROCEDURE:

With the patient either supine or sitting, instruct the patient to cross one leg over the other (Fig. 13.18). With your index and middle finger, palpate the lateral collateral ligament from the lateral epicondyle of the femur to the head of the fibula. Note any pain, tenderness, or defect. Pain and tenderness may indicate a strain or calcification of the ligament. A defect secondary to trauma may indicate a tear or avulsion of the lateral collateral ligament. Next, palpate the entire length of the iliotibial band from halfway between the hip and knee on the lateral aspect to the lateral condyle of the tibia (Fig. 13.19). Note any pain, tenderness, or defects of the iliotibial band. Pain and tenderness may indicate a strain of the band. A defect secondary to trauma may indicate a tear or avulsion of the band from the lateral condyle of the tibia.

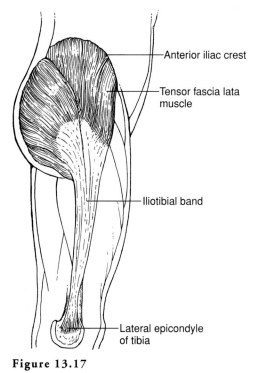

Figure 13.17

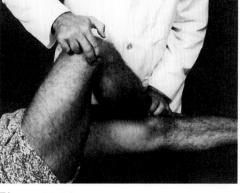

Figure 13.18

13

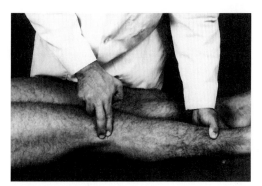

Figure 13.19

Posterior Aspect

Popliteal Fossa and Associated Structures

DESCRIPTIVE ANATOMY:

The popliteal fossa is surrounded by the biceps femoris tendon on the superior lateral border, and the tendons of the semimembranosus and semitendinosus on the superior medial border. The inferior borders are bound by the two heads of the gastrocnemius muscles. The posterior tibial nerve, popliteal artery, and vein cross the popliteal fossa (Fig. 13.20).

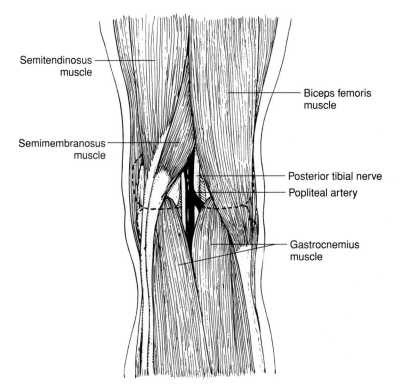

Semitendinosus muscle

Semimembranosus muscle

Biceps femoris muscle

Posterior tibial nerve

Popliteal artery

Gastrocnemius muscle

Figure 13.20

PROCEDURE:

With the knee slightly flexed, palpate the popliteal fossa for swelling or tenderness (Fig. 13.21). These signs may indicate a Baker's cyst, which is a pressure diverticulum of the synovial sac protruding through the joint capsule of the knee. Next, palpate the biceps femoris tendon (Fig. 13.22), semimembranosus tendon, semitendinosus tendon (Fig. 13.23), and both heads of the gastrocnemius muscle (Fig. 13.24) for tenderness, swelling, or continuity. This tenderness and swelling may indicate a strain of the respective tendons or muscles. Loss of continuity may indicate an avulsion of the respective muscles or tendons.

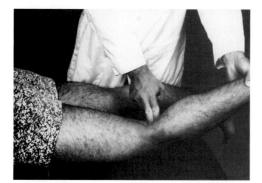

Figure 13.21

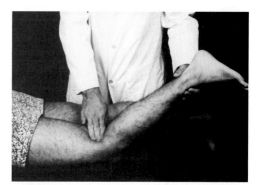

Figure 13.22

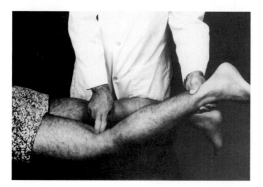

Figure 13.23

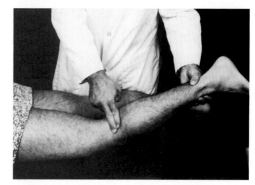

Figure 13.24

13

KNEE RANGE OF MOTION

Flexion (1)

With the patient in the prone position and the leg extended, place the goniometer in the sagittal plane with the center at the knee joint (Fig. 13.25). Instruct the patient to flex his leg as far as possible while following the leg with one arm of the goniometer (Fig. 13.26).

NORMAL RANGE (2):

141 ± 6.5 degrees or greater from the 0 or neutral position.

Muscles Involved in Action	*Nerve Supply*
1. Biceps femoris	Sciatic
2. Semimembranosus	Sciatic
3. Semitendinosus	Sciatic
4. Gracilis	Obturator
5. Sartorius	Femoral
6. Popliteus	Tibial
7. Gastrocnemius	Tibial
8. Plantaris	Superior gluteal

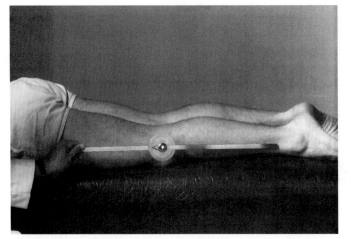

Figure 13.25

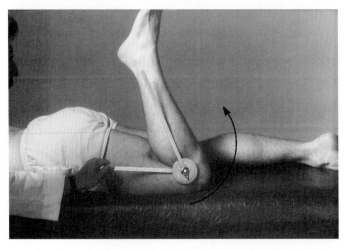

Figure 13.26

Extension (1)

With the patient in the seated position and the foot on the floor, place the goniometer in the sagittal plane with the center at the knee joint (Fig. 13.27). Instruct the patient to extend his leg as far as possible while following the leg with one arm of the goniometer (Fig. 13.28). Note that we are starting with the leg in 90 degrees of flexion and we want the knee to extend to the 0 or neutral position.

NORMAL RANGE (2):

0 to −2 degrees.

Muscles Involved in Action	Nerve Supply
1. Rectus femoris	Femoral
2. Vastus medialis	Femoral
3. Vastus intermedius	Femoral
4. Vastus lateralis	Femoral

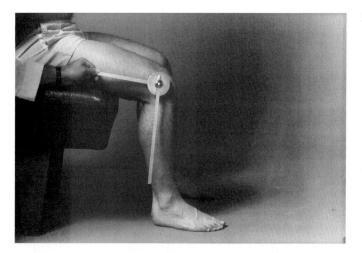

Figure 13.27

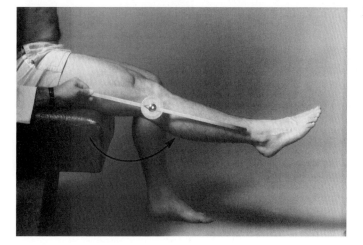

Figure 13.28

13

MENISCUS INSTABILITY

Apley's Compression Test (3)

PROCEDURE:

With the patient prone, flex his leg to 90 degrees. Stabilize the patient's thigh with your knee. Place downward pressure on the patient's heel while you internally (Fig. 13.29) and externally (Fig. 13.30) rotate the foot.

NOTE:

If the patient also has an ankle injury, grasp the distal aspect of the leg and internally and externally rotate the leg with downward pressure. This modified maneuver is performed to avoid further ankle injury.

RATIONALE:

The meniscus, which are asymmetric fibrocartilaginous disks, separate the tibial condyles from the femoral condyles. When the knee is flexed, the meniscus distorts to maintain the congruence between the tibial and femoral condyles. By flexing the knee, downward pressure with internal and external rotation stress is applied to the already distorted meniscus. Pain on either side of the knee is indicative of a meniscus injury on the respective side.

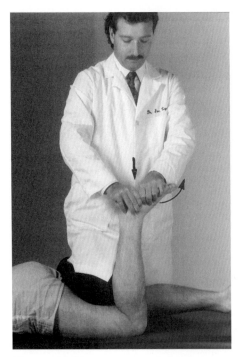

Figure 13.29

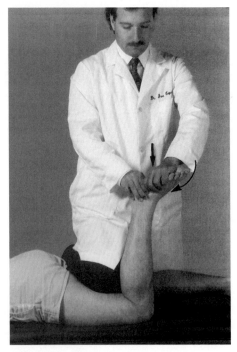

Figure 13.30

McMurray's Test (4)

PROCEDURE:

With the patient in the supine position, flex his leg (Fig. 13.31). Externally rotate the leg as you extend (Fig. 13.32); internally rotate as you extend (Fig. 13.33).

RATIONALE:

Flexion and extension of the knee distorts the meniscus to maintain the congruence between the tibial and femoral condyles. Flexing and extending the knee with an internal and external rotation stress further stresses the already distorted meniscus. A palpable or audible click is indicative of an injury of the meniscus.

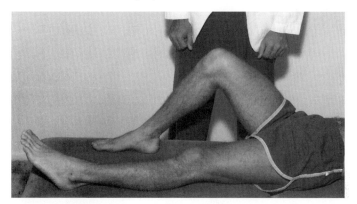

Figure 13.31

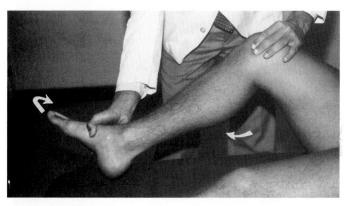

Figure 13.32

13

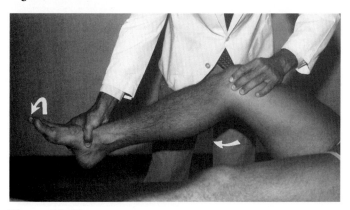

Figure 13.33

Bounce Home Test (5)

PROCEDURE:

With the patient in the supine position, instruct the patient to flex his leg. When the leg is flexed, cup your hand around the patient's heel (Fig. 13.34) and instruct him to passively extend his knee (Fig. 13.35).

RATIONALE:

Extension of the knee involves the medial rotation of the femur on the tibia. If injury to the meniscus has occurred, rotation of the femur on the tibia may be blocked and the patient may not be able to fully extend his knee. If the end feel is rubberlike on full extension, this is also a sign of a positive test.

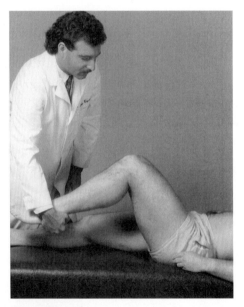

Figure 13.34

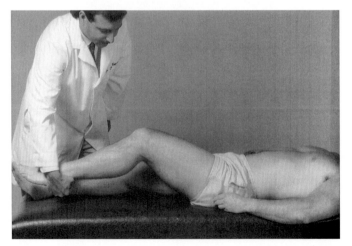

Figure 13.35

Steinman's Tenderness Displacement Test (6)

PROCEDURE:

With the patient in the supine position, flex the patient's hip and knee to 90 degrees. Place your thumb and index finger on the medial and lateral knee joint lines, respectively (Fig. 13.36). With your opposite hand, grasp the patient's ankle and alternately flex and extend the knee while palpating the entire joint line (Fig. 13.37).

RATIONALE:

When the knee is extended, the meniscus moves anteriorly, and when the knee is flexed, the meniscus moves posteriorly. If the pain seems to move anteriorly when the knee is extended or posteriorly when the knee is flexed, then a tear or injury of the meniscus is suspect.

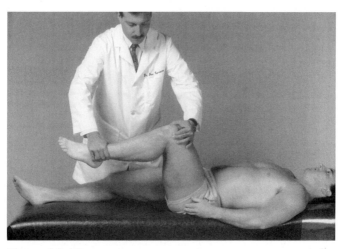

Figure 13.36

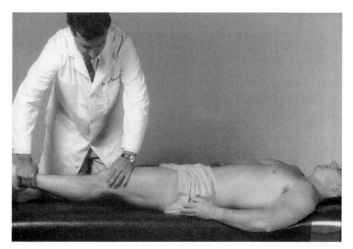

13

Figure 13.37

Retreating Meniscus Test (7)

PROCEDURE:

With the patient in the supine position and the patient's hip and leg flexed to 90 degrees, palpate the meniscus on the medial joint line anterior to the medial collateral ligament. With your opposite hand, rotate the leg medially and laterally while noting if the meniscus that you are palpating is still present or has disappeared (Figs. 13.38, 13.39).

RATIONALE:

When the knee is flexed to 90 degrees, the femur should rotate medially on the tibia. If the meniscus does not disappear while rotating the leg, then a torn meniscus is suspect because rotation of the tibia is blocked.

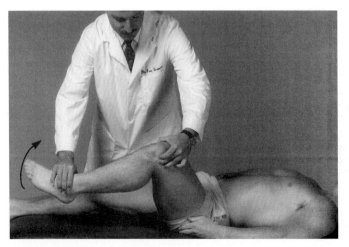

Figure 13.38

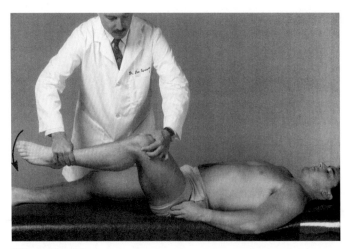

Figure 13.39

Modified Helfet's Test (7)

PROCEDURE:

With the patient in the seated position and his foot on the floor, note the location of the tibial tuberosity in relation to the midline (Fig. 13.40). Passively extend the patient's leg and again note the location of the tibial tuberosity in relation to the patella (Fig. 13.41).

RATIONALE:

In the normal knee, the tibial tuberosity is at the midline when the knee is in 90 degrees of flexion. When the knee is extended, the tibial tuberosity moves in line with the lateral border on the patella. If this does not occur, then a tear of the meniscus is suspect because rotation of the tibia is blocked.

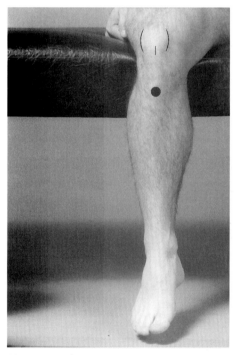

Figure 13.40

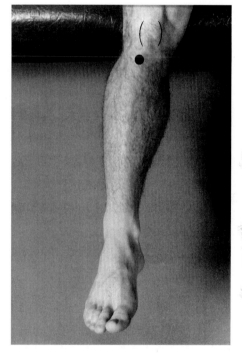

Figure 13.41

13

Payr's Test (8)

PROCEDURE:

With the patient in the supine position, abduct the patient's hip and have the patient cross his leg in the "Figure 4" position (Fig. 13.42). With one hand, grasp the ankle and pull it in a superior direction. With the opposite hand, palpate the medial joint line (Fig. 13.43).

RATIONALE:

By placing the knee in the "Figure 4" position, stress is applied to the medial and posterior part of the meniscus. Pain in the medial aspect of the knee may indicate a medial or posterior meniscal tear.

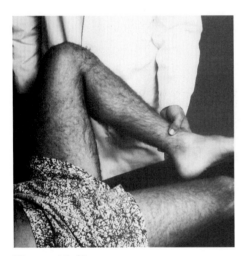

Figure 13.42

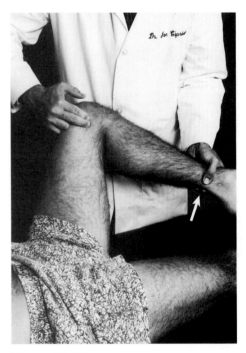

Figure 13.43

Cabot's Popliteal Sign (8)

PROCEDURE:

With the patient in the supine position, instruct the patient to abduct his thigh and cross the leg of the affected knee (Fig. 13.44). Grasp the ankle with one hand, and with the other hand palpate the joint line with your thumb and index finger (Fig. 13.45). Ask the patient to isometrically straighten out the knee against examiner resistance.

RATIONALE:

Resisting extension of the knee in the "Figure 4" position stresses the meniscus. Pain on the joint line indicates a tear or pathology of the meniscus.

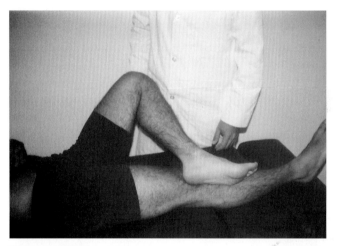

Figure 13.44

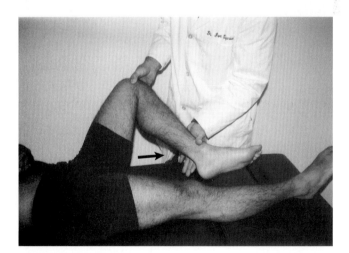

Figure 13.45

13

Bohler's Sign (8)

PROCEDURE:

With the patient in the supine position, stabilize the medial thigh with one hand and place a valgus force on the lateral aspect of the leg with your opposite hand (Fig. 13.46). Next, stabilize the lateral knee and place a varus force on the medial aspect of the leg (Fig. 13.47).

RATIONALE:

Placing a lateral or medial pressure on the knee distracts the joint capsule and meniscus on the opposite side of the pressure. Pain on the opposite side of joint pressure may indicate a lesion of the joint capsule or meniscus.

NOTE:

This test is similar to the adduction and abduction stress test for collateral ligament defect. If this test is positive, evaluate for collateral ligament defect opposite the side of pressure.

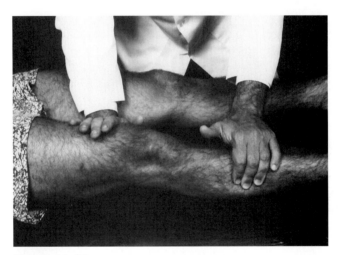

Figure 13.46

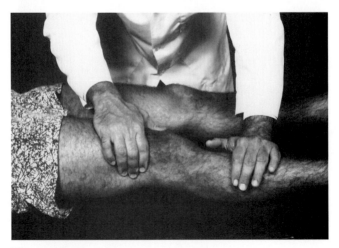

Figure 13.47

Anderson Medial-Lateral Grind Test (9)

PROCEDURE:

With the patient in the supine position, grasp the leg of the affected knee and place it between your trunk and arm. With your opposite thumb and index finger, palpate the anterior lateral and medial joint lines. Place a valgus stress on the knee as it is flexed passively (Fig. 13.48) and a varus stress on the knee as the knee is extended passively (Fig. 13.49). This movement should be circular, and valgus and varus stresses should be increased after each complete circle.

RATIONALE:

This movement stresses the meniscus on the medial side with valgus stress and on the lateral side with varum stress. Pain and/or grinding on movement may indicate a meniscus tear or pathology.

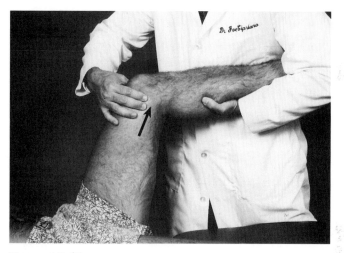

Figure 13.48

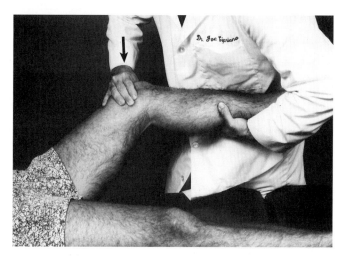

Figure 13.49

13

PLICA TESTS

Mediopatella Plica Test (10)

PROCEDURE:

With the patient in the supine position, flex the affected leg to 30 degrees. With the other hand, move the patella medially (Fig. 13.50).

RATIONALE:

Moving the patella medially with the leg in 30 degrees of flexion causes the plica to be pinched between the medial femoral condyle and the patella. Pain may indicate that the plica is attached to the patella and is inflamed. The plica is the remnant of an embryonic septum that makes up the knee joint capsule.

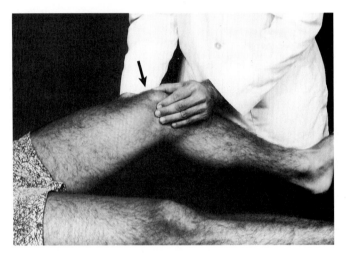

Figure 13.50

Hughston Plica Test (11)

PROCEDURE:

With the patient in the supine position, grasp the patient's leg. Flex and medially rotate the leg. With your opposite hand, move the patella medially with the heel of your hand and palpate the medial femoral condyle with the fingers of the same hand (Fig. 13.51). Flex and extend the knee while feeling for "popping" of the plical band under your fingers (Fig. 13.52).

RATIONALE:

Popping underneath your fingers may indicate that the plica may be attached to the patella and may be inflamed. The incidence of patella plica varies from 18% to 60% of the population according to different authors.

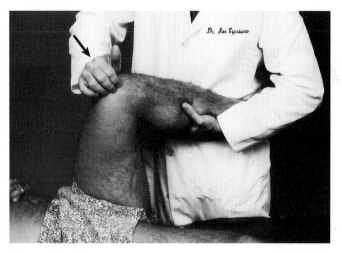

Figure 13.51

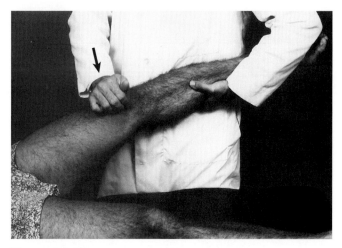

Figure 13.52

13

LIGAMENTOUS INSTABILITY

Drawer's Sign (12,13)

PROCEDURE:

With the patient in the supine position, flex the leg and place the foot on the table (Fig. 13.53). Grasp behind the flexed knee and exert a pulling (Fig. 13.54) and pushing (Fig. 13.55) pressure on the leg. The hamstring tendons must be relaxed to perform this test accurately.

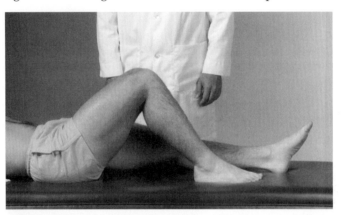

Figure 13.53

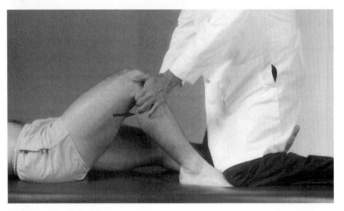

Figure 13.54

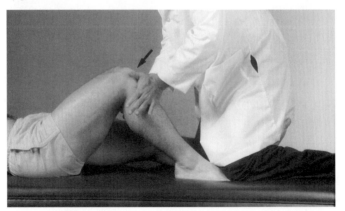

Figure 13.55

RATIONALE:

If there is more than 5 mm of tibial movement on the femur when the leg is pulled, an injury of some degree to one or more of the following structures is indicated:

1. Anterior cruciate ligament (Fig.13.56)
2. Posterolateral capsule
3. Posteromedial capsule
4. Medial collateral ligament (if more than 1 cm of movement)
5. Iliotibial band
6. Posterior oblique ligament
7. Arcuate-popliteus complex

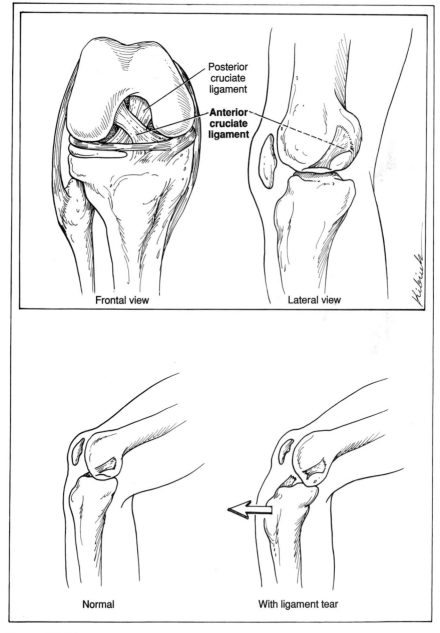

Figure 13.56

If excessive movement occurs when the leg is pushed, an injury to one of the following structures is indicated:

1. Posterior cruciate ligament (Fig. 13.57)
2. Arcuate-popliteus complex
3. Posterior oblique ligament
4. Anterior cruciate ligament

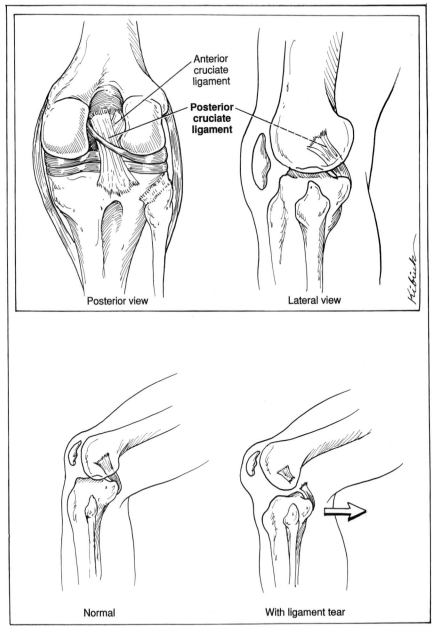

Figure 13.57

Lachman's Test (14)

PROCEDURE:

With the patient in the supine position and the knee in 30 degrees of flexion, grasp the patient's thigh with one hand to stabilize it. With the opposite hand, grasp the tibia and pull it forward (Fig. 13.58).

RATIONALE:

If a softened feel and anterior translation of the tibia is present when the tibia is moved forward, then instability of any of the following ligaments is suspect:

1. Anterior cruciate ligament
2. Posterior oblique ligament

This is the most reliable test for anterior cruciate ligament rupture because the knee does not need to flex to 90 degrees like the anterior drawer sign, there is less meniscal impingement, and the hamstrings are less likely to spasm.

Figure 13.58

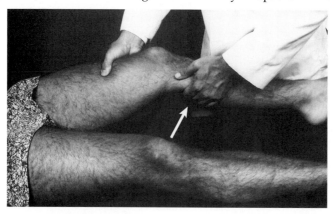

Reverse Lachman's Test (8)

PROCEDURE:

With the patient in the prone position, flex the leg to 30 degrees. With one hand, stabilize the posterior thigh, making sure that the hamstring muscles are relaxed. With your opposite hand, grasp the tibia and push it in a posterior direction (Fig. 13.59).

RATIONALE:

By placing a posterior pressure on the tibia, the posterior cruciate ligament is stressed. A soft end-feel and a posterior translation of the tibia indicates an injury to the posterior cruciate ligament.

Figure 13.59

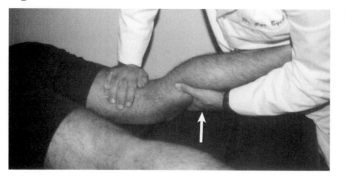

Slocum Test (15)

PROCEDURE:

With the patient in the supine position, place the patient's foot on the examination table in 30 degrees of internal rotation. Stabilize the patient's foot with your knee, grasp the tibia with your hand, and pull the tibia towards you (Fig. 13.60).

RATIONALE:

This test is similar to an anterior drawer's sign except, in this test, the foot is in 30 degrees of internal rotation. If tibial translation and a soft end-feel exists when the tibia is drawn forward, then suspect instability of any of the following ligaments:

1. Anterior cruciate
2. Posterolateral capsule
3. Fibular collateral ligament
4. Posterior cruciate ligament
5. Iliotibial band

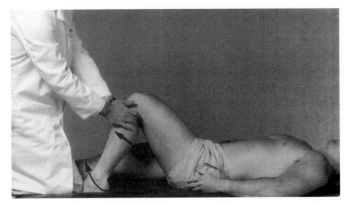

Figure 13.60

Losee Test (16)

PROCEDURE:

With the patient in the supine position, grasp the patient's leg with one hand, externally rotate it, and brace it against your abdomen. Flex the leg 30 degrees to relax the hamstring muscles (Fig. 13.61). With your opposite hand, grasp the knee with your thumb behind the fibular head and your fingers over the patella. Place a valgus force against the lateral aspect of the knee and a forward pressure behind the fibular head while extending the knee (Fig. 13.62).

RATIONALE:

By externally rotating the leg in 30 degrees of flexion and applying a valgus force, the structure in the lateral compartment of the knee is compressed. This compression may accentuate an anterior subluxation of the tibia. While extending the knee and applying a valgus force, look for a palpable "clunk." This clunk may indicate an anterior subluxation of the tibia, which is a reproduction of the patient's previous instability experience. It indicates injury to one or more of the following structures:

1. Anterior cruciate ligament
2. Posterolateral joint capsule
3. Arcuate-popliteus complex
4. Lateral collateral ligament
5. Iliotibial band

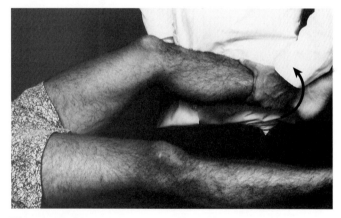

Figure 13.61

13

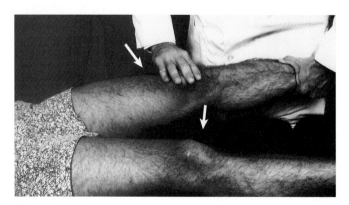

Figure 13.62

Apley's Distraction Test (17)

PROCEDURE:

With the patient in the prone position, flex his leg to 90 degrees. Stabilize the patient's thigh with your knee. Pull on the patient's foot while internally (Fig. 13.63) and externally (Fig. 13.64) rotating the leg.

NOTE:

If the patient also has an ankle injury, grasp the distal aspect of the leg and internally and externally rotate the leg with upward pressure. This modified maneuver is performed to avoid further ankle injury.

RATIONALE:

Distraction of the knee takes pressure off the meniscus and puts strain on the medial and lateral collateral ligaments. Pain on distraction is indicative of nonspecific ligament injury or instability.

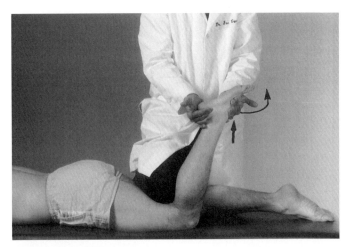

Figure 13.63

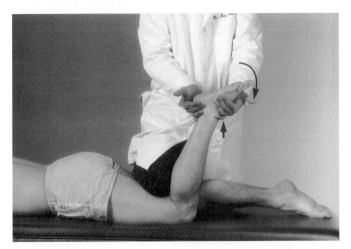

Figure 13.64

Adduction Stress Test (5)

PROCEDURE:

With the patient in the supine position, stabilize the medial thigh. The examiner grasps the leg and pushes it medially (Fig. 13.65). Also perform this test with the knee in 20 to 30 degrees of flexion (Fig. 13.66).

RATIONALE:

If the tibia moves an excessive amount away from the femur (see medial stability rating scale) (Fig. 13.67) when the knee is in full extension, there may be instability of any of the following ligaments:

1. Tibial collateral ligament
2. Posterior meniscofemoral ligament
3. Posterior medial capsule
4. Anterior cruciate ligament
5. Posterior cruciate ligament

If the foregoing is positive when the knee is flexed 20 to 30 degrees, then any of the following ligaments may be unstable:

1. Tibial collateral ligament
2. Posterior meniscofemoral ligament
3. Posterior cruciate ligament

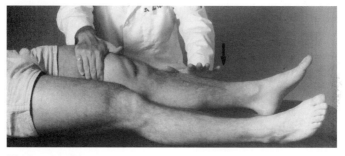

Figure 13.65

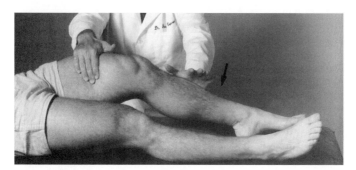

Figure 13.66

13

Grade 0 = no joint opening
Grade 1+ = less than 0.5cm joint opening
Grade 2+ = 0.5 to 1.0cm joint opening
Grade 3+ = more than 1 cm joint opening

Figure 13.67   Medial Stability Rating Scale.

Abduction Stress Test (5)

PROCEDURE:

With the patient in the supine position, stabilize the lateral thigh. Grasp the leg and pull it laterally (Fig. 13.68). Then perform this test in 20 to 30 degrees of flexion (Fig. 13.69).

RATIONALE:

If the tibia moves an excessive amount away from the femur (see lateral instability rating scale) (Fig. 13.70) when the knee is in full extension, there may be instability of any of the following ligaments:

1. Fibular collateral ligament
2. Posterolateral capsule
3. Posterior cruciate ligament
4. Anterior cruciate ligament

If the foregoing is positive when the knee is flexed 20 to 30 degrees, then the following ligaments may be unstable:

1. Fibular collateral ligament
2. Posterolateral capsule
3. Iliotibial band

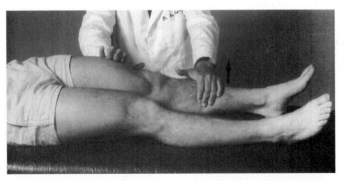

Figure 13.68

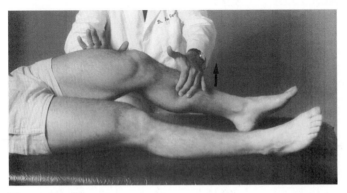

Figure 13.69

Grade 0 = no joint opening
Grade 1+ = less than 0.5cm joint opening
Grade 2+ = 0.5 to 1.0cm joint opening
Grade 3+ = more than 1cm joint opening

Figure 13.70   Lateral Stability Rating Scale.

PATELLA TESTS

Patella Grinding Test

PROCEDURE:

With the patient in the supine position, move the patella medially and laterally while exerting downward pressure (Fig. 13.71).

RATIONALE:

Pain under the patella is indicative of either chondromalacia patella, retropatellar arthritis, or a chondral fracture. Osteochondritis of the patella will also elicit pain on the patella. Pain over the patella may indicate prepatella bursitis.

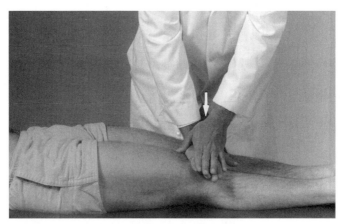

Figure 13.71

Patella Apprehension Test (17)

PROCEDURE:

With the patient in the supine position, manually displace the patella laterally (Fig. 13.72).

RATIONALE:

A look of apprehension on the patient's face and a contraction of the quadriceps muscle indicates a chronic tendency toward frequent lateral patella dislocation. Pain also is accompanied with this test.

13

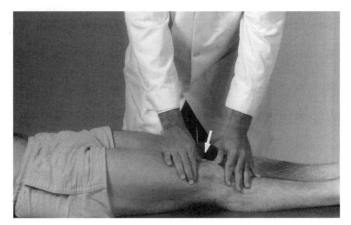

Figure 13.72

Dreyer's Test

PROCEDURE:

With the patient in the supine position, instruct him to raise his leg actively (Fig. 13.73). If the patient is unable to raise the leg, stabilize the quadriceps tendon just above the knee. At this point, instruct the patient to raise his leg again (Fig. 13.74).

RATIONALE:

If the patient is able to raise his leg the second time, suspect a fracture of the patella secondary to trauma. The rectus femoris muscle, which is a primary hip flexor, is attached to the patella by the quadriceps tendon. If the patella is fractured, the quadriceps tendon is not stabilized. By stabilizing the quadriceps tendon manually, hip flexion can occur.

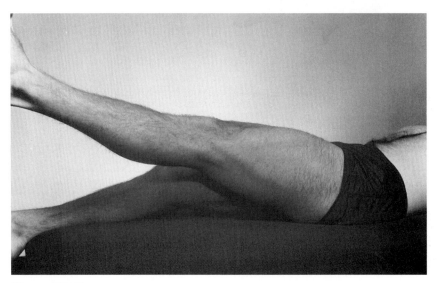

Figure 13.73

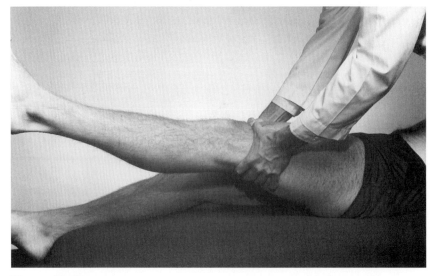

Figure 13.74

Waldron Test (18)

PROCEDURE:

Instruct the patient to perform several slow deep knee bends while you palpate the patella (Fig. 13.75).

RATIONALE:

Upon deep knee bending, the patella slides on the femoral condyles while being seated upon them. If pain and crepitus occur simultaneously, then chondromalacia patella is suspect.

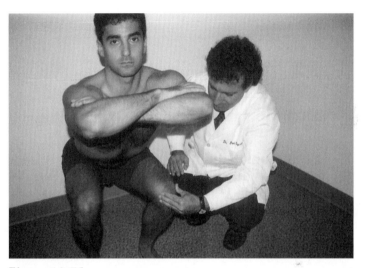

Figure 13.75

13

KNEE JOINT EFFUSION

Patella Ballottement Test

PROCEDURE:

With one hand, encircle and place downward pressure above the superior aspect of the patella. With the other hand, push the patella against the femur with your finger (Fig. 13.76).

RATIONALE:

If fluid is present in the knee, the patella will elevate when pressure is applied. When the patella is pushed down, it will strike the femur with a palpable tap.

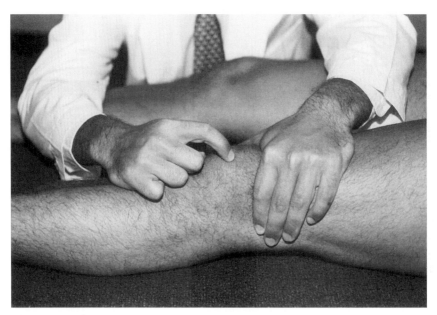

Figure 13.76

Stroke Test (5)

PROCEDURE:

With the patient in the supine position, stroke the medial side of the patella upward toward the suprapatellar pouch two or three times with your fingers and simultaneously stroke the lateral aspect of the patella downward with your opposite hand (Fig. 13.77).

RATIONALE:

If a wave of synovial fluid is present, it will concentrate to the inferior medial border of the patella; subsequently, the area will be bulged.

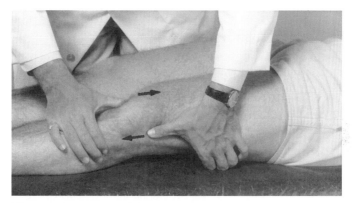

Figure 13.77

Fluctuation Test (5)

PROCEDURE:

With the patient in the supine position, grasp the thigh at the suprapatella pouch with one hand and grasp the leg just below the patella with your opposite hand (Fig. 13.78). Alternately, place downward pressure with each hand.

RATIONALE:

If synovial fluid is present, you will feel it fluctuate alternately under your hand. This fluctuation indicates significant joint effusion.

13

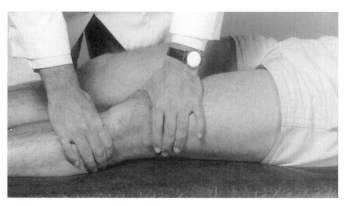

Figure 13.78

References

1. American Academy of Orthopaedic Surgeons. The clinical measurement of joint motion. Chicago: American Academy of Orthopaedic Surgeons, 1994.
2. Boone DC, Azen SP. Normal range of motion of the joints in male subjects. J Bone Joint Surg Am 1979;61:756–759.
3. Apley AG. The diagnosis of meniscus injuries: some new clinical methods. J Bone Joint Surg 1947;29:78.
4. McMurray TP. The semilunar cartilages. Br J Surg 1942;29:407.
5. McGee DJ. Orthopedic physical assessment. 2nd ed. Philadelphia: WB Saunders, 1992.
6. Ricklin P, Ruttiman A, Del Buono MS. Meniscal lesions: diagnosis, differential diagnosis, and therapy. 2nd ed. Mieller NH, trans. New York: Theme Stratton, 1983.
7. Helfet A. Disorders of the knee. Philadelphia: JB Lippincott, 1974.
8. Strobel M, Stedtfeld HW. Diagnostic evaluation of the knee. Berlin: Springer-Verlag, 1990.
9. Anderson AF, Lipscomb AB. Clinical diagnosis of meniscal tears—description of a new manipulative test. Am J Sports Med 1988;14:291.
10. Mital MA, Hayden J. Pain in the knee in children: the medial plica shelf syndrome. Orthop Clin North Am 1979;10:713.
11. Houghston JC, Walsh WM, Puddu G. Patella subluxation and dislocation. Philadelphia: WB Saunders, 1984.
12. Butler DL, Noyes FR, Grood ES. Ligamentous restraints to anterior-posterior drawer in the human knee. J Bone Joint Surg Am 1980;62:259.
13. Fukybayashi T, Torzilli PA, Sherman MF, et al. An in vitro biomechanical evaluation of anterior posterior motion of the knee. J Bone Joint Surg Br 1972;54:763.
14. Jonsson TB, Althoff L, Peterson J, et al. Clinical diagnosis of ruptures of the anterior cruciate ligament: a comparative study of the Lachman test and the anterior drawer sign. Am J Sports Med 1982;10:100.
15. Slocum DB, James SL, Larson RL, et al. A clinical test for anterolateral rotary instability of the knee. Clin Orthop 1976;118;63.
16. Loose RE, Jenning TR, Southwich WO. Anterior subluxation of the lateral tibial plateau: a diagnostic test and operative review. J Bone Joint Surg Am 1978;60:1015.
17. Hoppenfeld S. Physical examination of the spine and extremities. New York: Appleton-Century-Crofts, 1976:127.
18. Waldron VD. A test for chondromalacia patella. Orthop Rev 1983;12:103.

General References

Bloom MH. Differentiating between meniscal and patellar pain. Phy Sports Med 1989;17(8):95–108.

Butler DL, Noyes FR, Grood ES. Ligamentous restraints to anterior-posterior drawer in the human knee. J Bone Joint Surg Am 1980;62:259.

Cailliet R. Knee pain and disability. Philadelphia: FA Davis Co, 1973.

Cipriano J. Post traumatic knee injuries. Today's Chiropractic 1985;13(5):49–51.

Clancy WG. Evaluation of acute knee injuries. American Association of Orthopedic Surgeons. Symposium on sports medicine: the knee. St. Louis: Mosby, 1985.

Clancy WG, Keene JS, Goletz TH. The symptomatic dislocation of the anterior horn of the medial meniscus. Am J Sports Med 1984;12:57–64.

Cyriax J. Textbook of orthopaedic medicine. Vol. 1. Diagnosis of soft tissue lesions. London: Bailliere Tindall, 1982.

Frankel VH, Burstein AH, Brooks DB. Biomechanics of internal derangement of the knee. J Bone Joint Surg Am 1971;53:945.

Hardaker WT, Whipple TL, Bassett FH. Diagnosis and treatment of the plica syndrome of the knee. J Bone Joint Surg Am 1980;62:221–255.

Johnson T, Althoff B, Peterson L, et al. Clinical diagnosis of ruptures of the anterior cruciate ligament: a comparative study of the Lachman test and the anterior drawer sign. Am J Sports Med 1982;10:100.

Kapandji LA. The physiology of the joints. Vol. 2. Lower limb. New York: Churchill Livingstone, 1970.

Katz KW, Fingeroth RF. The diagnostic accuracy of ruptures of the anterior cruciate ligament comparing the Lachman test, the anterior drawer sign and the pivot shift test in acute and chronic knee injuries. Am J Sports Med 1986;14:88.

Nottage WM, Sprague NF, Auerbach BJ, et al. The medial patellar plica syndrome. Am J Sports Med 1983;11:211–214.

Pickett JC, Radin EL. Chondromalacia of the patella. Baltimore: Williams & Wilkins, 1983.

Slocum DB, Larson RL. Rotary instability of the knee. J Bone Joint Surg Am 1968;50:211.

Stickland A. Examination of the knee joint. Physiotherapy 1984;70:144.

Torg JS, Conrad W, Nalen V. Clinical diagnosis of anterior cruciate ligament instability in the athlete. Am J Sports Med 1976;4:84.

14
Ankle Orthopaedic Tests

14

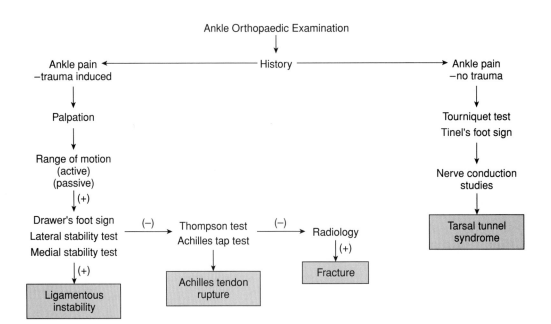

PALPATION

Medial Aspect

Medial Malleolus and Deltoid Ligament

DESCRIPTIVE ANATOMY:

The medial malleolus is a distal-most prominence of the tibia. It embraces the medial aspect of the talus and gives the ankle joint bony stability. Attached to the malleolus is the strong deltoid ligament that connects with three tarsal bones: the talus, navicular, and calcaneus. This ligament is a four-part ligament that is named according to its attachments: tibionavicular, anterior and posterior tibiotalar, and tibiocalcaneal (Fig. 14.1). The deltoid ligament strengthens and provides medial stability to the ankle joint and holds the calca-neus and navicular bones against the talus. A common injury is a forceful eversion of the foot that causes an avulsion fracture of the deltoid ligament on the medial malleolus.

PROCEDURE:

With the patient either supine or nonweight-bearing, palpate the medial malleolus and deltoid ligament for tenderness and/or swelling (Fig. 14.2). Tenderness and/or swelling secondary to trauma may indicate periosteal contusion, strain, or avulsion of the deltoid ligament.

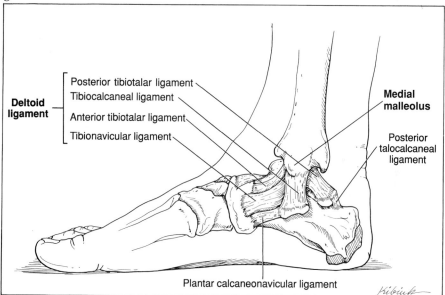

Deltoid ligament
- Posterior tibiotalar ligament
- Tibiocalcaneal ligament
- Anterior tibiotalar ligament
- Tibionavicular ligament

Medial malleolus

Posterior talocalcaneal ligament

Plantar calcaneonavicular ligament

Figure 14.1

14

Figure 14.2

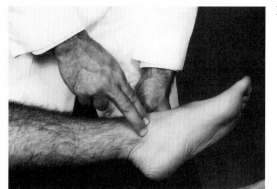

Tibialis Posterior, Flexor Digitorum Longus, and Flexor Hallucis Longus Tendons

DESCRIPTIVE ANATOMY:

The posterior tibial tendon passes medial to the medial malleolus and inserts into the tuberosity of the navicular bone (Fig. 14.3). The action of the muscle and tendon is to plantar flex the ankle and evert the foot. The flexor digitorum longus tendon is posterior to the posterior tibial tendon and closely follows the tibia, and it passes behind the medial malleolus (Fig. 14.3). It inserts into the distal phalanges of the lateral four digits. The action of the muscle and tendon is to plantar flex the ankle and flex all the joints of the last four toes. The flexor hallucis longus tendon is posterior to the flexor digitorum longus tendon, and it passes behind the ankle joint, not posterior to the medial malleolus. It inserts into the base of the distal phalanx of the great toe (Fig. 14.3). Its action is to flex the great toe.

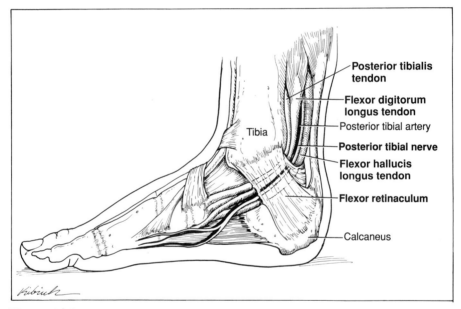

Figure 14.3

Procedure:

To palpate the tibialis posterior tendon, invert and plantar flex the patient's foot. Palpate medial to the tibia around the medial malleolus (Fig. 14.4). Note the continuity of the tendon and any tenderness or swelling. Tenderness and/or swelling may indicate a strain secondary to trauma or tendinitis of the tendon. Loss of continuity and a valgus foot secondary to trauma may indicate a ruptured tendon.

Palpate the flexor digitorum longus tendon, which is posterior to the tibialis posterior tendon. With one hand, resist flexion of the patient's toes, and with the other hand palpate the tendon (Fig. 14.5). Note any tenderness, swelling, or crepitus. These signs may indicate a strain or tendinitis of the tendon.

The flexor hallucis longus tendon is not palpable and will not be described.

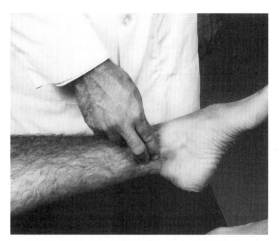

Figure 14.4

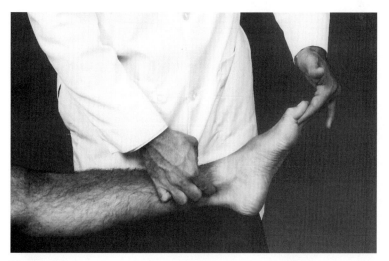

Figure 14.5

14

Posterior Tibial Artery and Tibial Nerve

DESCRIPTIVE ANATOMY:

The posterior tibial artery is located between the tendons of the flexor digitorum longus and flexor hallucis longus muscles. This artery is the major blood supply to the foot. The tibial nerve is a branch of the sciatic nerve. It runs with the posterior tibial artery underneath the flexor retinaculum of the ankle and posterior to the medial malleolus (Fig. 14.6). The flexor retinaculum may become constricted and cause a neurovascular deficit to the foot similar to carpal tunnel in the wrist.

PROCEDURE:

Using light pressure with your middle and index finger, palpate the posterior tibial artery (Fig. 14.7). Note the amplitude and compare bilaterally. A decrease in the pulse amplitude may indicate a compression of the posterior tibial artery. The tibial nerve is difficult at best to palpate and will not be discussed. It is an important nerve supply to the sole of the foot.

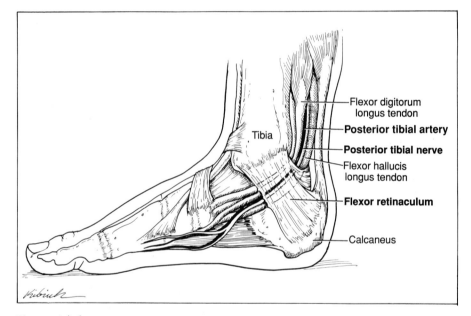

Figure 14.6

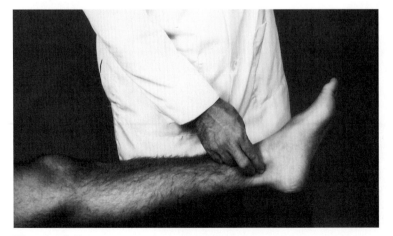

Figure 14.7

338

Lateral Aspect

Lateral Malleolus and Attached Ligaments

DESCRIPTIVE ANATOMY:

The lateral malleolus is the protuberance at the distal end of the fibula. Attached to the malleolus are three clinically important ligaments. They are as follows:

1. Anterior talofibular ligament
2. Calcaneofibular ligament
3. Posterior talofibular ligament

These ligaments provide lateral support to the ankle but they are not as strong as the deltoid ligament on the medial aspect (Fig. 14.8). These ligaments are prone to defects in inversion injuries.

PROCEDURE:

Palpate the lateral malleolus with your index and middle fingers (Fig. 14.9). Note any tenderness and/or swelling. These signs may indicate periosteal contusion, fracture, avulsion fracture, or inversion sprain of any of the previously mentioned ligaments secondary to trauma.

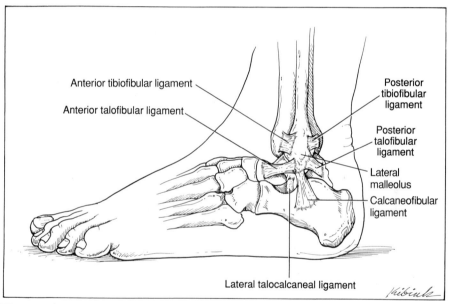

Anterior tibiofibular ligament

Anterior talofibular ligament

Posterior tibiofibular ligament

Posterior talofibular ligament

Lateral malleolus

Calcaneofibular ligament

Lateral talocalcaneal ligament

Figure 14.8

14

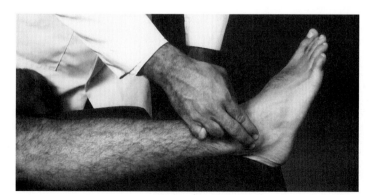

Figure 14.9

Peroneus Longus and Brevis Tendons

DESCRIPTIVE ANATOMY:

The peroneus tendons travel together behind the lateral malleolus and are held in place by the peroneal retinaculum (Fig. 14.10). The action of the muscles and tendons are to evert the foot.

PROCEDURE:

With the patient in non-weight bearing position, palpate behind the lateral malleolus with one hand, and passively invert (Fig. 14.11) and evert (Fig. 14.12) the foot with the other hand. Note any tenderness, swelling, or snapping. Tenderness and/or swelling may indicate a tenosynovitis of either or both tendons. Tenderness with snapping may indicate a defect of the peroneal retinaculum that causes the peroneal tendons to subluxate or dislocate.

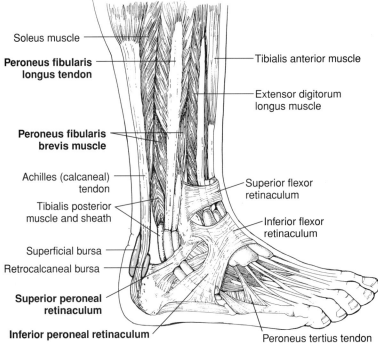

Soleus muscle

Peroneus fibularis longus tendon

Tibialis anterior muscle

Extensor digitorum longus muscle

Peroneus fibularis brevis muscle

Achilles (calcaneal) tendon

Tibialis posterior muscle and sheath

Superficial bursa

Retrocalcaneal bursa

Superior peroneal retinaculum

Inferior peroneal retinaculum

Superior flexor retinaculum

Inferior flexor retinaculum

Peroneus tertius tendon

Figure 14.10

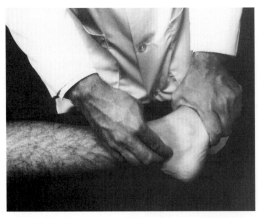

Figure 14.11

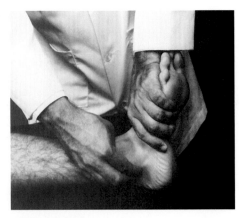

Figure 14.12

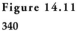

Anterior Aspect

Tibialis Anterior, Extensor Hallucis Longus, and Extensor Digitorum Longus Tendons

DESCRIPTIVE ANATOMY:

The tibialis anterior tendon lies against the anterior surface of the tibia under the extensor retinaculum. It attaches to the medial cuneiform bone and first metatarsal (Fig. 14.13). Its action is to dorsiflex the ankle and invert the foot. The extensor hallucis longus tendon passes under the superior and inferior extensor retinacula. It inserts into the dorsal aspect of the great toe (Fig. 14.13). The action of the muscle is to dorsiflex the ankle and extend the great toe. The extensor digitorum longus tendon lies lateral to the tibialis anterior. It inserts into the middle and distal phalanges of the lateral four toes. It passes under the superior and inferior flexor retinacula (Fig. 14.13). Its action is to dorsiflex the ankle, evert the foot, and extend the lateral four toes.

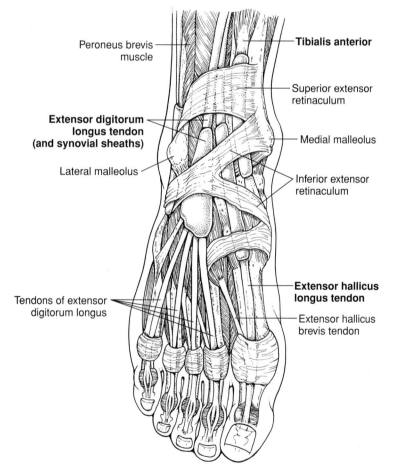

Figure 14.13

14

PROCEDURE:

To palpate the tibialis anterior, instruct the patient to dorsiflex and invert the foot. The tendon should become prominent. Palpate the tendon for point tenderness (Fig. 14.14). Tenderness may be caused by overpronation, especially in runners. Tendinitis or a strain of the tendon also may be suspect. This muscle and tendon support the longitudinal arch of the foot.

To palpate the extensor hallucis longus tendon, instruct the patient to extend the great toe (Fig. 14.15). The tendon should be prominent. Palpate the tendon for point tenderness. This may indicate tendinitis or strain of the tendon.

To palpate the extensor digitorum longus tendon, instruct the patient to extend the toes. Palpate the tendon first were it crosses the ankle (Fig. 14.16) then when it divides into four parts (Fig. 14.17) which insert into the middle phalanx. Tenderness may indicate tendonitis or tenosynovitis from overuse, especially in the runner.

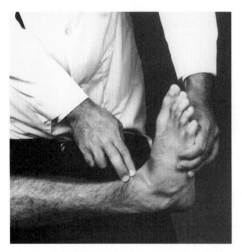

Figure 14.14

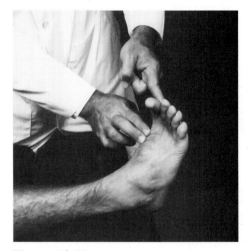

Figure 14.15

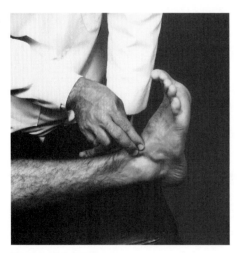

Figure 14.16

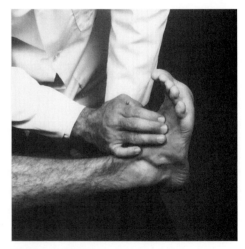

Figure 14.17

Posterior Aspect

Achilles Tendon, Calcaneal Bursa, and Retrocalcaneal Bursa

DESCRIPTIVE ANATOMY:

The Achilles tendon attaches the gastrocnemius muscle to the calcaneus. It is the strongest tendon in the body but the one most frequently ruptured. Two bursa surround this tendon: the calcaneal bursa, which is located superficial to the Achilles tendon and below the skin; and the retrocalcaneal bursa, which is located deep to the Achilles tendon (Fig. 14.18). These bursa are normally nonpalpable unless they are inflamed.

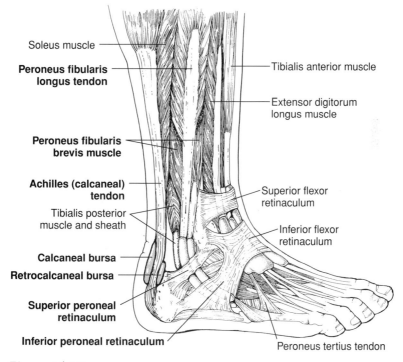

Figure 14.18

PROCEDURE:

With the ankle in the neutral position, palpate the Achilles tendon with your thumb and index finger (Fig. 14.19). Next, place anterior to posterior pressure on the Achilles tendon with your thumb (Fig. 14.20). Note any pain, tenderness, increase in temperature, swelling, crepitus, and/or continuity of the tendon. Pain, tenderness, and an increase in temperature may indicate tendinitis, a strain, or a partial tear of the tendon. Loss of continuity of the tendon may indicate a complete rupture of the tendon. This is rare but can occur, especially in patients with a history of chronic Achilles tendinitis. Pain, tenderness, and inflammation deep to the Achilles tendon may indicate retrocalcaneal bursitis. Pain, tenderness, and swelling over the Achilles tendon and below the skin are indicative of calcaneal bursitis.

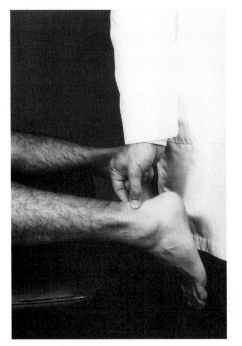

Figure 14.19

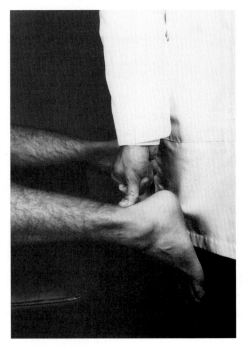

Figure 14.20

ANKLE RANGE OF MOTION

Dorsiflexion (1)

With the patient in the supine position, place the goniometer in the sagittal plane with the center at the lateral malleolus (Fig. 14.21). Instruct the patient to flex his foot backwards while following the foot with one arm of the goniometer (Fig. 14.22).

NORMAL RANGE (2):

13 ± 4.4 degrees or greater from the 0 or neutral position.

Muscles Involved in Action	*Nerve Supply*
1. Tibialis anterior	Deep peroneal
2. Extensor digitorum longus	Deep peroneal
3. Extensor hallucis longus	Deep peroneal
4. Peroneus tertius	Deep peroneal

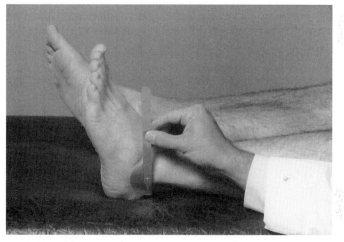

Figure 14.21

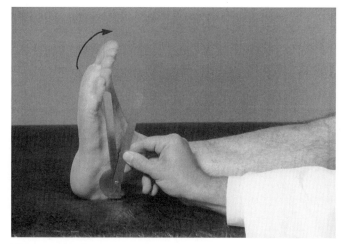

Figure 14.22

14

Plantar Flexion (1)

With the patient in the supine position, place the goniometer in the sagittal plane with the center at the lateral malleolus (Fig. 14.23). Instruct the patient to flex his foot forward while following the foot with one arm of the goniometer (Fig. 14.24).

NORMAL RANGE (2):

56 ± 6.1 degrees or greater from the 0 or neutral position.

Muscles Involved in Action	Nerve Supply
1. Gastrocnemius	Tibial
2. Soleus	Tibial
3. Plantaris	Tibial
4. Flexor digitorum longus	Tibial
5. Peroneus longus	Superficial peroneal
6. Peroneus brevis	Superficial peroneal
7. Flexor hallucis longus	Tibial
8. Tibialis posterior	Tibial

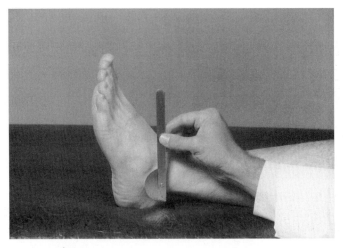

Figure 14.23

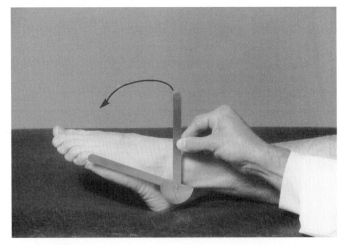

Figure 14.24

Inversion (1)

With the patient in the prone position and the knee flexed, place the inclinometer at the base of the heel and zero out the inclinometer (Fig. 14.25). Instruct the patient to invert the foot, and record the measurement (Fig. 14.26).

NORMAL RANGE (2):

37 ± 4.5 degrees or greater from the 0 or neutral position.

Muscles Involved in Action	*Nerve Supply*
1. Tibialis posterior	Tibial
2. Flexor digitorum longus	Tibial
3. Flexor hallucis longus	Tibial
4. Tibialis anterior	Deep peroneal
5. Extensor hallucis longus	Deep peroneal

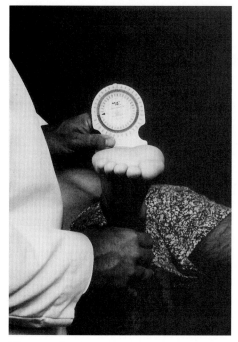

Figure 14.25

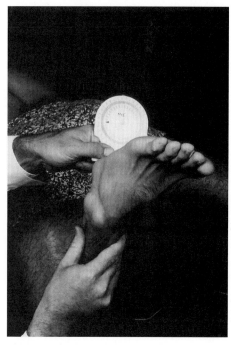

Figure 14.26

14

Eversion (1,2)

With the patient in the prone position and the knee flexed, place the inclinometer at the base of the heel and zero out the inclinometer (Fig. 14.27). Instruct the patient to evert the foot and record the measurement (Fig. 14.28).

NORMAL RANGE:

21 ± 5.0 degrees or greater from the 0 or neutral position.

Muscles Involved in Action	Nerve Supply
1. Peroneus longus	Superficial peroneal
2. Peroneus brevis	Superficial peroneal
3. Peroneus tertius	Deep peroneal
4. Extensor hallucis longus	Deep peroneal

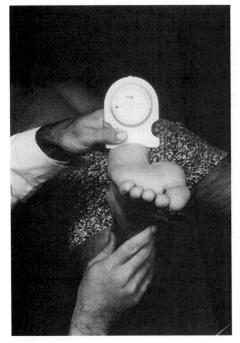

Figure 14.27

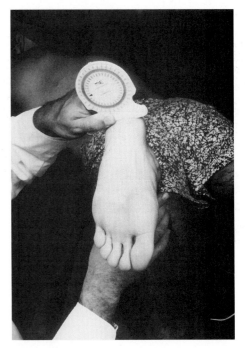

Figure 14.28

LIGAMENTOUS INSTABILITY

Drawer's Foot Sign (3)

PROCEDURE:

With the patient in the supine position, stabilize the ankle with one hand. With your opposite hand, grasp and exert a pushing pressure on the tibia (Fig. 14.29). Next, grasp the anterior aspect of the foot. Grasp the posterior aspect of the tibia and pull (Fig. 14.30).

RATIONALE:

If gapping occurs secondary to trauma when the tibia is pushed, a tear of the anterior talofibular ligament is indicated. If gapping occurs when the tibia is pulled, a posterior talofibular ligament tear is indicated (Fig. 14.31).

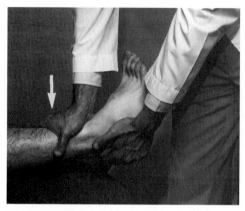

Figure 14.29

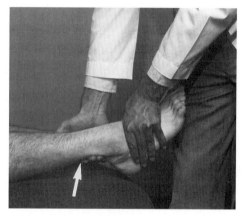

Figure 14.30

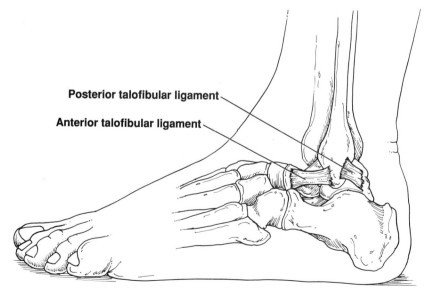

Posterior talofibular ligament
Anterior talofibular ligament

Figure 14.31

14

PROCEDURE:

With the patient in the supine position, grasp the patient's foot and passively invert it (Fig. 14.32).

RATIONALE:

If gapping is present secondary to trauma, suspect a tear of the anterior talofibular and/ or calcaneofibular ligament (Fig. 14.33).

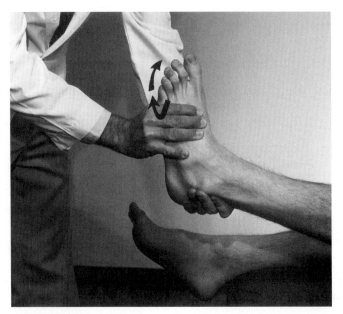

Figure 14.32

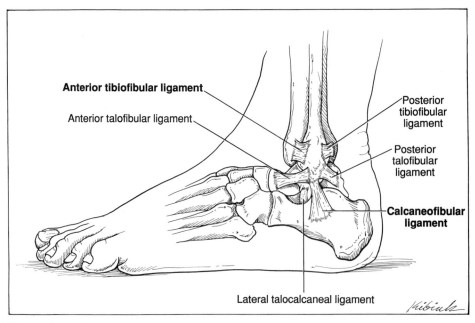

Anterior tibiofibular ligament

Anterior talofibular ligament

Posterior tibiofibular ligament

Posterior talofibular ligament

Calcaneofibular ligament

Lateral talocalcaneal ligament

Figure 14.33

Medial Stability Test (3)

PROCEDURE:

With the patient in the supine position, grasp the foot and passively evert it (Fig. 14.34).

RATIONALE:

If gapping is present secondary to trauma, suspect a tear of the deltoid ligament (Fig. 14.35).

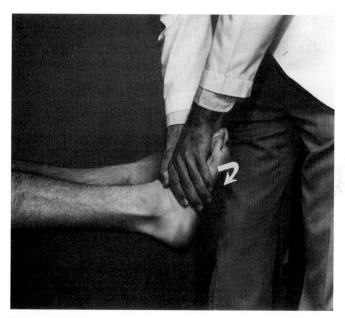

Figure 14.34

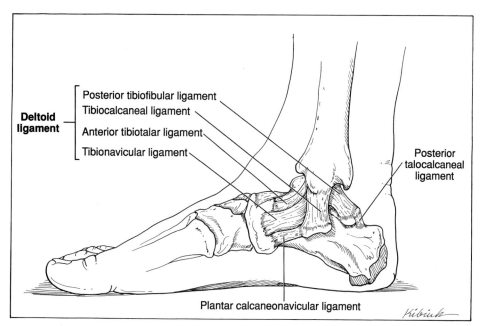

14

Figure 14.35

TARSAL TUNNEL SYNDROME

Tourniquet Test (4)

PROCEDURE:

Wrap a sphygmomanometer cuff around the affected ankle and inflate it to just above the patient's systolic blood pressure. Hold for 1 to 2 minutes (Fig. 14.36).

RATIONALE:

Tarsal tunnel syndrome is the compression of the posterior tibial nerve beneath the flexor retinaculum at the ankle (Fig. 14.37). Compression of the area by the cuff accentuates the narrowing of the tunnel, thus increasing the patient's pain. If pain is elicited or existing pain is exacerbated, then suspect a compromise of the tarsal tunnel.

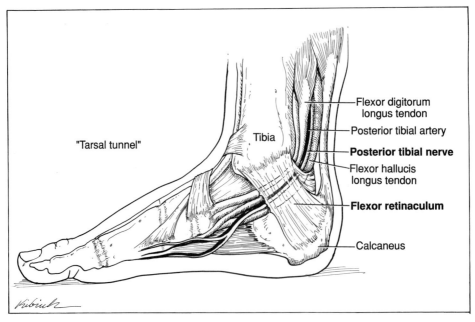

Figure 14.36

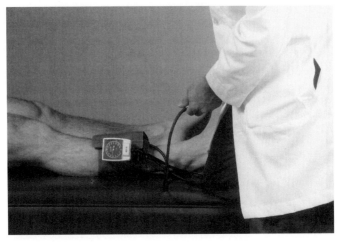

Figure 14.37

Tinel's Foot Sign

PROCEDURE:

Tap the area over the posterior tibial nerve with a neurological reflex hammer (Fig. 14.38).

RATIONALE:

Paresthesias radiating to the foot is indicative of an irritation to the posterior tibial nerve that may be caused by a constriction of the tarsal tunnel.

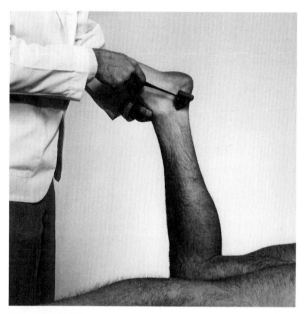

Figure 14.38

14

ACHILLES TENDON RUPTURE

Thompson's Test (5)

PROCEDURE:

With the patient in the prone position, instruct the patient to flex his knee. Squeeze the calf muscles against the tibia and fibula (Fig. 14.39)

RATIONALE:

When the calf muscles are squeezed, mechanical contraction of the gastrocnemius and soleus muscles occurs. These muscles are attached to the Achilles tendon, which in turn plantar flexes the foot. If the Achilles tendon is ruptured, then contraction of the gastrocnemius and soleus muscles will not plantar flex the foot.

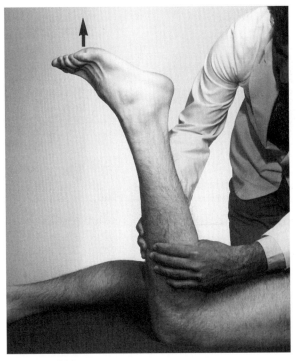

Figure 14.39

Achilles Tap Test

PROCEDURE:

Tap the Achilles tendon with a neurological reflex hammer (Fig. 14.40).

RATIONALE:

Exacerbation of pain and a loss of plantar flexion is indicative of an Achilles tendon rupture.

NOTE:

The patient must be neurologically sound for this test to be valid.

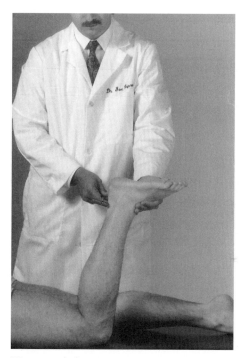

Figure 14.40

14

References

1. American Academy of Orthopaedic Surgeons. The clinical measurement of joint motion. Chicago: American Academy of Orthopaedic Surgeons, 1994.
2. Boone DC, Azen SP. Normal range of motion of joint in male subjects. J Bone Joint Surg Am 1979;61:756–759.
3. Hoppenfeld S. Physical examination of the spine and extremities. New York: Appleton-Century-Crofts, 1976:127.
4. McRae R. Clinical orthopedic examination. New York: Churchill Livingstone, 1976.
5. Thompson T, Doherty J. Spontaneous rupture of the tendon of Achilles: a new clinical diagnostic test. Anat Res 1967;158:126.

General References

Colter JM. Lateral ligamentous injuries of the ankle. In: Hamilton WC, ed. Traumatic disorders of the ankle. New York: Springer-Verlag, 1984.

Cox JS, Brand RL. Evaluation and treatment of lateral ankle sprains. Sports Med 1977;5:51.

Kapandji LA. The physiology of the joints. Vol. 2. Lower limb. New York: Churchill Livingstone, 1970.

Lam SJ. Tarsal tunnel syndrome. Lancet 1962; 2:1354.

Mennell JM. Foot pain. Boston: Little, Brown, 1969.

Post M. Physical examination of the musculoskeletal system. Chicago: Year Book Medical Publishers, 1987.

15
MISCELLANEOUS ORTHOPAEDIC TESTS

15

ARTERIAL INSUFFICIENCY

Buerger's Test

PROCEDURE:

With the patient in the supine position, instruct him to elevate one leg at a time. The patient must consecutively dorsiflex and plantar flex the foot in the raised position for a minimum of 2 minutes (Figs. 15.1, 15.2). The leg is then lowered and hung off the side of the table with the patient seated (Fig. 15.3).

RATIONALE:

Elevating the foot and consecutively flexing the foot causes the blood flow in the lower extremity to diminish. When the leg is then lowered and hung off the table, the lower leg and foot should fill with blood. This turns the foot a reddish, cyanotic color, and the veins distend. This process takes less than 1 minute. If it takes longer than 1 minute for the foot to turn a reddish, cyanotic color, the test is positive for arterial compromise to the lower extremity.

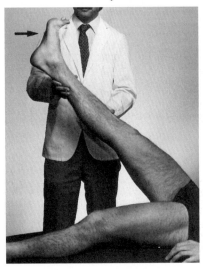

Figure 15.1

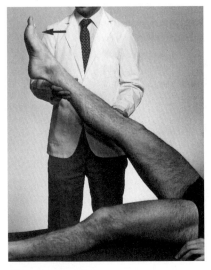

Figure 15.2

Figure 15.3

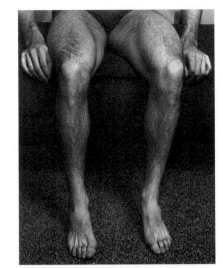

Allen's Test (1,2)

With the patient in the seated position, instruct the patient to raise his arm and open and close his fist. Have him do this for 1 minute (Figs. 15.4, 15.5). At that point, lower the patient's arm while occluding the radial artery (Fig. 15.6), and then the ulnar artery (Fig. 15.7), at the wrist.

RATIONALE:

Raising the arm and consecutively opening and closing the fist causes the blood flow in the upper extremity to diminish. When the arm is then lowered and one of the arteries is occluded, the hand should fill with blood, which turns it a reddish, cyanotic color, and the veins then distend. A delay of more than 10 seconds in returning a reddish, cyanotic color to the hand is indicative of either ulnar artery insufficiency or radial artery insufficiency. The artery being tested is the one not being occluded manually.

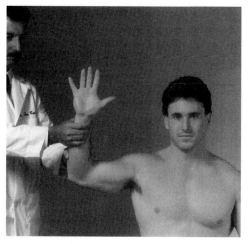

Figure 15.4

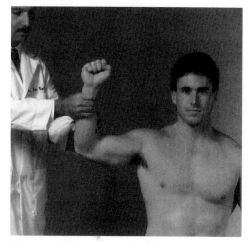

Figure 15.5

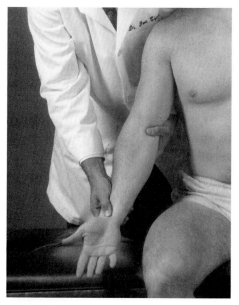

Figure 15.6

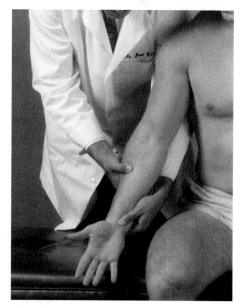

Figure 15.7

15

THROMBOPHLEBITIS

Homan's Sign

PROCEDURE:

With the patient in the supine position, dorsiflex the patient's foot and squeeze the calf (Fig. 15.8) (3).

RATIONALE:

Deep-seated pain at the posterior leg or calf may be indicative of thrombophlebitis. Dorsiflexing the foot places a dynamic stretch on the gastrocnemius muscle and tension of the deep veins. The addition of squeezing the calf compresses the surrounding tissue against the thrombus, thereby stimulating a nociceptive response.

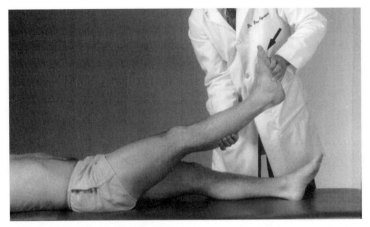

Figure 15.8

SYMPTOM MAGNIFICATION ASSESSMENT

Hoover's Sign (3,4)

PROCEDURE:

With the patient in the supine position, instruct him to lift the affected leg while you place one hand under the patient's heel on the nonaffected side (Fig. 15.9).

RATIONALE:

If the patient is magnifying his symptoms, he will not raise the affected leg and no pressure will be put on the nonaffected heel. If the patient is genuinely trying to raise his leg but is unable to do so, the examiner will feel pressure from the nonaffected heel.

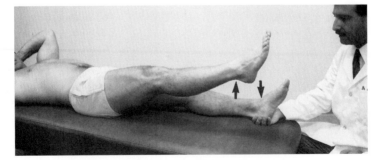

Figure 15.9

Burn's Bench Test

PROCEDURE:

Instruct the patient to kneel on the examination table. Have the patient bend to touch the floor while you stabilize the legs (Fig. 15.10).

RATIONALE:

Patients with low back pain will be able to perform this test because no strenuous activity of the back is involved. The stress is placed on the posterior leg muscles. If the patient with low back pain cannot perform the test, suspect a patient magnifying his symptoms.

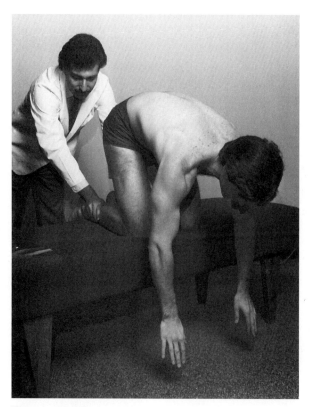

Figure 15.10

15

Sitting Lasègue's Test

PROCEDURE:

With the patient in the seated position, instruct him to extend alternately one leg at a time (Fig. 15.11).

RATIONALE:

This test is performed on the patient who reports sciatic radiculopathy. When the patient is seated and the leg is flexed, the traction on the sciatic nerve is reduced. If the patient has true sciatic pain when the leg is extended, the patient will experience increased pain. To reduce this pain, the patient will lean back on the table (Fig. 15.12). If the patient does not lean back and he reports a radicular component to the extended extremity, then the patient may be magnifying his symptoms.

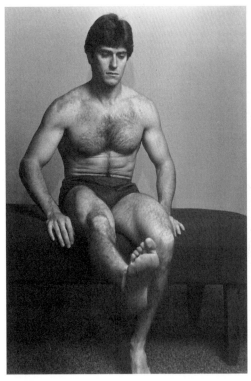

Figure 15.11

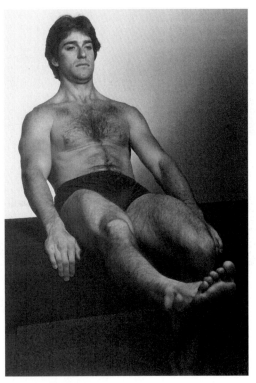

Figure 15.12

Magnuson's Test

PROCEDURE:

With the patient sitting, instruct him to point to the site of his pain (Fig. 15.13). Next, distract the patient by performing some irrelevant test. Then instruct the patient to point to the site of the pain again (Fig. 15.14).

RATIONALE:

The patient who experiences real pain will point to the specific site of pain both times. The patient who is magnifying his symptoms usually will not be able to locate the exact site twice.

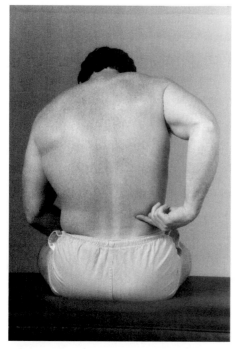

Figure 15.13

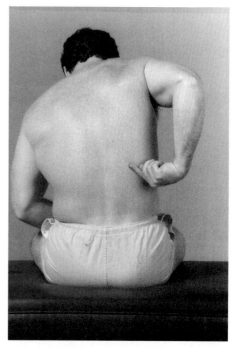

Figure 15.14

15

Mannkopf's Maneuver

PROCEDURE:

With the patient in the seated position, obtain the patient's resting pulse rate (Fig. 15.15). Then irritate the patient's complaint by poking at it with your finger (Fig. 15.16). Next, retake the pulse rate.

RATIONALE:

The sympathetic system controls vasoconstriction and heart rate. When the area of pain is provoked, the patient with true pain will experience a flight or flight phenomenon, increasing the heart rate and blood pressure. In the patient who has true pain, the pulse rate will increase by 10% or more. This reaction is carried out below the conscious level and is not under patient control. If the heart rate does not increase, then the patient may be magnifying his symptoms.

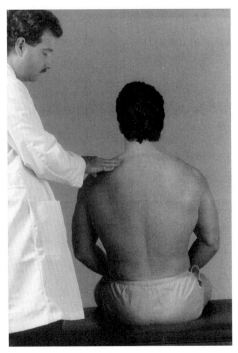

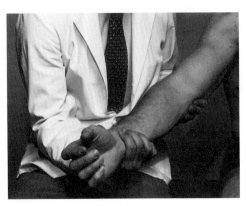

Figure 15.15

Figure 15.16

HYPERSENSITIVITY

Libman's Test

PROCEDURE:

With the patient in the seated position, place bilateral pressure on the mastoid processes (Fig. 15.17).

RATIONALE:

Placing pressure on the mastoid processes on a patient with no reports of headaches, occipital pain, or mastoid pain should not cause pain or discomfort on the mastoids. If the patient reports pain, he may have a low pain threshold.

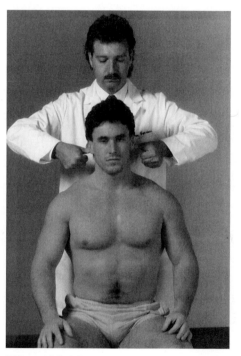

Figure 15.17

15

MENINGEAL IRRITATION

Kernig's Test (5–7)

PROCEDURE:

With the patient in the supine position, instruct him to flex his hip and knee to 90 degrees with his leg parallel to the table (Fig. 15.18). Then instruct the patient to extend the leg on the side that is being tested (Fig. 15.19).

RATIONALE:

With the hip flexed and the knee flexed, the sciatic nerve and the dural sac are relaxed. When the knee is extended, this action tractions the sciatic nerve, ultimately tractioning the dural sac or meninges. Inability to straighten the leg or pain while straightening the leg is indicative of meningeal irritation or nerve root involvement.

NOTE:

If bacterial meningitis is suspect, the patient may experience head pain that is increased with sudden neck movements, neck stiffness, nuchal rigidity, and an elevated temperature. This test will also elicit radicular pain in the patient with sciatic radiculopathy.

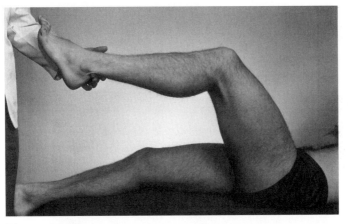

Figure 15.18

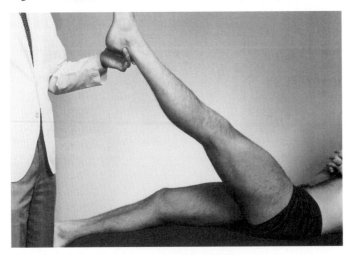

Figure 15.19

Brudzinski's Sign (8)

PROCEDURE:

With the patient supine, flex the patient's neck to his chest (Fig. 15.20).

RATIONALE:

When the patient flexes the neck, the dural sac and spinal cord are tractioned. Irritation of the dural sac will cause pain at the level of irritation. Flexing the knees reduces the traction on the spinal cord and meninges. If the patient flexes his knees, the test is positive and is indicative of meningeal irritation or nerve root involvement (Fig. 15.21).

NOTE:

Bacterial meningitis is suspect if the patient experiences head pain that is increased with sudden neck movements, neck stiffness, nuchal rigidity, and an elevated temperature. This test will also elicit radicular pain in the patient with sciatic radiculopathy.

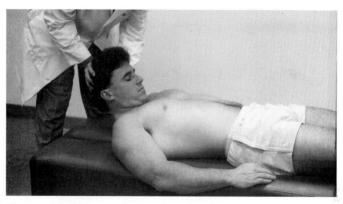

Figure 15.20

15

Lhermitte's Sign

PROCEDURE:

With the patient in the sitting position, passively flex the patient's head to his chest (Fig. 15.21).

RATIONALE:

The action of flexing the neck stretches the spinal cord and meninges. Sharp pain radiating down the spine or into the upper or lower extremities may indicate nerve root, dural, or meningeal irritation. It also may be indicative of cervical myelopathy or multiple sclerosis.

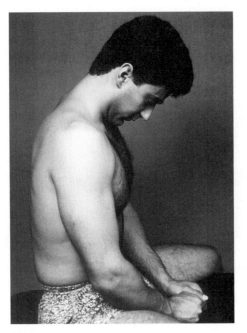

Figure 15.21

LEG MEASUREMENTS

Actual Leg Length

PROCEDURE:

With the patient standing, take a tape measure and measure bilaterally from the anterior superior iliac spine to the floor (Fig. 15.22).

RATIONALE:

This is a true measurement of the patient's lower extremity. Compare the measurements. Any difference is indicative of an anatomic short leg.

Figure 15.22

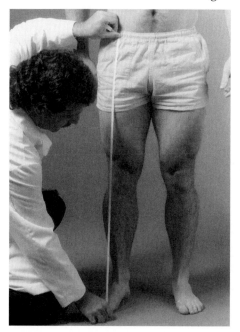

Apparent Leg Length

PROCEDURE:

With the patient in the supine position, measure bilaterally the distance between the umbilicus and the medial malleolus (Fig. 15.23).

RATIONALE:

Any difference in the two measurements indicates a functional leg deficiency that may be caused by muscular or ligamentous contracture deformities.

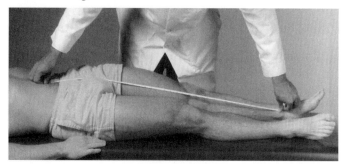

Figure 15.23

References

1. Allen EV, Barker NW, Hines EA Jr. Peripheral vascular disease. 4th ed. Philadelphia: WB Saunders, 1972:37–38.
2. Allen EV. Thromboangiitis obliterans: methods of diagnosis of chronic occlusive arterial lesions distal to the wrist. Am J Med Sci 1929;178:238–239.
3. Arieff AJ, Tigay EI, Kurtz JF, et al. The Hoover sign: an objective sign of pain and/or weakness in the back or lower extremities. Arch Neurol 1961;5:673.
4. Hoover CF. A new sign for the detection of malingering and functional paralysis of the lower extremities. JAMA 1928;51:746–749.
5. Kernig W. Concerning a little noted sign of meningitis. Arch Neurol 1969;21:216.
6. Wartenberg R. The signs of Brudzinski and of Kernig. J Pediatr 1950;37:679.
7. Brody IA, Williams KH. The sign of Kernig and Brudzinski. Arch Neurol 1969;21:215.
8. Brudzinski J. A new sign of the lower extremities in meningitis of children (neck sign). Arch Neurol 1969;21:215.

General References

American Society for Surgery of the Hand. The hand—examination and diagnosis. Aurora, CO: American Society for Surgery of the Hand, 1978.

Edgar VA, Barker NW, Hines EA Jr. Peripheral vascular disease. Philadelphia: WB Saunders, 1946:57–58.

Hoppenfeld S. Physical examination of the spine and extremities. New York: Appleton-Century-Crofts, 1976:127.

Woerman AL, Binder-Macleod SA. Leg-length discrepancy assessment: accuracy and precision in five clinical methods of evaluation. J Orthop Sports Phys Ther 1984;5:230.

16
CRANIAL NERVES

16

There are 12 pairs of cranial nerves that exit from the brain and brainstem. These nerves innervate the face, head, and neck. They control all motor and sensory functions in these areas, including the senses of vision, hearing, smell, and taste.

The cranial nerves may be affected by cranial trauma, infections, aneurysm, stroke, degenerative diseases (multiple sclerosis), upper motor neuron lesions, lower motor neuron lesions, increased intracranial pressure, and abnormal masses or tumors.

An important anatomic feature of cranial nerves is bilateral and unilateral innervation. In bilateral innervation, relatively equal distributions of right and left brain hemisphere innervation govern the function of a specific facial part. Movements that are performed in bilateral synchrony, such as swallowing or moving the forehead, are innervated bilaterally. In unilateral innervation, the contralateral hemisphere innervates the specific body part. Fine movements of the face are examples of unilateral cranial nerve innervation.

Multiple cranial nerve lesions with a number of different syndromes may also be present. A unilaterally affected cranial nerve V, VII, and VIII may indicate a cerebellopontine angle lesion. A unilaterally affected cranial nerve III, IV, V, and VI may indicate a cavernous sinuous lesion. A unilaterally affected cranial nerve IX, X, and XI may indicate a jugular foramen syndrome. A combined, bilaterally affected cranial nerve X, XI, and XII may indicate bulbar or pseudobulbar palsy. Multiple cranial nerve abnormalities are shown in Figure 16.1.

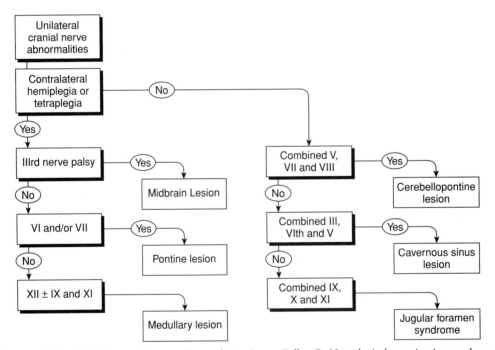

Figure 16.1 Multiple cranial nerve abnormalities. From: Fuller G. Neurological examination made easy. London: Churchill Livingstone, 1993.

OLFACTORY NERVE (I)

PROCEDURE:

The olfactory nerve is responsible for the sense of smell. To test this nerve, obtain some aromatic substances, i.e., coffee, tobacco, or peppermint oil. Instruct the patient to close one of his nostrils. Place the substance underneath the open nostril and ask if he can smell anything and, if so, ask him to identify the smell (Fig. 16.2). Repeat the procedure for the opposite nostril.

RATIONALE:

If the patient is unable to smell or identify the smell unilaterally, a lesion of the olfactory nerve may be suspect. If the patient is unable to smell or identify the smell bilaterally, consider a nonorganic problem or a bilateral cranial nerve I lesion.

NOTE:

A diminished or almost absent sense of smell is common in elderly patients or patients. It will be apparent if loss of smell is bilateral and no trauma has been induced to the cranium. Other non-neurogenic lesions, such as sinus infection, deviated septum, and lesions caused by smoking, may also cause a loss of smell, either unilaterally or bilaterally.

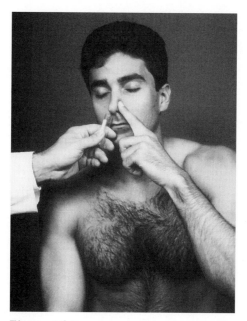

Figure 16.2

16

OPTIC NERVE (II)

Procedure:

The optic nerve is responsible for visual acuity and peripheral vision. To test for visual acuity, ask the patient to cover one eye and read the smallest print he can on a Snellen chart (Fig. 16.3). Repeat the test with the opposite eye. Note the results. We are not testing visual acuity for refractive error. We are testing the acuity for optic nerve involvement. This test may be performed with the patient wearing his glasses or contact lenses.

To test for peripheral vision, ask the patient to cover one eye with his hand and instruct the patient to keep a fixed gaze on your nose with the uncovered eye. Directly motion a large cross with your finger from superior to inferior and from right to left (Fig. 16.4). Instruct the patient to tell you when he begins to see your finger. Repeat with the opposite eye and record the results.

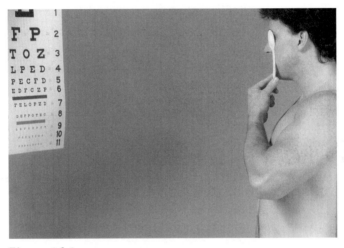

Figure 16.3

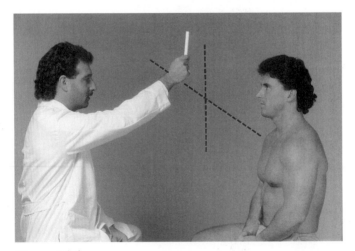

Figure 16.4

RATIONALE:

Any loss of vision, from complete unilateral or bilateral loss of vision to loss of half fields of vision (hemianopsia) or a partial defect in the field of vision (scotoma), is indicative of an optic nerve lesion. Temporal lobe lesions can produce superior contralateral quadrantanopsia. Occipital lobe lesions can produce a contralateral homonymous hemianopsia with macular sparing. Figure 16.5 shows a schematic of the neural pathway from the brain to the retina and demonstrates the location of the lesion and its effect on vision. Also associated with the schematic is a flow chart of field defects (Fig. 16.6).

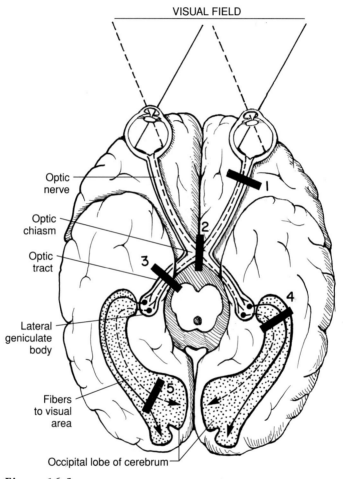

VISUAL FIELD

Optic nerve

Optic chiasm

Optic tract

Lateral geniculate body

Fibers to visual area

Occipital lobe of cerebrum

Figure 16.5

16

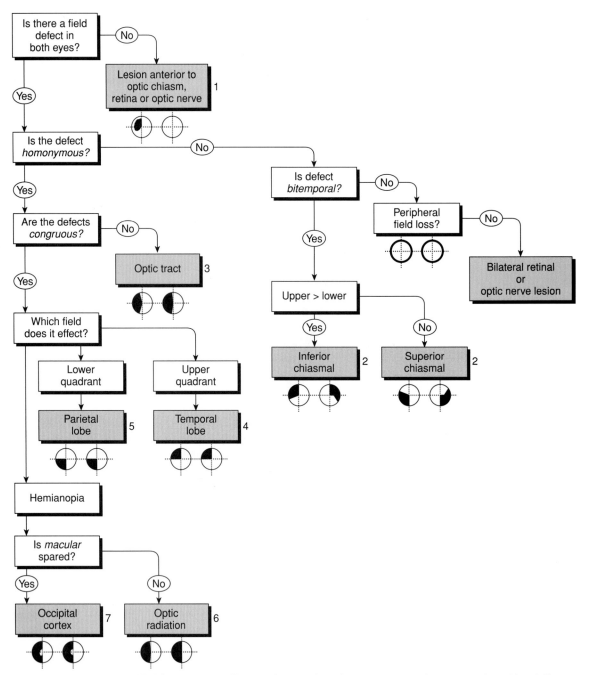

Figure 16.6 Field defects. From: Fuller G, ed. Neurological examination made easy. London: Churchill Livingstone, 1993.

Ophthalmoscopic Exam

PROCEDURE:

With an ophthalmoscope, look into the patient's eye. Bring the scope 1 to 2 cm from the eye and encourage the patient to fix his gaze at a distant point (Fig. 16.7). Use the focus ring to correct for your vision and the patient's vision. If you or the patient is myopic and is not using glasses or contacts, turn the focus ring dial counterclockwise to focus on the eye. If you or the patient is presbyopic, turn the focus dial clockwise to focus on the eye. Look at the optic disc, blood vessels, and retinal background.

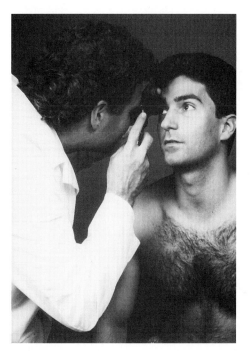

Figure 16.7

16

RATIONALE:

Visualize the optic nerve, the optic disc, and the optic cup for swelling and atrophy (see Fig. 16.8).

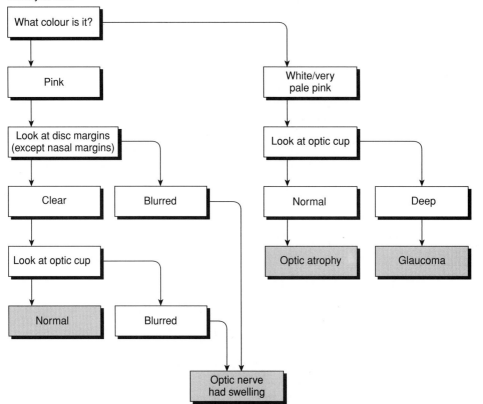

Figure 16.8 Optic disc abnormalities. From: Fuller G. Neurological examination made easy. London: Churchill Livingstone, 1993.

Oculomotor, Trochlear, and Abducens Nerves (III, IV, VI)

PROCEDURE:

Cranial nerves III, IV, and VI are all associated with ocular and pupillary motility and are tested together for simplicity. Cranial nerve III also innervates the levator palpebrae muscles, which are responsible for movement of the eyelids. First, look at the patient's eyelids and note any ptosis. After inspection of the eyelids, inspect the eye globes for alignment. Dysfunction of cranial III, IV, or VI may be responsible for deviations of eye alignment. Next, inspect the pupils and determine their size and shape. Then test the pupillary reflex by flashing a light into one of the patient's eyes (Fig. 16.9). Look at both pupils one at a time for contraction or dilation.

To test the ocular movements, have the patient follow either your finger or a moving object through the entire field of vision in all axes. Observe for nystagmus and/or the inability to move the eye in a particular axis (Fig. 16.10). Also, test for convergence by having the patient look at a distant object and continue to focus on it as you move that object closer to the patient. The pupil should constrict and converge as the object approaches. Look at both pupils in both instances.

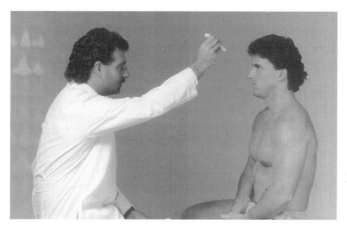

Figure 16.9

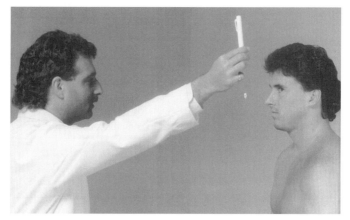

Figure 16.10

16

RATIONALE:

An oculomotor nerve lesion will present with ptosis of the eyelid with inability to open the lid. Eye alignment may be down and lateral. Also, inability to move the eyeball upward, inward, or downward because of weakness of the medial, superior, and inferior rectus muscles and the inferior oblique muscle will be observed. The pupil is usually dilated, and the pupillary reflex is absent. The most frequent cause of a cranial nerve III paralysis is an aneurysm in the circle of Willis. Other conditions may also cause the pupil to dilate and the pupillary reflex to become absent (Fig. 16.11).

A trochlear nerve lesion will present with a deviation of the eye superior and lateral and with inability to move the eyeball downward and inward because of weakness of the superior oblique muscle.

An abducens nerve lesion will present with medial eye alignment an inability to move the eyeball outward because of weakness of the lateral rectus muscle (Fig. 16.12).

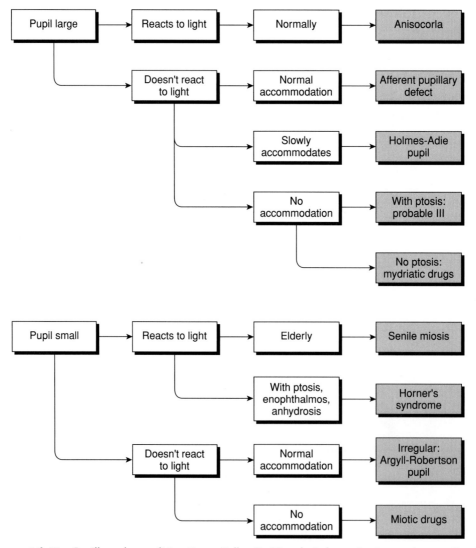

Figure 16.11 Pupillary abnormalities. From: Fuller G. Neurological examination made easy. London: Churchill Livingstone, 1993.

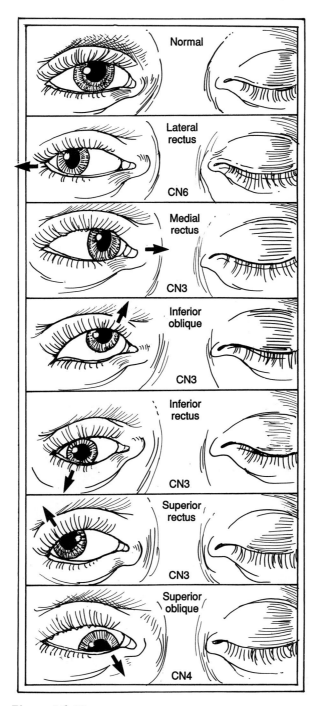

Figure 16.12

16

TRIGEMINAL NERVE (V)

The trigeminal nerve is composed of motor and sensory portions. The motor portion innervates the muscles of mastication. These muscles are the masseter, pterygoid, and temporal muscles. The sensory portion is divided into three branches: the ophthalmic (V1), maxillary (V2), and mandibular branches (V3).

Motor

PROCEDURE (MASSETER, PTERYGOID, TEMPORALIS MUSCLES):

To test the motor portion that innervates the masseter muscle, instruct the patient to simulate a bite while you palpate the masseter muscle and attempt to open the patient's jaw with your thumbs (Fig. 16. 13). To test the pterygoid muscle, instruct the patient to deviate his jaw against your resistance (Fig. 16.14). To test the temporalis muscle, instruct the patient to clench his jaw while you palpate the temporalis muscles with your fingers (Fig. 16.15). Note symmetrical muscle contraction.

RATIONALE:

The presence of a weak muscle when testing the masseter and pterygoid muscles may indicate a trigeminal nerve lesion. A difference in muscle tension of the temporalis muscle is also an indication of a trigeminal motor lesion. In bilateral paralysis, the jaw may not close tightly. In unilateral lesions, the jaw will deviate toward the side of the lesion when the patient opens his mouth.

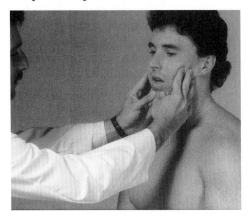

Figure 16.13

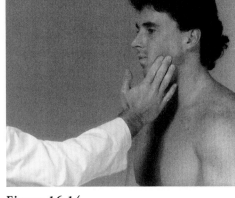

Figure 16.14

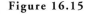

Figure 16.15

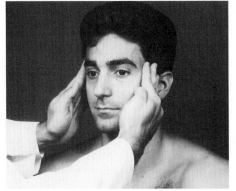

382

Reflex

Corneal Reflex

PROCEDURE:

Instruct the patient to gaze upward and inward while you touch the cornea with a strand of cotton, approaching from the lateral side (Fig. 16.16). Care must be taken not to touch the eyelash or conjunctiva. The patient should blink when the cornea is touched. The corneal reflex has sensory fibers from the trigeminal nerve and motor fibers from the facial nerve.

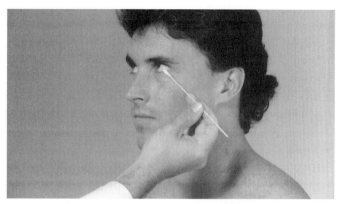

Figure 16.16

Jaw Reflex

PROCEDURE:

Instruct the patient to slightly open his mouth. Place your thumb or index finger just lateral to the midline of the patient's chin, and place downward pressure. With a neurological reflex hammer, tap downward on your finger to open the jaw (Fig. 16.17). The normal response is to close the jaw rapidly.

RATIONALE:

The corneal and jaw jerk reflexes have a sensory component from the trigeminal nerve. The jaw jerk reflex has a motor component to the trigeminal nerve. The corneal reflex has a motor component from the facial nerve. If the corneal reflexes are absent, then suspect a lesion of either the sensory portion of the trigeminal nerve or the motor component of the facial nerve. If the jaw jerk reflex is absent, suspect a lesion of the trigeminal nerve.

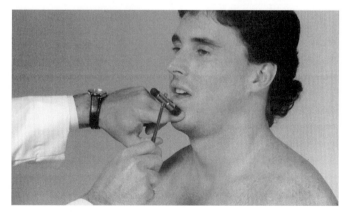

Figure 16.17

16

Sensory

PROCEDURE:

To test for sensory deficit, instruct the patient to close his eyes. Touch the forehead, cheek, and chin with a pin for pain sensation; a piece of cotton for the sensation of light touch; and small test tubes of hot and cold water for thermal sensation (Figs. 16.18, 16.19, 16.20).

Perform these procedures to both sides of the face and ask the patient to compare bilaterally. Next, instruct the patient to open his mouth and touch the tongue, the inside of both cheeks, and the hard palate with a wooden tongue depressor (Fig. 16.21). Instruct the patient to give a signal, such as raising his hand, when he feels the sensation.

RATIONALE:

A decrease in the sensation of light touch, pain, and/or temperature from one side to the other is indicative of a lesion of the sensory portion of the affected branch of the trigeminal nerve. Lesions of the ophthalmic, maxillary, or mandibular branches of the trigeminal nerve will produce decreased sensation of the forehead, cheek, or chin, respectively.

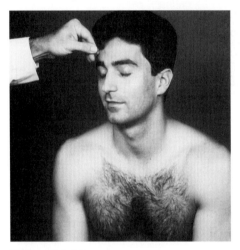

Figure 16.18

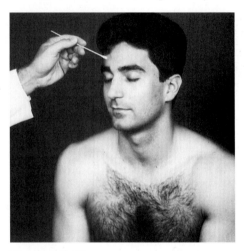

Figure 16.19

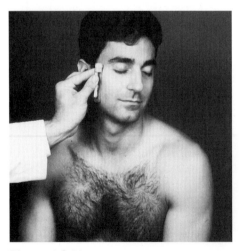

Figure 16.20

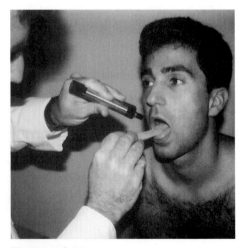

Figure 16.21

FACIAL NERVE (VII)

Motor

PROCEDURE:

The facial nerve has both motor and sensory fibers. The motor fibers innervate the muscles of the face and platysma. Observe the patient's face for abnormal movements, such as tics or tremors. Note the degree of expressional change or lack of change.

To test for motor function, observe the face in a reposed or neutral position. Then instruct the patient to frown, raise the eyebrows, close the eyes, show the teeth, smile, and whistle or puff the cheeks (Figs.16.22–16.25).

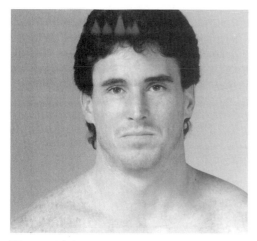

Figure 16.22

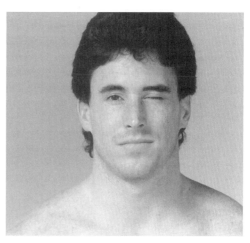

Figure 16.23

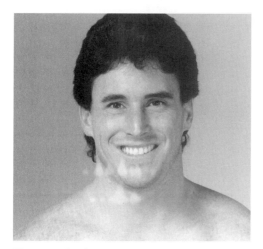

Figure 16.24

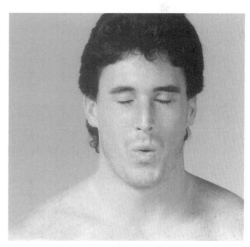

Figure 16.25

16

RATIONALE:

Facial nerve lesions may stem from upper motor neurons or lower motor neurons. These neurons may be distinguished by the various facial expressions. In an upper motor neuron lesion, there is generally no effect on the forehead and eyelids. In a lower motor neuron lesion, when the eyebrows are raised and lowered, wrinkling of the forehead is absent. Showing the teeth and whistling are absent in both upper and lower motor neuron lesions. Smiling may not elevate the mouth in a lower motor neuron lesion, but a symmetrical smile may occur in an upper motor neuron lesion. Inability of the patient to perform these movements indicates a lesion of the motor portion of the facial nerve (Fig. 16.26).

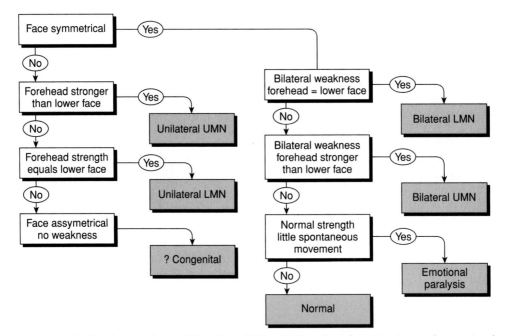

Figure 16.26   Facial nerve abnormalities. From: Fuller G. Neurological examination made easy. London: Churchill Livingstone, 1993.

Sensory

PROCEDURE:

Instruct the patient to close his eyes and protrude his tongue. Apply solutions of sugar, salt, and/or vinegar to one side and on the anterior two-thirds of the tongue (Fig. 16.27). Instruct the patient to identify each substance without retracting his tongue. This can be done by having the patient point to a list of various substances on a card or on a sheet of paper. Instruct the patient to rinse his mouth, then apply another substance on the opposite side.

RATIONALE:

Inability to taste and/or identify the substances may indicate a lesion of the sensory portion of the facial nerve.

NOTE:

Complete loss of taste in facial nerve lesions is rare. It is most common for the patient to present with a spontaneous or perverted taste as opposed to complete loss of taste. If complete loss of taste is noted, then you should consider non-neurogenic causes, such as viral infection, aging, smoking, and toxic or metabolic disease.

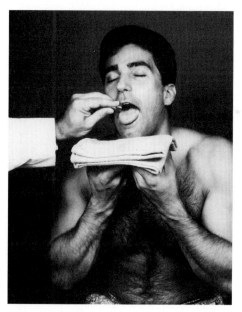

Figure 16.27

16

AUDITORY NERVE (VIII)

The auditory nerve is responsible for hearing. It is composed of a cochlear portion and a vestibular portion. The cochlear portion is responsible for hearing and the vestibular portion is responsible for balance. The cochlear portion is tested by evaluating the patient's hearing. The most accurate way to test hearing is with an audiometer. If one is not available, place a ticking watch close to the patient's ear and see if he can hear it. Weber's and Rinne's tests are indicative of cochlear lesions. Vestibular lesions are also determined by veering and past pointing tests and by observing the patient for nystagmus.

Weber's Test (Cochlear)

PROCEDURE:

Place a vibrating 256 tuning fork on the vertex of the patient's head (Fig. 16.28). Ask the patient if he hears the sound equally in both ears.

RATIONALE:

The test is normal if the patient hears the sound equally in both ears. If the sound is louder in one ear than in the other, suspect a conduction problem, such as a blockage of the ear canal or middle ear disease on the side of the louder sound. If a nerve lesion is suspected, the sound will be heard only in the normal ear. This hearing problem could be caused by otosclerosis, Meniere's disease, meningitis, cerebellopontine tumors, trauma, or demyelinating lesions.

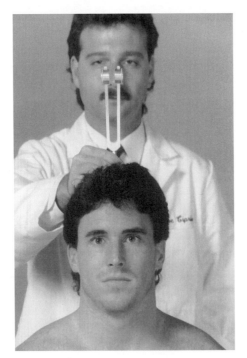

Figure 16.28

Rinne's Test (Cochlear)

PROCEDURE:

Place a vibrating tuning fork on the mastoid process (Fig 16.29). Ask the patient to identify when the sound disappears. After the sound disappears, place the tuning fork next to, but not touching, the external acoustic meatus (Fig. 16.30). Ask the patient again to identify when the sound disappears.

RATIONALE:

Normally, air conduction is two times greater than bone conduction—this is termed a Rinne positive. In conduction lesions or non-neurogenic lesions, bone conduction is greater than air conduction—this is termed a Rinne negative. In auditory nerve lesions, air conduction is greater than bone conduction.

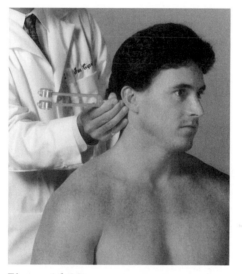

Figure 16.29

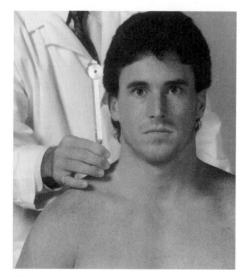

Figure 16.30

16

Veering Test (Vestibular)

PROCEDURE:

Instruct the patient to walk with his eyes closed (Fig. 16.31).

RATIONALE:

Veering in walking or a positive Romberg's test is indicative of a unilateral vestibular lesion. See Chapter 18 for Romberg's Test.

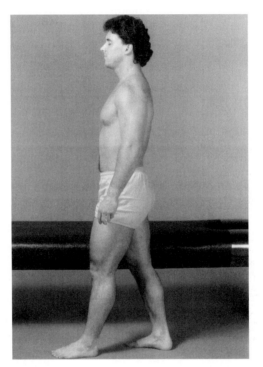

Figure 16.31

Past Pointing Test (Vestibular)

PROCEDURE:

With the patient's eyes opened, instruct the patient to elevate his extended arm over his head with his index finger extended (Fig. 16.32). Next, instruct the patient to touch your extended index finger, which is placed near the patient at the level of his hip (Fig. 16.33). Repeat the test with the patient's eyes closed.

RATIONALE:

If the patient has a vestibular lesion, the patient's arm will drift, and he will have difficulty placing his finger on yours with his eyes closed.

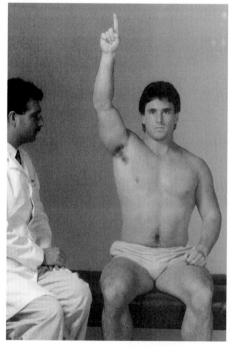

Figure 16.32

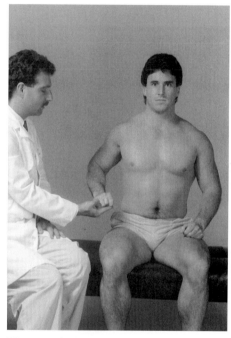

Figure 16.33

16

Labyrinthine Test for Positional Nystagmus

PROCEDURE:

With the patient in the seated position, inspect the eyes and note any nystagmus (Fig. 16.34). Nystagmus is a slow drift of the eye in one direction with a fast correction in the opposite direction. It is described in the direction of the fast phase. Next, have the patient lie supine and inspect for nystagmus for 30 seconds (Fig. 16.35). Next, assist the patient to turn to one side and stabilize his head. Note any nystagmus for 30 seconds (Fig. 16.36). Repeat with the patient turned to the opposite side. Next, have the patient extend his head over the examination table, and inspect for nystagmus for 30 seconds (Fig. 16.37). Allow sufficient time between tests for the patient with nystagmus to recover.

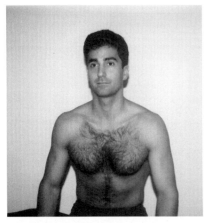

Figure 16.34

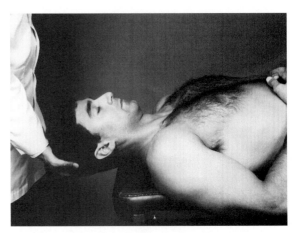

Figure 16.35

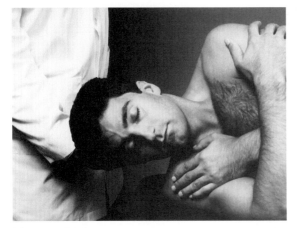

Figure 16.36

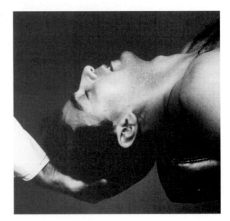

Figure 16.37

A patient with persistent nystagmus that changes direction with changes in the head position and that appears on repeated maneuvers suggests a brain stem or posterior fossa pathology. A delayed, mild, rapidly disappearing response that produces nystagmus in only one direction and cannot be repeated suggests benign postural vertigo (Fig. 16.38).

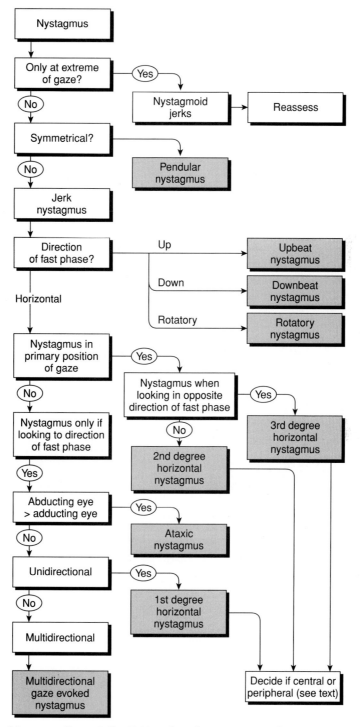

Figure 16.38 Nystagmus. From: Fuller G. Neurological examination made easy. London: Churchill Livingstone, 1993.

GLOSSOPHARYNGEAL AND VAGUS NERVES (IX, X)

The glossopharyngeal and vagus nerves are clinically inseparable because the fibers of both nerves overlap and are therefore tested together. The glossopharyngeal nerve conveys taste from the posterior tongue and has sensory innervation to the tonsillar pillars, soft palate, and pharyngeal wall. The vagus nerve overlaps the functions of the glossopharyngeal nerve and innervates the larynx. Note any hoarseness or change in voice tone.

The vagus nerve controls activity in the cardiac, respiratory, and gastrointestinal systems; however, these functions are difficult to assay because of the variable suprasegmental and hormonal influences.

Motor function is assessed by having the patient say "AHH" and observing the palate for deviation. Place a tongue depressor on the patient's tongue and observe palatal deviation (Fig. 16.39). If deviation exists, it will be toward the normal side. Next, ask the patient to swallow rapidly while you palpate the trachea (Fig. 16.40). Fatigue on continued swallowing may be seen in a patient who has myasthenia gravis. You may also ask the patient to puff his cheeks with air (Fig. 16.41). Leakage through the nose indicates a weakness in the muscle of the soft palate. This weakness is also a sign of a cranial nerve IX or X lesion. The leakage can be stopped by pinching the nose.

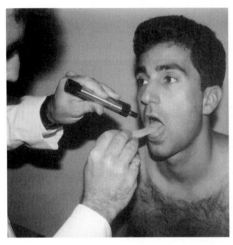

Figure 16.39

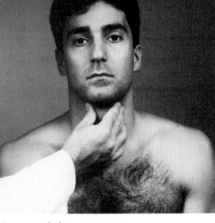

Figure 16.40

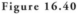

Figure 16.41

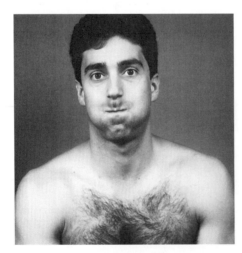

Sensory

PROCEDURE:

Instruct the patient to close his eyes and protrude his tongue. Apply a bitter-tasting solution on one side and on the posterior one-third of the tongue (Fig. 16.42). Instruct the patient to identify each substance without retracting his tongue. This can be done by having the patient point to a list of various substances on a card or on a sheet of paper.

RATIONALE:

Inability to taste and/or identify the substances indicates a lesion of the sensory portions of the glossopharyngeal and/or vagus nerves.

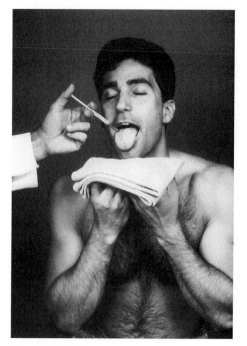

Figure 16.42

16

Reflex

Gag Reflex

PROCEDURE:

With a throat stick, touch the posterior pharyngeal wall, first on one side and then on the other (Fig. 16.43). Observe the movement of the palate and the patient when he gags. Also, ask the patient if the stimulus feels the same on both sides or is stronger on one side than on the other.

RATIONALE:

Deviation of the palate to one side and/or an asymmetrical feeling of the stimulus is indicative of a lesion of the glossopharyngeal and/or vagus nerves. If the patient has had a tonsillectomy, a slight asymmetry of palatal movement may be normal.

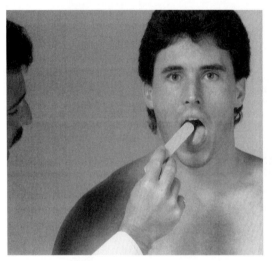

Figure 16.43

SPINAL ACCESSORY NERVE (XI)

The spinal accessory nerve innervates the trapezius and the sternocleidomastoideus muscles. To assess the spinal accessory nerve, muscle test the trapezius and sternocleidomastoideus muscles.

Trapezius Muscle Test

PROCEDURE:

With the patient seated, apply pressure to the patient's shoulders bilaterally and ask him to shrug his shoulders against your resistance (Fig. 16.44). Grade each side according to the muscle grading chart in Chapter 3.

RATIONALE:

A grade 0 to 4 is indicative of a spinal accessory nerve lesion. A strained or weak trapezius muscle is suspect if the sternocleidomastoideus muscle is of reasonably normal strength.

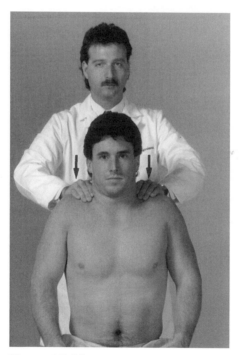

Figure 16.44

16

Sternocleidomastoideus Muscle Test

PROCEDURE:

With the patient seated, place your hand on the lateral aspect of the patient's jaw and instruct him to turn his head toward your hand against resistance (Fig. 16.45). Grade each side according to the muscle grading chart in Chapter 3.

RATIONALE:

A grade 0 to 4 is indicative of a spinal accessory nerve lesion. A strained or weak sternocleidomastoideus muscle is suspect if the trapezius muscle is of reasonably normal strength.

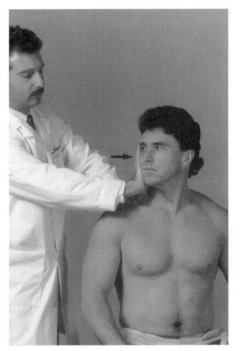

Figure 16.45

HYPOGLOSSAL NERVE (XII)

The hypoglossal nerve is purely motor and is responsible for the movement of the tongue.

PROCEDURE:

Place your hand on the patient's cheek and instruct the patient to press the tip of his tongue against his cheek under your hand (Fig. 16.46). Have the patient do this bilaterally. Instruct the patient to protrude his tongue (Fig. 16.47).

RATIONALE:

If the pressure under your hand by the patient's tongue is unequal, suspect a unilateral hypoglossal nerve lesion. A unilateral hypoglossal nerve lesion will exhibit a deviation of the tongue toward the side of the lesion.

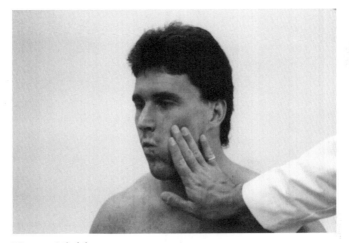

Figure 16.46

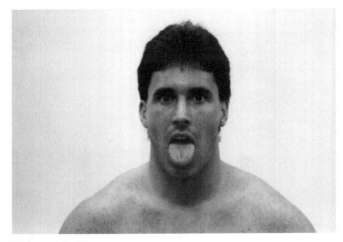

Figure 16.47

16

General References

Barrows HS. Guide to neurological assessment. Philadelphia: JB Lippincott, 1980.

Bickerstaff ER. Neurological examination in clinical practice. 4th ed. Boston: Blackwell Scientific Publications, 1980.

Chusid JG. Correlative neuroanatomy and functional neurology. 16th ed. Los Altos: Lange Medical Publishers, 1976.

Colling RD. Illustrated manual of neurologic diagnosis. 2nd ed. Philadelphia: JB Lippincott, 1982.

DeJong RN. The neurologic examination. 4th ed. Hagerstown, MD: Harper & Row, 1979.

DeMyer W. Technique of the neurologic examination: a programmed text. 3rd ed. New York: McGraw-Hill, 1980.

Devinsky O, Feldmann E. Examination of the cranial and peripheral nerves. New York: Churchill Livingstone, 1988.

Fuller G. Neurological examination made easy. London. Churchill Livingstone, 1993.

Mancall E. Essentials of the neurologic examination. 2nd ed. Philadelphia: FA Davis, 1981.

Merritt HH. A textbook of neurology. 4th ed. Philadelphia: Lea & Febiger, 1967.

VanAllen MW, Rodnitzky RL. Pictorial manual of neurologic tests. 2nd ed. Chicago: Year Book Medical Publishers, 1981.

17
Reflexes

17

PATHOLOGIC (UPPER EXTREMITY REFLEXES)

This chapter discusses various pathologic reflexes that usually are present in corticospinal disease and higher cortical dysfunction, such as stroke, tumor, demyelinating diseases, or vasculitis. If corticospinal pathology or other higher cortical dysfunction is not present, these reflexes should be absent. These reflexes are not graded on the Wexler scale but are referred to as being either present or absent. A Babinski and/or a Rossolimo's foot sign may be present in infants and is considered normal.

Hoffman's Sign

PROCEDURE:

With the patient's wrist in the prone position, grasp the patient's hand and middle finger. With your opposite hand, flick the distal end of the patient's middle finger, stretching the flexor and eliciting a stretch reflex (Fig. 17.1).

RATIONALE:

A present sign is elicited if the patient flexes his thumb and forefinger (Fig. 17.2). A present sign is indicative of a hyperactive reflex only. If this sign is present, it may be one indicator of pyramidal tract disease.

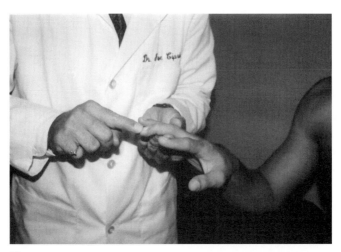

Figure 17.1

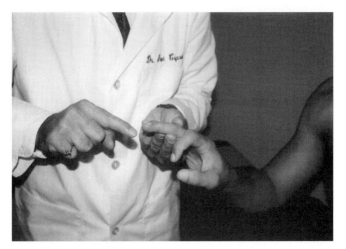

Figure 17.2

17

Tromner's Sign

PROCEDURE:

Grasp the patient's wrist and tap the plantar surface of the tip of the index and middle digits (Fig. 17.3).

RATIONALE:

A present sign is elicited if the patient flexes all of his fingers (Fig. 17.4). A present sign is indicative of a hyperactive reflex only. If this sign is present, it may be one indicator of corticospinal tract disease.

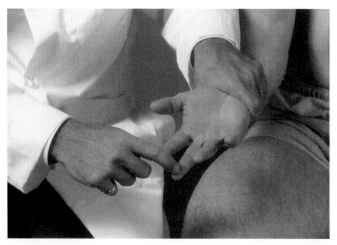

Figure 17.3

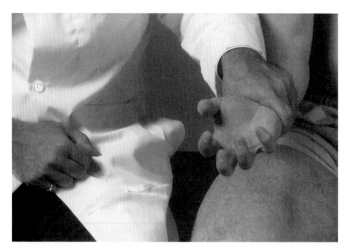

Figure 17.4

Rossolimo's Hand Sign

PROCEDURE:

With a neurological reflex hammer, percuss the palmar surface of the metacarpal-phalangeal joint (Fig. 17.5).

RATIONALE:

A present sign is elicited if the patient flexes all of his fingers (Fig. 17.6). This sign is present in pyramidal tract disease.

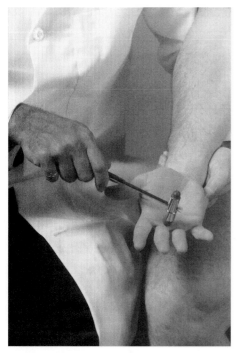

Figure 17.5

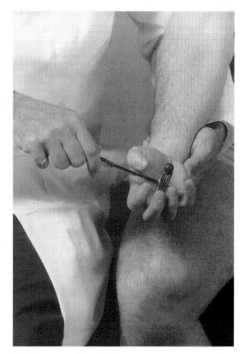

Figure 17.6

17

Chaddock's Wrist Sign

PROCEDURE:

Grasp the patient's wrist by putting pressure on the palmaris longus tendon (Fig. 17.7).

RATIONALE:

A present sign is elicited if the patient flexes his wrist and extends his fingers (Fig. 17.8). This sign is present in pyramidal tract disease.

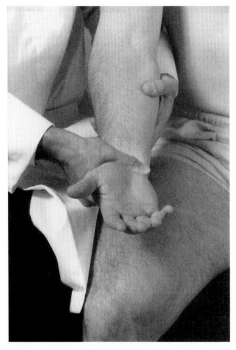

Figure 17.7

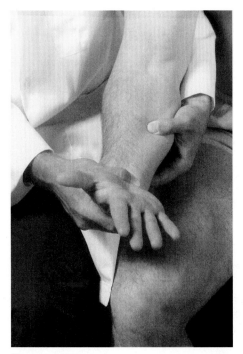

Figure 17.8

Gordon's Wrist Sign

PROCEDURE:

With the patient's fingers flexed, grasp the patient's wrist and squeeze the region of the pisiform bone (Fig. 17.9).

RATIONALE:

A present sign is elicited if the patient extends his flexed fingers (Fig. 17.10). This sign is present in pyramidal tract disease.

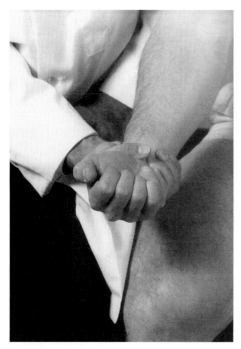

Figure 17.9

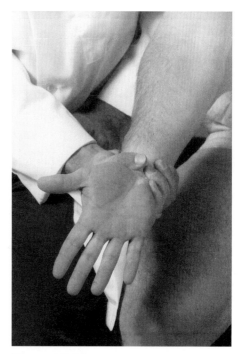

Figure 17.10

17

PATHOLOGIC (LOWER EXTREMITY REFLEXES)

Babinski's Sign

PROCEDURE:

With the patient in the supine position, stroke the sole of the foot with a blunt object like the handle of a neurological reflex hammer. Begin with the lateral aspect of the heel and move superiorward and medial to the big toe (Fig. 17.11).

RATIONALE:

This sign is very important in the neurological examination. A present sign is evident if the patient dorsiflexes his great toe and fans the rest of his digits (Fig. 17.12). If present, this sign is a classic indication of a corticospinal motor system lesion. This sign may be present in normal infants aged 12 to 16 months.

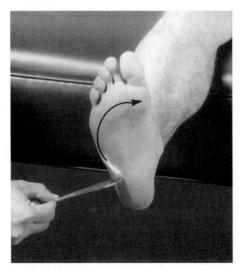

Figure 17.11

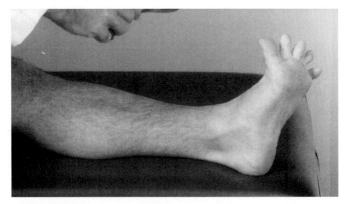

Figure 17.12

Oppenheim's Sign

PROCEDURE:

With the patient in the supine position, stroke the medial side of the tibia with a blunt object (Fig. 17.13).

RATIONALE:

Extension of the great toe is indicative of a present sign (Fig. 17.14). If this reflex is present, suspect a corticospinal motor system lesion.

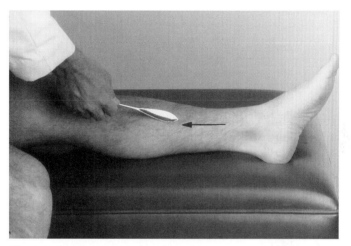

Figure 17.13

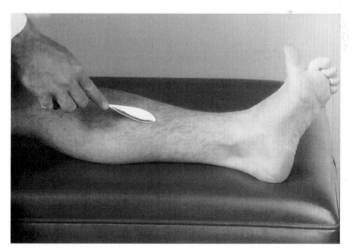

Figure 17.14

17

Chaddock's Foot Sign

PROCEDURE:

With the patient in the supine position, stroke the lateral malleolus with a blunt object (Fig. 17.15).

RATIONALE:

Extension of the great toe is indicative of a present sign (Fig. 17.16). If this reflex is present, suspect a corticospinal motor system lesion.

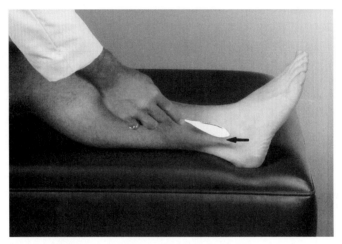

Figure 17.15

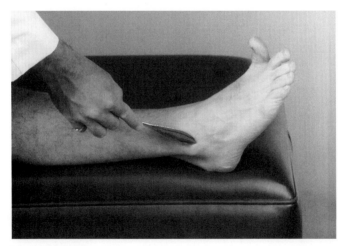

Figure 17.16

Rossolimo's Foot Sign

PROCEDURE:

With the patient in the supine position, tap the balls of the patient's feet with a neurological reflex hammer (Fig. 17.17).

RATIONALE:

Plantar flexion of the toes is indicative of a present sign (Fig. 17.18). This sign may be present in children from 2–3 months to 2–3 years of age and is then considered normal. In other age groups, if this sign and a Babinski sign are present, then pyramidal tract disease is suspect.

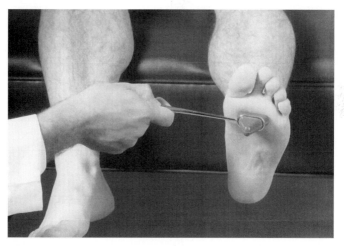

Figure 17.17

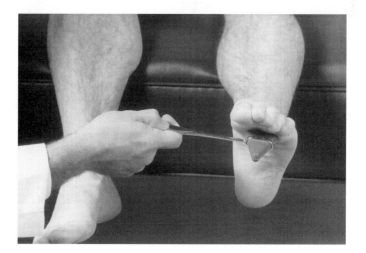

Figure 17.18

17

Mendel-Bechterew's Sign

PROCEDURE:

With the patient in the supine position, tap the lateral aspect of the dorsum of the foot (Fig. 17.19).

RATIONALE:

Plantar flexion of the toes is indicative of a present sign (Fig. 17.20). If this sign is present, suspect a pyramidal tract lesion.

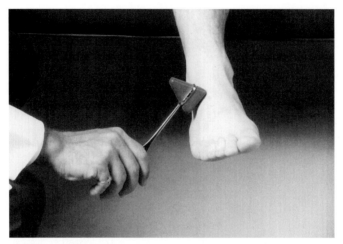

Figure 17.19

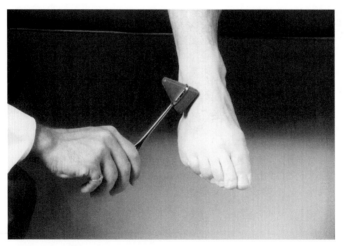

Figure 17.20

Schaeffer's Sign

PROCEDURE:

With the patient in the supine position and the feet overhanging the examination table, squeeze the Achilles tendon (Fig. 17.21).

RATIONALE:

Extension of the great toe is a present sign (Fig. 17.22). If this sign is present, then suspect a lesion of the pyramidal tract.

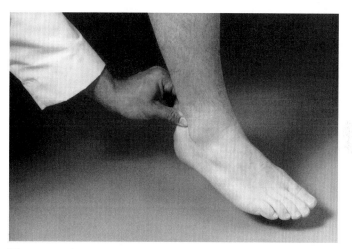

Figure 17.21

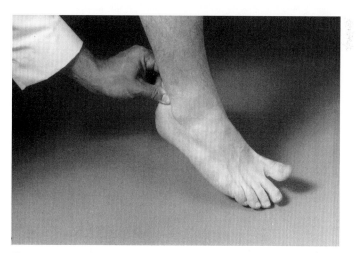

Figure 17.22

17

SUPERFICIAL CUTANEOUS REFLEXES

Superficial cutaneous reflexes are polysynaptic. They are mediated through a reflex arc but are controlled inherently by the corticospinal system. These reflexes are also not graded by the Wexler scale but are either present or absent. Unlike the pathologic reflexes, these reflexes are normally present if there is no lesion of the corticospinal tract. The superficial corneal, pharyngeal, and palatal reflexes belong in this group but are tested in the Cranial Nerve chapter.

Upper Abdominal Reflex

PROCEDURE:

With the patient in the supine position, scrape the skin from medial to lateral above the umbilicus with the blunt end of a neurological reflex hammer (Fig. 17.23) and evaluate bilaterally.

RATIONALE:

A deviation of the umbilicus to the stroked side is a normal response. If the umbilicus does not move unilaterally or if the response is delayed, this is a sign of an absent response. The reflex may be absent in obese patients and pregnant women. This absent reflex is normal, but only if it is absent bilaterally. An absent unilateral response is indicative of a T7-T9 nerve root lesion or disease of the corticospinal system. If the latter is suspect, perform other corticospinal system tests to verify your findings.

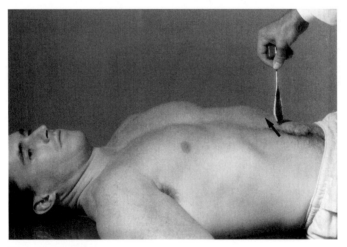

Figure 17.23

Lower Abdominal Reflex

PROCEDURE:

With the patient in the supine position, scrape the skin from medial to lateral below the umbilicus with the blunt end of a neurological reflex hammer (Fig. 17.24) and evaluate bilaterally.

RATIONALE:

A deviation of the umbilicus to the stroked side is a normal response. If the umbilicus does not move unilaterally or if the response is delayed, this is a sign of an absent response. The reflex may be absent in obese patients and pregnant women. This absence is normal, but only if the reflex is absent bilaterally. An absent unilateral response is indicative of a T10-T12 nerve root lesion or disease of the corticospinal system. If the latter is suspect, perform other corticospinal system tests to verify your findings.

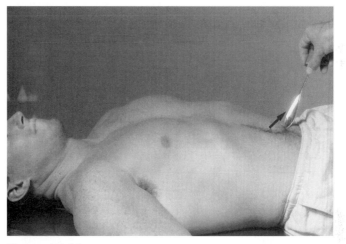

Figure 17.24

17

Cremasteric Reflex

PROCEDURE:

With the patient in the supine position, stroke the patient's inner thigh with the blunt end of a neurological reflex hammer (Fig. 17.25).

RATIONALE:

A normal response is the ipsilateral elevation of the testicle. If no response is elicited, then an L1 or L2 spinal nerve root lesion or a disease of the corticospinal system is suspect. If the latter is suspect, then perform other corticospinal system tests to confirm your findings.

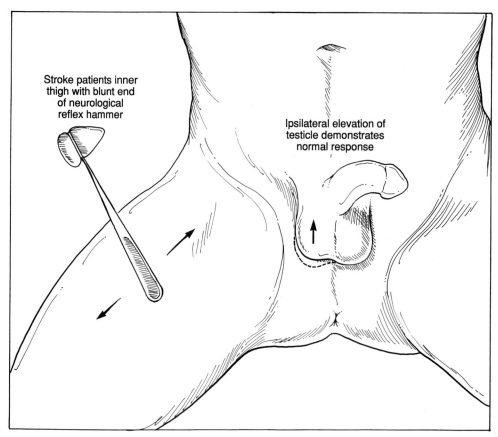

Stroke patients inner thigh with blunt end of neurological reflex hammer

Ipsilateral elevation of testicle demonstrates normal response

Figure 17.25

Superficial Gluteal Reflex

PROCEDURE:

With the patient in the prone position, scrape the buttock with the blunt end of a neurological reflex hammer (Fig. 17.26). Perform this test bilaterally.

RATIONALE:

A contraction of the gluteal muscle on the side of the scraping is a normal response. If the reflex is absent unilaterally, then an L4 or L5 nerve root lesion or a corticospinal system lesion is suspect. If the latter is suspect, then perform other corticospinal system tests to verify your evaluation.

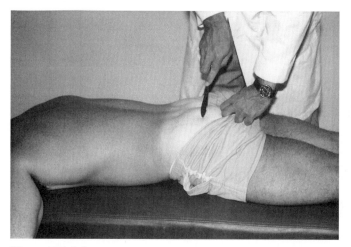

Figure 17.26

17

Superficial Anal Reflex

PROCEDURE:

With the patient in the prone position, prick the perianal fascia with a pin (Fig. 17.27).

RATIONALE:

A normal response is the contraction of the anal sphincters. If no response is elicited, then a lesion of the S5 and coccygeal nerve roots is suspect.

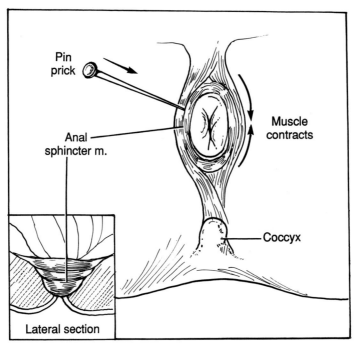

Figure 17.27

Bulbocavernosus Reflex

PROCEDURE:

With the patient in the supine position, pinch the glans penis with your fingers (Fig. 17.28).

RATIONALE:

A contraction of the bulbocavernosus muscle that can be seen or felt at the base of the penis is a normal response. If the reflex is absent, then suspect a S3-S4 nerve root lesion. This reflex is valuable in assessing bladder function in paraplegics.

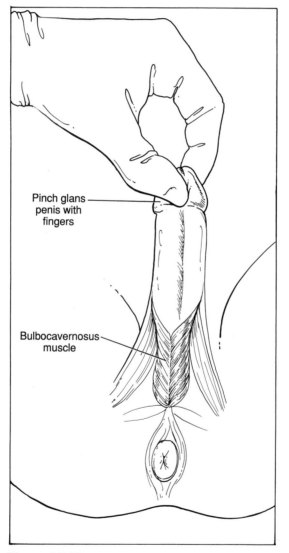

Pinch glans
penis with
fingers

Bulbocavernosus
muscle

Figure 17.28

17

Corneal Reflex

See Chapter 16.

Pharyngeal Reflex

See Chapter 16.

Palatal Reflex

See Chapter 16.

General References

Barrows HS. Guide to neurological assessment. Philadelphia: JB Lippincott, 1980

Bickerstaff ER. Neurological examination in clinical practice. 4th ed. Boston: Blackwell Scientific Publications, 1980.

Bronisch FW. The clinically important reflexes. New York: Grune & Stratton, 1952.

Chusid JG. Correlative neuroanatomy and functional neurology. 16th ed. Los Altos, CA: Lange Medical Publications, 1976.

Colling RD. Illustrated manual of neurologic diagnosis. 2nd ed. Philadelphia: JB Lippincott, 1982.

DeJong RN. The neurologic examination. 4th ed. Hagerstown, MD: Harper & Row, 1979.

DeMyer W. Technique of the neurologic examination: a programmed text. 3rd ed. New York: McGraw-Hill, 1980.

Devinsky O, Feldmann E. Examination of the cranial and peripheral nerves. New York: Churchill Livingstone, 1988.

Heilman NM, Watson RT, Green M. Handbook for differential diagnosis of neurologic signs and symptoms. New York: Appleton-Century-Crofts, 1977.

Lapides J, Babbitt JM. Diagnostic value of bulbocavernosus reflex. JAMA 1956;162:971.

Mancall E. Essentials of the neurologic examination. 2nd ed. Philadelphia: FA Davis, 1981.

Merritt HH. A textbook of neurology. 4th ed. Philadelphia: Lea & Febiger, 1967.

Swanson P. Signs and symptoms in neurology. Philadelphia: JB Lippincott, 1989.

VanAllen MW, Rodnitzky RL. Pictorial manual of neurologic tests. 2nd ed. Chicago: Year Book Medical Publishers, 1981.

18
Cerebellar Function Tests

18

Cerebellar dysfunction is an interruption of the integration of sensory feedback and motor output. Loss of joint position sense can produce some incoordination, which can be made substantially worse when the eyes are closed. The following tests attempt to evaluate the patient's coordination and joint position sense.

If any of the tests are positive unilaterally, then suspect an ipsilateral cerebellar syndrome. This syndrome may be caused by demyelination, vascular diseases, trauma, tumors, or abscesses. If any of the tests are positive bilaterally, suspect a bilateral cerebellar syndrome. This syndrome may be caused by alcohol consumption, demyelination, or vascular diseases.

UPPER EXTREMITY

Finger-Nose Test

PROCEDURE:

With the patient standing or sitting and his eyes closed, ask him to touch each index finger simultaneously to his nose (Fig. 18.1).

RATIONALE:

This procedure should be performed smoothly and easily by the patient. If the patient is unable to perform this procedure, then cerebellar function is impaired.

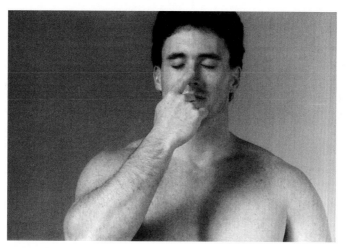

Figure 18.1

18

Finger-Finger Test

PROCEDURE:

Ask the patient to place his finger on your finger. Repeat this several times with the patient's eyes open and closed (Figs. 18.2, 18.3).

RATIONALE:

This procedure should be performed smoothly and easily by the patient. If the patient is unable to perform this procedure, then cerebellar function is impaired.

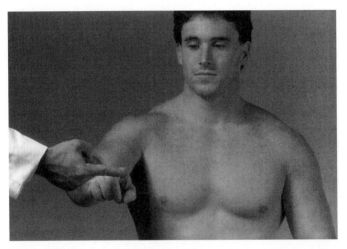

Figure 18.2

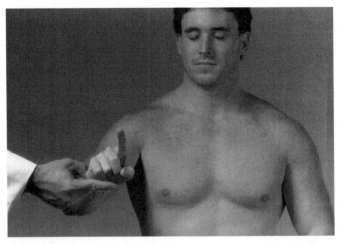

Figure 18.3

Pronation-Supination Test

PROCEDURE:

With the patient standing, ask him to extend his arms in front of him. Next, ask the patient to pronate and supinate his arms rapidly (Figs. 18.4, 18.5).

RATIONALE:

The patient should be able to perform these movements smoothly and with an even rhythm. If the patient is unable to perform the movements or if he performs them in a spastic or uncoordinated manner, then cerebellar dysfunction is suspect.

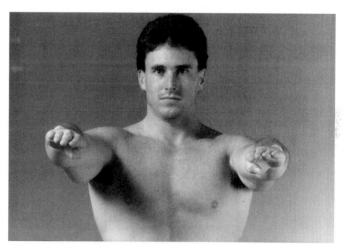

Figure 18.4

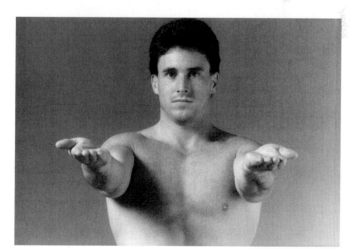

Figure 18.5

18

Patting Test

PROCEDURE:

With the patient seated, instruct him to pat his hand rapidly and repeatedly on his thigh (Fig. 18.6).

RATIONALE:

The patient should be able to perform this movement briskly and with equal amplitude. If he is unable to perform this movement or if he performs it in a slow, spastic, or uncoordinated manner, then cerebellar dysfunction is suspect.

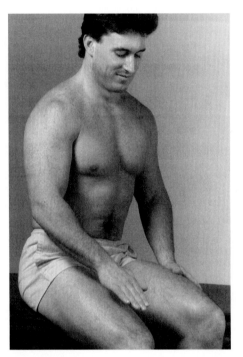

Figure 18.6

Dexterity Test

PROCEDURE:

Ask the patient to touch each fingertip with the thumb of the same hand sequentially (Figs. 18.7, 18.8).

RATIONALE:

These movements are usually done in a smooth and coordinated manner. If the patient is unable to perform these movements or if he performs them in a spastic or uncoordinated manner, then cerebellar dysfunction is suspect.

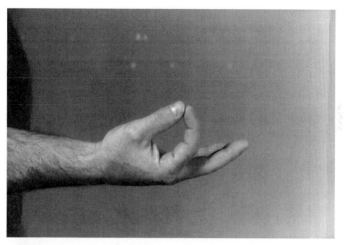

Figure 18.7

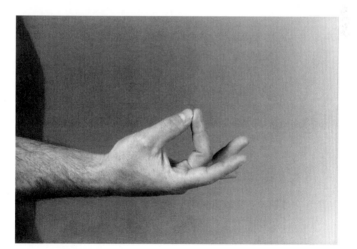

Figure 18.8

18

Lower Extremity

Heel-Knee Test

PROCEDURE:

With the patient in the supine position, ask the patient to place one foot on the opposite knee (Fig. 18.9). Then ask the patient to slide his foot down the shin (Fig. 18.10).

RATIONALE:

These movements are usually done in a smooth and coordinated manner. If the patient is unable to perform these movements or if he performs them in a spastic or uncoordinated manner, then cerebellar dysfunction is suspect.

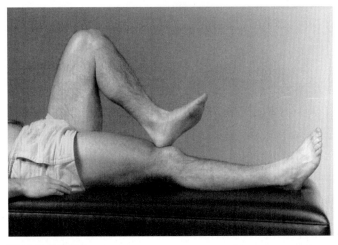

Figure 18.9

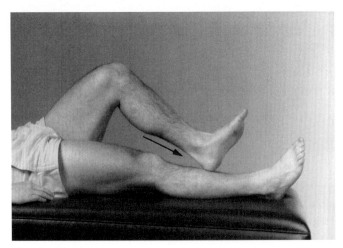

Figure 18.10

Patting Test

PROCEDURE:

Ask the patient to pat his foot rapidly and repeatedly on the floor (Figs. 18.11, 18.12).

RATIONALE:

The patient should be able to perform this movement briskly and with equal amplitude. If he is unable to perform this movement or if he performs it in a slow, spastic, or uncoordinated manner, then cerebellar dysfunction is suspect.

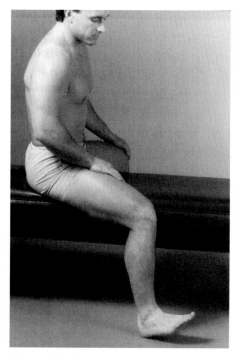

Figure 18.11

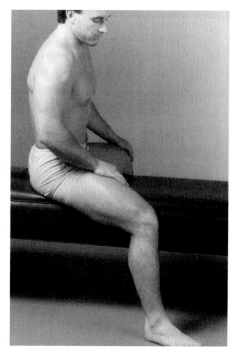

Figure 18.12

18

Figure-of-Eight Test

PROCEDURE:

With the patient in the supine position, ask the patient to draw a figure-of-eight in the air with his great toe (Fig. 18.13).

RATIONALE:

These movements are usually done in a smooth and coordinated manner. If the patient is unable to perform these movements or if he performs them in a spastic or uncoordinated manner, then cerebellar dysfunction is suspect.

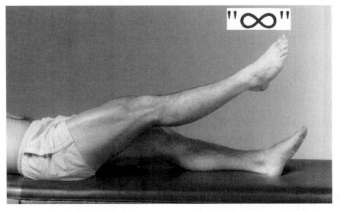

Figure 18.13

PROCEDURE:

Instruct the patient to stand. Observe the patient for any swaying. While the patient is still standing, instruct him to close his eyes (Fig. 18.14).

RATIONALE:

This test is not a cerebellar test per se, but if the patient sways when his eyes are closed, a posterior column disorder is suspected. A patient with a cerebellar dysfunction will sway with his eyes open, but the swaying will be exaggerated with his eyes closed.

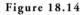

Figure 18.14

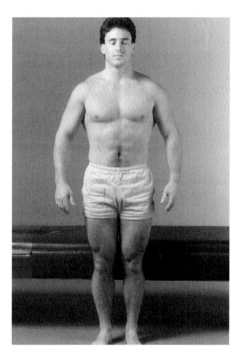

General References

Barrows HS. Guide to neurological assessment. Philadelphia: JB Lippincott, 1980.

Bickerstaff ER. Neurological examination in clinical practice. 4th ed. Boston: Blackwell Scientific Publications, 1980.

Chusid JG. Correlative neuroanatomy and functional neurology. 16th ed. Los Altos, CA: Lange Medical Publications, 1976.

Colling RD. Illustrated manual of neurologic diagnosis. 2nd ed. Philadelphia: JB Lippincott, 1982.

DeJong RN. The neurologic examination. 4th ed. Hagerstown, MD: Harper & Row, 1979.

Greenberg DA, Aminoff MJ, Simon RP. Clinical neurology. 2nd ed. Norwalk: Appleton & Lang, 1993.

Heilman NM, Watson RT, Green M. Handbook for differential diagnosis of neurologic signs and symptoms. New York: Appleton-Century-Crofts, 1977.

Klein R, Mayer-Gross W. The clinical examination of patients with organic cerebral disease. Springfield, IL: Charles C Thomas, 1957.

Mancall E. Essentials of the neurologic examination. 2nd ed. Philadelphia: FA Davis, 1981.

Merritt HH. A textbook of neurology. 4th ed. Philadelphia: Lea & Febiger, 1967.

Scheinberg P. An introduction to diagnosis and management of common neurologic disorders. 3rd ed. New York: Raven Press, 1986.

Steegmann AT. Examination of the nervous system: a student's guide. Chicago: Year Book Medical Publishers, 1970.

Swanson P. Signs and symptoms in neurology. Philadelphia: JB Lippincott, 1989.

VanAllen MW, Rodnitzky RL. Pictorial manual of neurologic tests. 2nd ed. Chicago: Year Book Medical Publishers, 1981.

18

INDEX

Page numbers followed by t or f indicate tables or figures, respectively.